CRITICAL THINKING

CLINICAL JUDGMENT

WITHDRAWN

THIRD EDITION

CRITICAL THINKING AND CLINICAL JUDGMENT

A PRACTICAL APPROACH

Rosalinda Alfaro-LeFevre, RN, MSN

President, Teaching Smart/Learning Easy
Stuart, Florida
www.AlfaroTeachSmart.com

SAUNDERS

An Imprint of Elsevier

SAUNDERS
An Imprint of Elsevier

11830 Westline Industrial Drive
St. Louis, Missouri 63146

CRITICAL THINKING AND CLINICAL JUDGMENT   ISBN 0-7216-9729-1
Copyright © 2004, Elsevier (USA). All rights reserved.

NOTICE

Nursing is an ever-changing field. Standard safety precautions must be followed, but as new research and clinical experience broaden our knowledge, changes in treatment and drug therapy may become necessary or appropriate. Readers are advised to check the most current product information provided by the manufacturer of each drug to be administered to verify the recommended dose, the method and duration of administration, and contraindications. It is the responsibility of the licensed prescriber, relying on experience and knowledge of the patient, to determine dosages and the best treatment for each individual patient. Neither the publisher nor the author assumes any liability for any injury and/or damage to persons or property arising from this publication.

Previous editions copyrighted 1995, 1999.

International Standard Book Number 0-7216-9729-1

Executive Editor: Michael S. Ledbetter
Developmental Editor: Amanda Sunderman Politte
Publishing Services Manager: Catherine Jackson
Project Manager: Anne Gassett
Design Coordinator: Teresa Breckwoldt
Internal Design: GraphCom
Cover Art: Paul M. Fry

Printed in the United States.

Last digit is the print number: 9 8 7 6 5 4 3 2

DEDICATION

To my advisors, here in the United States and throughout the world,
and to two of the best minds I've had the privilege of knowing:

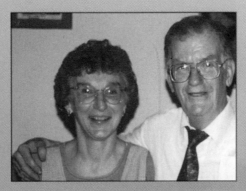

Nancy Flynn, RNC, MSN
July 6, 1932–May 1, 2001

"When you were born you cried and the world rejoiced…
Live your life so that when you die, the world cries and you rejoice. "

The mother of five and a nurse educator from 1953 to 2001, Nancy's wisdom,
humor, and compassion live on in her children, grandchildren,
and the many nurses and patients touched by her teaching and care.

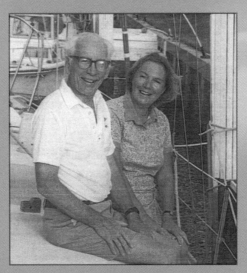

Nathaniel (Nat) Rochester
January 14, 1919–June 8, 2001

"Good minds discuss events. Great minds discuss ideas."

The father of four and stepfather of six, Nat was the chief architect
of the first IBM computer (701). He was a leader in computer design from 1948–1991,
had an ability to connect with people of all ages, and enjoyed working to find
useful solutions to everyday problems.

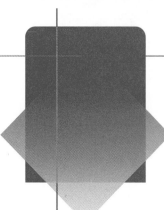

Contributor

Donna D. Ignatavicius, MS, RN, Cm
President, DI Associates, Inc.
Co-author of *Medical-Surgical Nursing: Critical Thinking for
   Collaborative Care* and *A Critical Thinking Approach to
   Skill Development and Competency Evaluation*
Hughesville, Maryland
"Managing Your Time" in Chapter 6

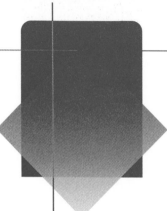

Advisors and Reviewers

UNITED STATES

Carol B. Allen, PhDc, RN
Instructor, Intercollegiate College of Nursing
Washington State University College of Nursing
Spokane, Washington

Gloria F. Antall, ND, APRN, BC
Assistant Professor
Frances Payne Bolton School of Nursing
Case Western Reserve University
Cleveland, Ohio

Ledjie Ballard, CRNA, MSN
Independent Practitioner, Out Patient & Office Anesthesia
Affiliate Clinical Faculty
University of Washington
Seattle, Washington

Suzanne C. Beyea, RN, PhD
Director of Research
Association of Operating Room Nurses
Denver, Colorado

Joyce Begley, MSN, MA, RN
Assistant Professor, Department of Nursing
Eastern Kentucky University
Richmond, Kentucky

Hilda H. Brito, RN, BC, MSN
Director of Education
Kendall Medical Center
Miami, Florida

Bette Case, PhD, RN, BC
Independent Consultant and President
Clinical Care Solutions
Chicago, Illinois

Beverly L. Emonds, MSN, RN
Nurse Recruitment and Retention Manager
Hospital of the University of Pennsylvania
Philadelphia, Pennsylvania

Frances Foster, MS, RN, CS
Advanced Practice Nurse
Massachusetts General Hospital, Bulfinch
   Medical Group
Boston, Massachusetts

Darnell Cockram-Cox, EdD, RN
Director of Education
Danville Regional Medical Center &
Danville Regional Medical Center School of
   Nursing
Danville, Virginia

Pam Di Vito-Thomas, RN, MS, PhD
Nursing Faculty
Anna Vaughn School of Nursing
Oral Roberts University
Tulsa, Oklahoma

Bonnie Eyeler, MSN, RN, JD
Boca Raton, Florida

Ann B. Fives, RN, MS
Professor Emeritus
Raritan Valley Community College
North Branch, New Jersey

Rebecca S. Frugé, RN, PhD
Director
Department of Bilingual Nursing
Inter American University of Puerto Rico
Metropolitan Campus
San Juan, Puerto Rico

Pauline McKinney Green, PhD, RN
Associate Professor
Howard University
College of Pharmacy, Nursing and Allied
   Health Sciences
Washington, D.C.

Esther Halvorson-Hill, RN, MN, MPA
Associate Professor, School of Nursing
Oregon Health Sciences University
Administrator, Halvorson-Hill Enterprises
Ashland, Oregon

Elizabeth E. Hand, MS, RN, CCRN
Acute Care Education Specialist
Hand-on Nursing, PLLC
Tulsa, Oklahoma

Diana Hankes, RN, PhD, CS
Professor of Nursing
Director of the Nursing Program
Carroll College
Waukesha, Wisconsin

Dan Hankison
Information Management and Computer
   Consultant
CONSULTING Dragons
Las Vegas, Nevada

Ruth Hansten, PhD, FACHE, MBA, BSN
President
Hansten Healthcare
Port Ludlow, Washington

Deborah J. Hess, PhD, RN
Assistant Professor
Xavier University
Department of Education
Cincinnati, Ohio

Millie Hill, MSN, RN
Clinical Nurse Educator
Staff Development & Patient Education
Paoli Memorial Hospital
Paoli, Pennsylvania

Taylor Hartman, PhD
CEO
Hartman Communications, Inc.
Midvale, Utah

Carol A. Hutton, EdD, ARNP
President
Hutton Associates
Boca Raton, Florida

Donna D. Ignatavicius, MS, RN, Cm
President, DI Associates, Inc.
Hughesville, Maryland

Marilynn Jackson, RN, PhD, MA, BSN
President
Intuitive Options
Tyler, Texas

Sharon Johnson, MSN, RNC, CNA
Director of Home Health, The Home Care
    Network
Jefferson Health System
Bryn Mawr, Pennsylvania

Suzanne Hall Johnson, MN, RN, C, CNS
Editor, *Nurse Author & Editor*
Lakewood, Colorado

Ann Kobs, RN, MS
President/CEO
Ann Kobs & Associates, Inc.
Goodyear, Arizona

Heidi Pape Laird, BA, MLA, Cert Ed.
Programmer
Highland Laboratories, Inc.
Ashland, Massachusetts

Jody M. Masterson, RN, MSN, CRRN
Adjunct Professor, College of Nursing
Villanova University
Villanova, Pennsylvania

Marycarol McGovern, PhD, RN
Assistant Professor
College of Nursing
Villanova University
Villanova, Pennsylvania

Judith C. Miller, MS, RN
President
Nursing Tutorial and Consulting Services
Clifton, Virginia

Barbara A. Musinski, RN, C, BS
Independent Nursing Consultant
West Palm Beach, Florida

Jan Nash, RN, MS, PhDc
Vice President, Patient Services
Paoli Memorial Hospital
Paoli, Pennsylvania

Terri Sue Patterson, RN, MSN, CRRN
President
Nursing Consultation Services and LifeTrak
Plymouth Meeting, Pennsylvania

William F. Perry, MA, RN
Informatics Consultant
Creekspace Informatics
Beavercreek, Ohio

Josy M. Petr, MS, RN
Lecturer & Educational Testing Director
Indiana University School of Nursing
Indiana University Northwest
Gary, Indiana

James Riley
Healthcare Informatics Specialist
Vice President
PayerPath
Richmond, Virginia

**Michael Riley, LMSW, LPC,
    EMT-Paramedic**
Director–St. Joseph Health Care Trust
Catholic Charities, Diocese of Fort Worth
Fort Worth, Texas

Rosalee J. Seymour, EdD, RN
Board Certified Informatics Nurse
Associate Professor, College of Nursing
PMNU Department
East Tennessee State University
Johnson City, Tennessee

Kathleen R. Stevens, RN, EdD, FAAN
Professor and Director
Academic Center for Evidence-based
    Practice (ACE)
The University of Texas Health Science
    Center at San Antonio
San Antonio, Texas

Karen M. Seyfert, RN, BSN
Staff Nurse
Coatesville Veteran's Administration
    Hospital
Coatesville, Pennsylvania

Jean Smith, RN, BSN
Staff Nurse
ICU/CCU
Paoli Memorial Hospital
Paoli, Pennsylvania

Carol Taylor, CSFN, RN, PhD
Director, Center for Clinical Bioethics
Assistant Professor, Nursing
Georgetown University
Washington, D.C.

Stephanie Thibeault
Student Advisor
Owner/Webmaster, The Student Nurse
    Forum
http://kcsun3.tripod.com
Merriam, Kansas

Denise Thornby, RN, MS
Director, Education & Professional
    Development
Virginia Commonwealth University Health
    System
Richmond, Virginia

Theresa M. Valiga, EdD, RN
Director of Research and Professional
    Development
National League for Nursing
New York, New York

Ervena Weingartner, MN, RN, CPNP
Professor of Nursing
University of Cincinnati Raymond Walters
    College
Cincinnati, Ohio

Beth Willmitch, RN, BSN
Business Systems Analyst
Baptist Health Systems of South Florida
Coral Gables, Florida

Toni C. Wortham, RN, BSN, MSN
Professor
Madisonville Community College–Health
    Campus
Madisonville, Kentucky

◆ INTERNATIONAL

Cecile Boisvert, RN, MScN
Consultant-Educator in Nursing
Lecturer, University of Paris (Bobigny)
International Liaison on AFEDIR Board
    (Association Francophone Europeenne
    des Diagnostics, Interventions et Resultats
    des Soins Infirmiers)
St. Aubin, France

Emilia Campos de Carvalho, RN, PhD
Professor
University of Sao Paulo at Ribeirao Preto
College of Nursing
Ribeirao Preto, Brazil

**Professor Dame June Clark, DBE, PhD,
    RN, RHV, FRCN**
Professor of Community Nursing
School of Health Science
University of Wales Swansea
Wales, United Kingdom

Judy Boychuk Duchscher, RN, BScN, MN
Faculty
Nursing Education Program of
  Saskatchewan
SIAST Kelsey Campus
Saskatoon, Saskatchewan, Canada

Ana M. Giménez, RN
Professor of Medical-Surgical Nursing
Puerta de Hierro School of Nursing
Universidad Autónoma de Madrid
Madrid, Spain

Maria Teresa Luis, RN
Professor of Medical-Surgical Nursing
School of Nursing, Pavelló de Govern
Campus de Bellvitge
L'Hospitalet del Llobregat
Barcelona, Spain

**Judith Manning, RN, RM, B, EdMa,
  FRCNA**
Clinical Skills Coordinator
Clinical Education Development Unit
North Western Adelaide Health Service
Adelaide, South Australia

**Brian McCarthy, RGN, RPN, Dip N
  Informatics**
Postgrad. student in Masters in Health
  Informatics
Dundrum, Dublin, Ireland

Jeanne Liliane Marlene Michel, RN, MSN
Assistant Professor, Department of Nursing
Universidade Federal de Sao Paulo
Technical-Administrative Coordinator
Nursing Direction, Hospital
Sao Paulo, Brazil

**Gail P. Mooney, MSc (Econ.), PG Dip.
  Soc. Res. Methods, RGN, SEN**
Lecturer, School of Health Science
University of Wales Swansea
Swansea
Wales, United Kingdom

Nico Oud, RN, MNSc, Dipl.N.Adm
Consultant and Trainer of Aggression
  Management
"CONNECTING"
Amsterdam, The Netherlands

Ann Paterson, RN, BApp Sci, MA
Senior Lecturer in Nursing
Department of Nursing and Midwifery,
  RMIT University
Bundoora, VIC, Australia

Anne Price, RN, HV, BSc (Hons)
Nurse Practitioner, The Ashgrove Surgery
Morgan Street, Pontypridd, Wales
Doctoral Student, University of Wales
  Swansea
Wales, United Kingdom

Joanne Profetto-McGrath, RN, MEd, PhD
Assistant Professor, Faculty of Nursing
University of Alberta
Edmonton, Alberta, Canada

**Catherine Jean Thorpe, RN, RM, DipIC,
  Dip. Nursing Admin and Community
  Health Nursing, BAdmin.**
Deputy Director: Nursing
Groote Schuur Hospital Observatory
Capetown, South Africa

Preface

WHAT'S PRACTICAL ABOUT THIS APPROACH?

Critical thinking—our capacity to focus our thinking to get the results we need—may be the single most important factor that determines whether nurses succeed or fail. Yet too often we redesign curricula and care delivery systems but fail to help students and nurses acquire the *thinking skills* needed to function in today's challenging health care setting. Thinking is not "like it always was." Today's problems can't be solved with yesterday's thinking. Focusing on what you need to do to think effectively at the bedside today, this book encourages you to identify strategies to improve thinking and performance in your own way.

Here's how the chapters are organized:

- **Chapters 1 and 2**, "What Is Critical Thinking and Why Do We Care?" and "How to Think Critically," examine critical thinking in daily life with some reference to nursing situations. Whether you want to improve your ability to handle personal or professional matters, these chapters help you focus your thinking to get results using your own particular talents and strengths.
- **Chapters 3 and 4**, "Critical Thinking and Clinical Judgment" and "Critical Thinking in Nursing: Beyond Clinical Judgment" are designed to help you meet the challenges of acquiring the knowledge, confidence, and thinking skills needed to succeed in six common nursing situations: reasoning in the clinical setting (clinical judgment), moral and ethical reasoning, nursing research, teaching others, teaching ourselves, and test-taking.
- **Chapter 5**, "Practicing Clinical Judgment Skills: Up Close and Clinical," provides opportunities to practice critical judgment (clinical reasoning) skills using case scenarios based on real nursing experiences.
- **Chapter 6**, "Applied Critical Thinking: Mastering Common Workplace Skills," helps you gain key skills you need to work in any position that's highly relational (any job that demands a lot of

interaction with others). This section helps you "work smarter, not harder" by teaching you things such as how to manage conflict and work with a diverse team.

WHAT'S NEW IN THIS EDITION

Here's what's new:

1. A new title! We now include *Clinical Judgment* in the title to reflect new content and a greater emphasis on promoting clinical judgment (clinical reasoning) skills.

2. Introduction of Critical Thinking Indicators™ (CTIs™). These are evidence-based descriptions of the behaviors that demonstrate the knowledge, characteristics, and skills that promote critical thinking.

3. Completely revised and updated, this book centers on the new realities of today's health care setting, including giving more on:
   ◆ The need to recognize that fostering, supporting, and rewarding critical thinking behaviors are crucial to recruitment and retention.
   ◆ How personality, upbringing, and culture affect thinking and teamwork.
   ◆ How multidisciplinary practice, use of computers, and critical paths affect thinking.
   ◆ The call for outcome-focused, evidence-based care.
   ◆ The importance of moving to a predictive model (*Predict, Prevent, Manage, Promote*) rather than focusing only on a more reactive *Diagnose and Treat* approach.
   ◆ How the nursing process continues to evolve to a more proactive and dynamic way of providing nursing care.
   ◆ The role of logic, intuition, and creativity in critical thinking and clinical judgment.
   ◆ How to use mind mapping (concept mapping) to promote critical thinking and learn more efficiently.

4. New, detailed information on key workplace skills such as how to:
   ◆ Set priorities and manage your time
   ◆ Access and use information
   ◆ Deal with and prevent mistakes
   ◆ Build empowered partnerships
   ◆ Manage conflict constructively

5. More interactive case scenarios based on real experiences.

6. In accordance with my belief that humor sends strong messages and is good for the soul, new cartoons have been added. (My comic strip, *HMO*, returns to this edition. This comic, also known as *Help Me Out*, addresses the funny and ridiculous things that happen to care-givers and receivers. If you have a story—one that involves the care of

a patient, friend, family member, or pet—to share, please contact me at the address given at the end of this preface.)

WHAT'S THE SAME ABOUT THIS EDITION

Like the first edition, this book is:

1. **User Friendly.** Great pains have been taken to include design elements that motivate you to want to read and allow you to use your own way of mastering content (see page xvii, The Best Way to Read This Book).
2. **Practical and Concise.** Provides lots of useful information and strategies in a concise format. Includes theory, strategies, and critical thinking and practice exercises.
3. **Motivational.** The writing style is informal, interactive, and designed to make you feel like you're "right there" having a personal discussion. The scenarios and exercises, based on real experience, are designed to simulate clinical nursing situations.*
4. **Solid.** Detailed coverage on critical thinking in the context of clinical practice and everyday life.
5. **Comprehensive.** Input from the interdisciplinary domestic and international advisory board continues to bring key expert, up-to-date insights.

A WORD ABOUT "PATIENT/CLIENT" AND "HE/SHE"

Whenever possible, a fictitious name, or "someone," "person," "consumer," or "individual" is used (instead of "patient" or "client") to help us keep in mind that each patient or client is an individual who has unique needs, values, perceptions, and motivations. *He* and she are used interchangeably to avoid the awkwardness of using "he/she."

PLEASE TELL US WHAT YOU THINK

We want to hear your struggles and concerns. Whether you're a student or faculty member, if you're having a problem with something, it's likely others are, too. Your problems are our opportunities to learn, improve, and help others with the same concerns. Please let us know what you think. Address comments to myself or to Michael Ledbetter, Nursing Editorial, Elsevier, 11830 Westline Industrial Drive, St. Louis, MO 63146.

Rosalinda Alfaro-LeFevre, RN, MSN
6161 SE Landing Way #9
Stuart, FL 34997
www.AlfaroTeachSmart.com

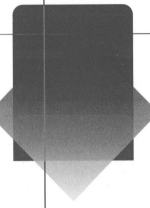

The Best Way to Read This Book

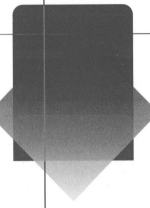 **THE BEST WAY TO READ THIS BOOK IS HOWEVER YOU CHOOSE TO READ IT**

1. For those of you who like the traditional approach, read it from beginning to end. You'll enjoy the narrative, logical approach, and numerous scenarios and examples designed to help you understand and *remember* content.
2. For those of you who like to use your own unique approach–for example, the *back to front* approach (read summaries before text), the *skip around to the stuff that looks interesting* approach, or the *read the stuff that will be on the test first* approach–here are some of the features that help you focus on what's most important.

PRECEDING EACH CHAPTER

♦ **This Chapter at a Glance:** Allows you to scan major headings.
♦ **Pre-chapter self-tests** help you focus on learning outcomes and decide where you stand in relation to what needs to be learned.
*Names and some facts are changed to provide anonymity.

FOLLOWING EACH CHAPTER

♦ **Key Points:** Provide a detailed summary of the most important content.
♦ **Critical Thinking Exercises and Practice Exercises:** Direct you to *use* content, helping you clarify understanding and move information into long-term memory.

OTHER FEATURES YOU NEED TO KNOW ABOUT

♦ **Glossary:** Provides definitions of key terms. If you don't understand words, look them up, or you may miss major points.

- **Critical Moments:** Give simple strategies that can make a BIG difference in results.
- **Other Perspectives:** Offer interesting (and sometimes amusing) points of view.
- **Response Key:** When appropriate, example responses for Critical Thinking and Practice Exercises are provided to help you evaluate your responses (all exercises that have an example response are marked with an asterisk). This is called a *response key,* rather than an *answer key,* to avoid implying that there's only one right answer to each question. In many cases, a variety of responses are acceptable (great minds don't always think alike). The main point of the exercises isn't necessarily to come up with the right response; rather, the point is to get in touch with the thinking that led you to your response and to be able to evaluate and correct your thinking as needed.

READING EFFICIENTLY

However you choose to read, keep in mind the following steps, which provide an organized and efficient way to master content.

- **Survey:** Scan the abstract, major headings, tables, and illustrations.
- **Question:** Turn major headings into questions.
- **Read:** Read, taking notes and answering your questions.
- **Review, Recite, and Re-read:** Review the chapter (or your notes), reciting key content out loud. Then ask yourself, "What's still not clear here?" Read the sections you don't understand again; raise questions to ask in class or discuss with your peers.

Acknowledgments

I want to thank my husband, Jim, for his love, support, and sense of humor and fun. I also want to thank the rest of my family—especially Daniel, Chelsey, and Chuck DeMarino—and the following people for their ongoing support and contribution to my personal and professional growth:

Grace and Frank Nola, Pat and Chuck Morgan, Mae and Bruce Franklin, Dan Hankison, Heidi Laird, Louise Rochester, Ledjie Ballard, Terri Patterson, Carol Taylor, Terry Valiga, Annette Sophocles, Melani (MiniMe) McGuire, Maria Sophocles Martin, Barbara Cohen, Patti Cleary, Carol Hutton, Bonnie Eyler, Lynda Carpenito, Charlie and Nancy Lindsay, Bill and Mary Jo Boyer, John Payne, the Villanova College of Nursing Faculty, and the past and present staff nurses of Paoli Memorial Hospital.

I can't thank those of you who have been willing to advise and give so freely of your time and expertise enough.

My special thanks go to the following people at Elsevier: Michael Ledbetter, executive editor; Amanda Politte, developmental editor; Anne Gassett, project manager; Joan Reinbott, copy editor; and the sales and marketing staff for their vital roles in making this book successful.

Rosalinda Alfaro-LeFevre RN, MSN
www.AlfaroTeachSmart.com

Assumptions and Promises

Before I began to write this book, I made some assumptions:
◆ You want to learn.
◆ Your time is valuable, and you don't want to waste it.
◆ You like to learn the most important things first.
◆ You learn better when you're motivated, know why information is relevant, and choose your own way of learning.
◆ It's inappropriate for *me to* tell *you* how to think.
◆ You feel a sense of accomplishment when you gain knowledge and skills that help you be more independent.

Because of these assumptions, I promise to:
◆ Let you know what's most important.
◆ Use lots of examples and present information in a usable way.
◆ Provide the "reasons behind the rules."
◆ Encourage you to *choose* what works for *you.*
◆ Help you gain or refine the skills required to be a better thinker, independent learner, and more effective nurse.

Contents

CHAPTER *1*

What Is Critical Thinking and Why Do We Care? xxx

WHY FOCUS ON CRITICAL THINKING? 2

HOW THIS BOOK HELPS YOU IMPROVE THINKING 3

WHAT'S THE DIFFERENCE BETWEEN THINKING AND CRITICAL THINKING? 3

CRITICAL THINKING: SOME DIFFERENT DESCRIPTIONS 4

    A Synonym 4

    Commonly Seen Descriptions of Critical Thinking 4

    Critical Thinking, Clinical Judgment, and Clinical Reasoning 5

    What about Common Sense? 6

WHAT DO CRITICAL THINKERS LOOK LIKE? 6

    Critical Thinking Indicators™ (CTIs™) 7

REFLECTION AND INSIGHT ("HEMMING AND HAWING" AND "AHA!") 9

WHAT'S FAMILIAR AND WHAT'S NEW 11

    What's Familiar 11

    What's New 13

KEY POINTS 15

CHAPTER *2*

How to Think Critically 20

GAINING INSIGHT AND SELF-AWARENESS 22

WHAT'S YOUR PERSONAL STYLE AND WHY DOES IT MATTER? 22

Understanding Learning Style Preferences 22

How Your Personality Affects Thinking 23

Effects of Upbringing and Culture 25

MENTORING AND BUILDING EMPOWERED PARTNERSHIPS 28

FACTORS INFLUENCING CRITICAL THINKING ABILITY 29

Personal Factors 30

Situational Factors 34

Habits Causing Barriers to Critical Thinking 35

Covey's 7 Habits of Highly Effective People® 37

OUTCOME-FOCUSED (RESULTS-ORIENTED) THINKING 38

Goals (Intent) versus Outcomes (Results) 38

Focusing on End Results 39

CRITICAL THINKING STRATEGIES 40

10 Key Questions 40

Using Logic, Intuition, and Trial and Error 43

Focusing on the Big and Small Pictures 44

Specific Strategies 44

KNOWLEDGE AND INTELLECTUAL SKILL INDICATORS 46

HOW TO READ MINDS 48

DEVELOPING CHARACTER, ACQUIRING KNOWLEDGE, AND PRACTICING SKILLS 49

KEY POINTS 51

CHAPTER *3*

Critical Thinking and Clinical Judgment 54

CRITICAL THINKING AND CLINICAL JUDGMENT 56

Applied Definition 56

Other Ways Nurses Describe Critical Thinking 57

What about Critical Thinking Indicators™ (CTIs™)? 60

GOALS AND OUTCOMES OF NURSING 60

Major Goals of Nursing 60

Major Outcomes of Nursing 60

What Are the Implications? 61

NOVICE VERSUS EXPERT THINKING 61

A NEW MINDSET 64

From "Diagnose and Treat" to a Predictive Approach 64

Predict, Prevent, Manage, Promote (PPMP) 65

Treating versus Managing 66

Outcome-Focused, Data-Driven, Evidence-Based Care 67

Clinical, Functional, and Other Outcomes 69

A CHANGING NURSING PROCESS 73

More Proactive and Dynamic 73

Is the Care Plan Dead? 75

What Do Nurses Diagnose? 76

Nursing Responsibilities Related to Diagnosis 77

DEVELOPING CLINICAL JUDGMENT (CLINICAL REASONING SKILLS) 83

Where Do Intuition and Logic Fit In? 84

What about Creativity? 85

Scope of Practice Decisions 86

Decision Making and Nursing Standards and Guidelines 88

How to Develop Effective Clinical Judgment 90

10 Strategies for Developing Clinical Judgment 91

MAKING SURE YOUR CHARTING REFLECTS CRITICAL THINKING 95

KEY POINTS 96

CHAPTER *4*

Critical Thinking in Nursing: Beyond Clinical Judgment 100

MORAL AND ETHICAL REASONING 102

Moral versus Ethical Reasoning 103

How Do You Decide? 103

Seven Ethical Principles 105

Standards, Ethics Codes, Patients' Rights, Advance Directives 105

Steps for Moral and Ethical Reasoning 108

NURSING RESEARCH 112

Frequently Asked Questions on Beginning Nurses' Research Role 112

Scanning Before Reading Research Articles 114

Getting Research into Practice 115

Quality Improvement 115

TEACHING OTHERS 120

TEACHING OURSELVES 123

Memorizing Effectively 123

TEST-TAKING 125

KEY POINTS 131

CHAPTER

Practicing Clinical Judgment Skills: Up Close and Clinical 134

CLINICAL JUDGMENT (CLINICAL REASONING) SKILLS: DYNAMIC AND INTERRELATED 136

WHAT'S THE POINT? 136

GENERAL INSTRUCTIONS 136

REQUIRED VOCABULARY FOR COMPLETING THIS CHAPTER 137

1. IDENTIFYING ASSUMPTIONS 138

Definition 138

Why This Skill Promotes Clinical Judgment 138

Guidelines: How to Identify Assumptions 138

Practice Exercises: Identifying Assumptions 139

2. ASSESSING SYSTEMATICALLY AND COMPREHENSIVELY 142

Definition 142

Why This Skill Promotes Clinical Judgment 142

Guidelines: How to Assess Systematically and Comprehensively 142

Clinical Judgment and Pre-Established Assessment Tools 142

Practice Exercises: Assessing Systematically and Comprehensively 143

Neurologic Focus Assessment Guide 145

3. CHECKING ACCURACY AND RELIABILITY (VALIDATING DATA) 146

Definition 146

Why This Skill Promotes Clinical Judgment 147

Guidelines: How to Check Accuracy and Reliability 147

Practice Exercises: Checking Accuracy and Reliability (Validating Data) 147

4. DISTINGUISHING NORMAL FROM ABNORMAL/IDENTIFYING SIGNS AND SYMPTOMS 148

Definition 148

Why This Skill Promotes Clinical Judgment 148

Guidelines: How to Distinguish Normal from Abnormal/Identify Signs and Symptoms 148

Practice Exercises: Distinguishing Normal from Abnormal/Identifying Signs and Symptoms 149

5. MAKING INFERENCES (DRAWING VALID CONCLUSIONS) 149

Definition 149

Why This Skill Promotes Clinical Judgment 150

Guidelines: How to Make Inferences (Draw Valid Conclusions) 150

Practice Exercises: Making Inferences (Drawing Valid Conclusions) 150

6. CLUSTERING RELATED CUES (DATA) 151

Definition 151

Why This Skill Promotes Clinical Judgment 151

Guidelines: How to Cluster Related Cues (Data) 151

Practice Exercises: Clustering Related Cues (Data) 152

7. DISTINGUISHING RELEVANT FROM IRRELEVANT 153

Definition 153

Why This Skill Promotes Clinical Judgment 153

Guidelines: How to Distinguish Relevant from Irrelevant 153

Practice Exercises: Distinguishing Relevant from Irrelevant 154

8. RECOGNIZING INCONSISTENCIES 155

Definition 155

Why This Skill Promotes Clinical Judgment 155

Guidelines: How to Recognize Inconsistencies 155

Practice Exercises: Recognizing Inconsistencies 156

9. IDENTIFYING PATTERNS 156

Definition 156

Why This Skill Promotes Clinical Judgment 157

Guidelines: How to Identify Patterns 157

Practice Exercises: Identifying Patterns 158

10. IDENTIFYING MISSING INFORMATION 158

Definition 158

Why This Skill Promotes Clinical Judgment 158

Guidelines: How to Identify Missing Information 158

Practice Exercises: Identifying Missing Information 159

11. PROMOTING HEALTH BY IDENTIFYING AND MANAGING RISK FACTORS* 159

Definition 159

Why This Skill Promotes Clinical Judgment 159

Guidelines: How to Identify and Manage Risk Factors 160

Practice Exercises: Promoting Health by Identifying and Managing Risk Factors 161

12. DIAGNOSING ACTUAL AND POTENTIAL (RISK) PROBLEMS 161

Definition 161

Why This Skill Promotes Clinical Judgment 162

Guidelines: How to Diagnose Actual and Potential Problems 162

Identifying Actual Problems 163

Predicting Potential Problems 165

Practice Exercises: Diagnosing Actual and Potential (Risk) Problems 165

13. SETTING PRIORITIES 167

Definition 167

Guidelines: How to Set Priorities 167

Practice Exercises: Setting Priorities 170

---

*This skill deals with identifying risk factors in healthy people. The next skill, *Diagnosing Actual and Potential (Risk) Problems*, deals with risk factors in the context of people with existing health problems.

14. DETERMINING CLIENT-CENTERED (PATIENT-CENTERED) EXPECTED OUTCOMES 171

Definition 171

Why This Skill Promotes Clinical Judgment 172

Guidelines: How to Determine Client-Centered (Patient-Centered) Expected Outcomes 172

Practice Exercises: Determining Client-Centered (Patient-Centered) Expected Outcomes 174

15. DETERMINING SPECIFIC INTERVENTIONS 175

Definition 175

Why This Skill Promotes Clinical Judgment 175

Guidelines: How to Determine Specific Interventions 175

Practice Exercises: Determining Specific Interventions 177

16. EVALUATING AND CORRECTING THINKING (SELF-REGULATING) 178

Definition 178

Why This Skill Promotes Clinical Judgment 178

Guidelines: How to Evaluate and Correct Thinking (Self-Regulate) 178

17. DETERMINING A COMPREHENSIVE PLAN/EVALUATING AND UPDATING THE PLAN 180

Definition 180

Why This Skill Promotes Clinical Judgment 180

Guidelines: How to Develop a Comprehensive Plan/Update the Plan 180

Practice Exercises: Determining a Comprehensive Plan/Updating the Plan 181

CHAPTER 6

Applied Critical Thinking: Mastering Common Workplace Skills 188

1. NAVIGATING AND FACILITATING CHANGE 190

Definition 190

Learning Outcomes 190

Thinking Critically about Change 190

How to Navigate and Facilitate Change 190

2. COMMUNICATING BAD NEWS 194

Definition 194

Learning Outcomes 194

Thinking Critically about Bad News 194

How to Communicate Bad News 194

3. DEALING WITH COMPLAINTS CONSTRUCTIVELY 196

Definition 196

Learning Outcomes 196

Thinking Critically about Complaints 196

How to Deal with Complaints 197

4. DEVELOPING EMPOWERED PARTNERSHIPS 199

Definition 199

Learning Outcomes 200

Thinking Critically about Empowered Partnerships 200

How to Develop Empowered Partnerships 200

5. GIVING AND TAKING FEEDBACK 204

Definition 204

Learning Outcomes 204

Thinking Critically about Giving and Taking Feedback 204

How to Give and Take Feedback 204

6. MANAGING CONFLICT CONSTRUCTIVELY 207

Definition 207

Learning Outcomes 207

Thinking Critically about Conflict 207

How to Manage Conflict Constructively 208

7. MANAGING YOUR TIME 213

Definition 213

Learning Outcomes 213

Thinking Critically about Managing Your Time 214

8. PREVENTING AND DEALING WITH MISTAKES CONSTRUCTIVELY 218

Definition 218

Learning Outcomes 219

Thinking Critically about Preventing and Dealing with Mistakes 219

How to Prevent and Deal with Mistakes Constructively 221

9. TRANSFORMING A GROUP INTO A TEAM 227

Definition 227

Learning Outcomes 227

Thinking Critically about Teamwork 227

How to Transform a Group into a Team 228

10. ACCESSING AND USING INFORMATION EFFECTIVELY 233

Definition 233

Learning Outcomes 233

Thinking Critically about Accessing and Using Information 233

How to Access and Use Information Effectively 234

11. OUTCOME-FOCUSED WRITING (WRITING TO GET RESULTS) 238

Definition 238

Learning Outcomes 238

Thinking Critically about Writing 238

How to Write to Get Results 239

10 Strategies for School Papers 240

Response Key for Chapters 1 to 5 Critical Thinking Exercises 246

APPENDIX *A* **Mind Mapping: Getting in the "Right" State of Mind** 260

APPENDIX *B* **American Nurses Association Standards for Practice and Code of Ethics** 263

APPENDIX *C* **Example Critical Pathway** 266

APPENDIX *D* **NANDA Nursing Diagnoses** 270

Glossary 280

Comprehensive Bibliography 286

Index 295

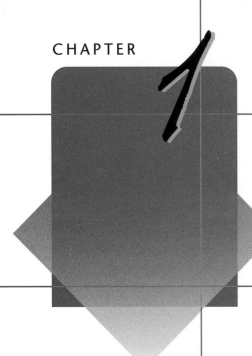

CHAPTER 1

What Is Critical Thinking and Why Do We Care?

THIS CHAPTER at a Glance ...

◆ Why Focus on Critical Thinking?
◆ How This Book Helps You Improve Thinking
◆ What's the Difference Between Thinking and Critical Thinking?
◆ Critical Thinking: Some Different Descriptions
    A Synonym
    Commonly Seen Descriptions of Critical Thinking
    Critical Thinking, Clinical Judgment, and Clinical
      Reasoning
    What about Common Sense?
◆ What Do Critical Thinkers Look Like?
    Critical Thinking Indicators™ (CTIs™)*
◆ Reflection and Insight ("Hemming and Hawing" and
  "Aha!")
◆ What's Familiar and What's New
    What's Familiar
    What's New
◆ Key Points

*The terms Critical Thinking Indicator™ and CTI™ are trademarks of Rosalinda Alfaro-LeFevre and Teaching Smart/Learning Easy, of Stuart, FL. The trademarks signify that the indicators are evidence-based. www.AlfaroTeachSmart.com

Read the following Learning Outcomes and decide whether you can readily achieve each one. If you can, you don't need to read this chapter and can go on to Chapter 2. Don't be concerned if you can't achieve any of the outcomes at this time. We'll come back to these outcomes later in the chapter, in Critical Thinking Exercises.

Suggestion: *Reading with a purpose* triggers your brain to get involved in what you're reading, carefully evaluating the material and making decisions about what's important and how you might use it. Study the outcomes at the beginning of each chapter, and then mark your book or take notes when you encounter relevant information.

Learning Outcomes

After studying this chapter, you should be able to:

◆ Describe critical thinking and clinical judgment using your own words, based on the definitions in this chapter.

◆ Give three reasons why critical thinking is essential for nurses.

◆ Explain the relationship between outcomes (results) and critical thinking.

◆ Clarify the term *critical thinking indicator*™ (CTI™).*

◆ Describe five critical thinking characteristics you'd like to develop or improve.

◆ Address how critical thinking is similar to and different from problem solving.

◆ Identify four principles of the scientific method that are evident in critical thinking.

WHY FOCUS ON CRITICAL THINKING?

Have you noticed how complicated life is these days? On a daily basis, we find ourselves dealing with information overload, multiple priorities, and new challenges that require us to learn and adapt. Critical thinking–your capacity to focus your thinking to get the results you need–may be the most important factor that determines whether you succeed or fail in this fast-paced world.

Whether you're trying to streamline a plan of care, resolve a conflict, or master new knowledge and skills, critical thinking–deliberate, informed thought–is the key. Yet thinking isn't "like it always was." We must learn to think in new ways. Consider the following reasons for focusing more on critical thinking:

◆ In communities, schools, and at work, we're expected to accept more responsibilities, collaborate with diverse individuals, and make more independent decisions (see Box 1-1). Acquiring critical thinking skills gives you the confidence to know when to act independently and when to say, "Wait. I'd better get help."

Box 1-1 WORKPLACE SKILLS*

To succeed in the workplace and as learners, you must know how to:
◆ **Take** ownership and responsibility.
◆ **Engage** in independent and group problem solving.
◆ **Use** resources: allocate time, money, materials, space, and human resources.
◆ **Establish** positive interpersonal relationships: work on teams, teach others, lead, negotiate, and work well with diverse individuals.
◆ **Acquire and evaluate** information: organize and maintain files, interpret and communicate, and use computers to process information.
◆ **Assess** social, organizational, and technologic systems: monitor and correct performance and design or improve systems.
◆ **Apply** professional and ethical standards to guide decision making.
◆ **Use** technology: select equipment and tools, apply technology to tasks, maintain and troubleshoot equipment.

Accomplishing the above requires you to have:
◆ **Basic skills:** reading, writing, mathematics, speaking, and listening.
◆ **Thinking skills:** knowing how to learn, reason, think creatively, generate and evaluate ideas, see things in the mind's eye, make decisions, and solve problems.
◆ **Personal qualities:** responsibility, self-esteem, self-confidence, self-management, sociability, and integrity.

*Recommended Reading: The Secretary's Commission on Achieving Necessary Skills (SCANS), The U.S. Department of Labor (1992). *Learning a living: a blueprint for high performance, a SCANS report for America 2000* (p. xiv). Washington, DC: Author. *A Vision for Nursing* (on-line) Available: http://nln.org/aboutnln/vision.htm. Assessed February 1, 2002 and The Pew Report in Sugars, D. O'Neil, and Bader, J. (Eds). (1991). *Healthy America: Practitioners for 2005, an Agenda for Action for U.S. Health Professional Schools.* Durham, NC: the Pew Health Professions Commission.

◆ Nurses are often involved in complex situations that require in-depth thinking. We must view ourselves as knowledge workers, who are thought-oriented rather than task-oriented.

◆ Critical thinking is the key to preventing and resolving problems. If you can't think critically, you become part of the problem.

◆ Critical thinking and test-taking skills are essential to passing the many tests we must take to formally demonstrate knowledge (e.g., certification tests and the National Council Licensure Examination, or NCLEX).

HOW THIS BOOK HELPS YOU IMPROVE THINKING

This book is based on the belief that thinking is like any skill (e.g., music, art, athletics)—we each have our own styles and innate or learned capabilities. And we can all improve by gaining insight, acquiring instruction and feedback, and consciously practicing to improve. Chapters are organized to encourage you to use your own thinking as a major tool for learning.

◆ **This chapter and Chapter 2** examine critical thinking in daily life with some reference to nursing situations. Whether you want to improve your ability to handle personal or professional matters, this section helps you focus your thinking to get results using your own particular talents.

◆ **Chapters 3 and 4** are designed to help you meet the challenges of acquiring the knowledge, confidence, and thinking skills required to succeed in six common nursing situations: reasoning in the clinical setting (clinical judgment), moral and ethical reasoning, nursing research, teaching others, teaching ourselves, and test taking.

◆ **Chapter 5** provides opportunities to practice critical judgment (clinical reasoning) skills using case scenarios based on real nursing experiences.

◆ **Chapter 6** helps you gain key skills needed to work in any position that's highly relational (any job that demands a lot of interaction with others). When you have key skills like managing conflict and working as a team, you can use your brainpower to resolve unique, rather than common "human nature" problems. This section also helps you learn to "work smarter, not harder," for example, how to set priorities and manage your time.

WHAT'S THE DIFFERENCE BETWEEN THINKING AND CRITICAL THINKING?

The key difference between thinking and critical thinking is *purpose* and *control.* Thinking refers to any mental activity—it can be "mindless," like when you're daydreaming or doing routine tasks like brushing your teeth.

On the other hand, critical thinking is controlled and purposeful; it focuses on using well-reasoned strategies to get the results you need.

CRITICAL THINKING: SOME DIFFERENT DESCRIPTIONS

Because critical thinking is a complex process that can be described in more than one way, there's no one right definition. Many authors (including myself) develop their own descriptions to complement and clarify someone else's (which is, by the way, a good example of thinking critically–critical thinking requires you to "personalize" information–to analyze it and decide what it means to you rather than simply memorizing someone else's words).

Think about the following synonym and commonly seen descriptions.

A Synonym

A good synonym for critical thinking is *reasoning*. If you were in elementary school today, you'd learn "four Rs" instead of three: reading, 'riting, 'rithmetic, and *reasoning*. Beginning in kindergarten, children learn the *how to*'s of effective reasoning. This fourth R is stressed throughout primary and secondary schools.

Now you know a synonym. But, since reasoning is a highly individualized, complex activity that involves distinct ideas, emotions, and perceptions, let's move on to a more substantial discussion.

Commonly Seen Descriptions of Critical Thinking

Here are some commonly seen descriptions of critical thinking:

◆ "Knowing how to learn, reason, think creatively, generate and evaluate ideas, see things in the mind's eye, make decisions, and solve problems."[1]
◆ "Reasonable, reflective thinking that focuses on what to believe or do."[2]
◆ "Purposeful and goal-directed thinking."[3]
◆ "The ability to solve problems by making sense of information using creative, intuitive, logical, and analytical mental processes ... and the process is continual."[4]
◆ "Thinking about your thinking, while you're thinking, to make it better, more clear, accurate, and defensible."[5]
◆ "The process of purposeful, self-regulatory judgment ... the cognitive engine that drives problem solving and decision making."[6]

All of these descriptions are helpful, and each one sheds more light on critical thinking. However, because critical thinking is contextual, meaning that we must look at the specific context in which thinking happens, let's look at some key points that describe what's involved in thinking critically in *nursing*.

Critical Thinking, Clinical Judgment, and Clinical Reasoning

The terms *critical thinking, clinical judgment,* and *clinical reasoning* are often used interchangeably. However, there is a slight difference in these terms:

◆ **Critical thinking** refers to purposeful, informed reasoning both *in* and *outside* the clinical setting (for example, determining the best way to write a class paper or present a topic, as well as the examples of clinical judgment and clinical reasoning that follow).

◆ **Clinical judgment and clinical reasoning** refer to using critical thinking in the clinical setting (for example, determining diagnoses, giving opinions, or making patient care decisions).

So what, exactly, do critical thinking and clinical judgment entail? Reflect on the following applied definition that focuses on critical thinking at the bedside.

Critical thinking and clinical judgment in nursing:

◆ Entails purposeful, informed, outcome-focused (results-oriented) thinking that requires careful identification of key problems, issues, and risks involved.
◆ Is driven by patient, family, and community needs.*
◆ Is based on principles of nursing process and scientific method (for example, making judgments based on evidence rather than guesswork).
◆ Uses both logic and intuition, based on knowledge, skills, and experience.
◆ Is guided by professional standards and ethics codes.
◆ Requires strategies that make the most of human potential (for example, using individual strengths) and compensate for problems created by human nature (for example, overcoming the powerful influence of personal views).
◆ Is constantly re-evaluating, self-correcting, and striving to improve.

We'll look at what clinical judgment entails in depth in Chapters 3 and 4. For now, keep in mind the following rule:

Rule: To think critically in any situation, you must answer two key questions: 1) What exactly are the results you need? and 2) What are the problems, issues, or risks that must be addressed to get the results? (Sometimes the results you *need* may be in conflict with the results you *want*. For example, you may *want* things done your way. But if you allow people to do things *their way*, you may get better results, and also promote independent problem-solving skills.)

---

*To think critically, nurses must be grounded in meeting patient and consumer needs. However, addressing nurses' and other disciplines' needs is often key to meeting patient and consumer needs. For example, streamlining charting for easy use improves communication and gives more time for patient care.

What about Common Sense?

Occasionally in my workshops someone asks, "Isn't critical thinking no more than *common sense*, something that can't be taught?" A statement like this takes a superficial look at what critical thinking is and at how you get "common sense." For example, you can put someone with a lot of common sense in a new or stressful situation, such as beginning a new job, and you're likely to see behaviors that don't seem like common sense. Think about the following scenario.

Case scenario
CRITICAL THINKING: SIMPLY COMMON SENSE?

I was an evening supervisor, and I stopped to check on a new graduate who was in charge for the first time. She appeared to be "in over her head," nervous and running around. Calmly, I asked how things were going. She replied, "Fine, except for the man in room 203. His temperature was 104 an hour ago. We drew blood cultures, gave aspirin, and started him on antibiotics." I asked, "What's the temperature now?" She replied, "We're not due to take it until eight" (three hours later). It seemed common sense to me that you would check the temperature more frequently when it was that high. Wanting to set a collaborative tone, I stressed the need to check it more frequently, and asked her to keep me informed. I also made sure I came back frequently to see how things were going. At the time I believed this nurse had no common sense, but she went on to be an excellent clinician with a track record of success. She was simply inexperienced, nervous, and overwhelmed in a new situation.

Although some people are blessed with an innate ability to focus on what's practical, useful, and helpful, a lot of common sense comes from knowledge, experience, and an ability to stay focused and pay attention. What may be common sense to you, based on your upbringing, schooling, or experience, may not be so to someone else. If you encounter someone who seems to have no common sense, don't jump to conclusions. Dig a little deeper to determine the real problems. For example, is there a knowledge, confidence, communication, or organizational skills problem? Is the person simply inexperienced or stressed by a new environment? Has the person become complacent? Could a learning disability be contributing to the problem? Like critical thinking, common sense often *can* be taught if you determine the underlying problems and do something about them. ◆

◆ WHAT DO CRITICAL THINKERS LOOK LIKE?

When we ask, "What do critical thinkers look like?" we mean, "What characteristics do we see in someone who thinks critically?"

Consider the following description:

The ideal critical thinker is habitually inquisitive, self-informed, trustful of reason, open-minded, flexible, fair-minded in evaluation, honest in facing personal biases, prudent in making judgments, willing to reconsider, clear about issues, orderly in complex matters, diligent in seeking relevant information, reasonable in selection of criteria, focused in inquiry, and persistent in seeking results that are as precise as the subject and the circumstances of inquiry permit.[7]

Now you have a somewhat lengthy description of what the ideal critical thinker looks like. Let's go on to the behaviors that promote critical thinking.

Critical Thinking Indicators™ (CTIs™)

Looking at how critical thinkers behave–what they *do and say*–gives us a picture of what things we can do to improve our ability to think critically. Box 1-2 shows behaviors that evidence suggests promotes critical thinking.* These behaviors are called critical thinking indicators (CTIs)™ because they *indicate* characteristics or attitudes of critical thinkers. Keep in mind that no one is perfect–there's no ideal critical thinker who demonstrates *all* of the characteristics. It's also possible to be a critical thinker, but not have some of the attributes *at all.* For example, you could have a critical thinking thief who isn't at all genuine, honest, or upright. Realize that even the best thinkers' characteristics vary, depending on circumstances such as comfort and familiarity with the people and situations at hand. What matters are *patterns* of behavior over time (is the behavior usually evident?). Also remember that CTIs™ focus on *clinical* nursing and critical thinking from a *nursing* perspective, which explains the inclusion of being self-disciplined and managing stress through healthy behaviors. If you're unhealthy or stressed out, you're likely to have trouble thinking critically.

In chapter 2, we'll address other CTIs™–indicators of knowledge and intellectual skills that promote critical thinking. For now, compare yourself with each indicator in Box 1-2 and rate how well you demonstrate the behavior using a scale of 0–10 (0 = I often have trouble demonstrating this indicator and 10 = I usually demonstrate this indicator). As you evaluate yourself, remember that some of you, due to your nature, will be harder on yourself than others (and vice versa). If you have some trusted

---

*The CTIs in this chapter and the next include behaviors addressed by key authors (See Donald, 2002, Facione and Facione, 1994, Paul and Elder, 2002, Scheffer and Rubenfeld, 2000, and Villaire, 1996, in the comprehensive bibliography on pages 286-293), as well as behaviors noted in key nursing documents (for example, *The Code of ethics for Nurses*, on page 264). The CTIs have been validated by expert and staff nurses in my workshops and via the Internet. CTIS are available at www.AlfaroTeachSmart.com.

Box 1-2 CRITICAL THINKING INDICATORS™ DEMONSTRATING
CRITICAL THINKING CHARACTERISTICS/ATTITUDES

The ideal critical thinking nurse is:

☐ **Self-aware:** Clarifies biases, inclinations, strengths, and limitations; acknowledges when thinking may be influenced by emotions or self-interest.

☐ **Genuine:** Shows authentic self; demonstrates behaviors that indicate stated values.

☐ **Self disciplined:** Promotes a healthy lifestyle; uses healthy behaviors to manage stress.

☐ **Autonomous and responsible:** Shows independent thinking and actions; begins and completes tasks without prodding; expresses ownership of accountability.

☐ **Careful and prudent:** Seeks help when needed; suspends or revises judgment as indicated by new or incomplete data.

☐ **Confident and resilient:** Expresses faith in ability to reason and learn; overcomes disappointments.

☐ **Honest and upright:** Seeks the truth, even if it sheds unwanted light; upholds standards; admits flaws in thinking.

☐ **Curious and inquisitive:** Looks for reasons, explanations, and meaning; seeks new information to broaden understanding.

☐ **Alert to context:** Looks for changes in circumstances that warrant a need to modify thinking or approaches.

☐ **Analytical and insightful:** Identifies relationships; expresses deep understanding.

☐ **Logical and intuitive:** Draws reasonable conclusions (if this is so, then it follows that ... because ...); uses intuition as a guide to search for evidence, acts on intuition only with knowledge of risks involved.

☐ **Open and fair-minded:** Shows tolerance for different viewpoints; questions how own viewpoints are influencing thinking.

☐ **Sensitive to diversity:** Expresses appreciation of human differences related to values, culture, personality, or learning style preferences; adapts to preferences as needed.

☐ **Creative:** Offers alternative solutions and approaches; comes up with useful ideas.

☐ **Realistic and practical:** Admits when things aren't feasible, looks for user-friendly solutions.

☐ **Reflective and self-corrective:** Carefully considers meaning of data and interpersonal interactions; asks for feedback, corrects own thinking, is alert to potential errors by self and others, finds ways to avoid future mistakes.

☐ **Proactive:** Anticipates consequences, plans ahead, acts on opportunities.

☐ **Courageous:** Stands up for beliefs, advocates for others, doesn't hide from challenges.

☐ **Patient and persistent:** Waits for right moment, perseveres to achieve best results.

☐ **Flexible:** Changes approaches as needed to get the best results.

☐ **Empathetic:** Listens well, shows ability to imagine others' feelings and difficulties.

☐ **Improvement-oriented (self, patients, systems):** (Self) Identifies learning needs, seeks new information, finds ways to overcome limitations. (Patients) Promotes health, maximizes function, comfort, and convenience. (Systems) Identifies risks and problems with health care systems, promotes safety, quality, satisfaction, and cost containment.

friends, peers, or family members, it's a good idea to get their input on how they see your behavior. You may be surprised—or reaffirmed!

Table 1-1 shows how other key authors describe critical thinking traits. These traits have been incorporated into the CTIs using simpler terms. Table 1-2 gives examples of what critical thinking is and what it's not.

REFLECTION AND INSIGHT ("HEMMING AND HAWING" AND "AHA!")

Once I asked a student how she went about answering test questions. She replied, "Usually I read the question, and then I hem and haw about what's being asked and what's the best response." Critical thinking requires reasonable, reflective thinking—it may require you to "hem and haw."

Another expression that is a key part of critical thinking is *aha!* We say "aha!" when we suddenly realize something or have our suspicions confirmed. We say aha! when we connect with something that was in the back of our minds but never put into words. Often, the greatest leaps in thinking come in these kinds of flashes of insight.

As you read this book, do some "hemming and hawing" (reflecting) about what you read. If you're not sure about something or want to give it more thought, write a brief question in the margin or on a piece of paper to remind yourself to come back to it. Then discuss your thoughts with a teacher or peer. You gain more from your reading when you discuss key questions with others, clarifying your thoughts and broadening your perspectives. You also retain what you read. Look for ahas. These moments of "light bulbs going off in your head" are energizing. They bring new ideas and stimulate you to learn more.

Critical Moments

QUESTIONS PLEASE
Socrates learned more from questioning others than he did from reading books. Seek others' opinions and question deeply to gain understanding.

Table 1-1 HOW OTHER AUTHORS DESCRIBE CRITICAL THINKING TRAITS

Paul and Elder's Intellectual Traits*	Facione and Facione's Critical Thinking Dispositions†	Scheffer and Rubenfeld's Habits of the Mind‡
Intellectual humility: Consciousness of limits of your knowledge; willingness to admit what you don't know	**Truthseeking:** A courageous desire for the best knowledge, even if such knowledge fails to support or undermines one's preconceptions, beliefs, or self-interest	**Confidence:** Assurance of one's reasoning abilities
Intellectual courage: Awareness of the need to face and fairly address ideas, beliefs, or viewpoints to which you haven't given serious hearing	**Open-mindedness:** Tolerance of divergence views, self-monitoring for possible bias	**Contextual perspective:** Consideration of the whole situation, including relationships, background, and environment relevant to some happening
Intellectual empathy: Consciousness of the need to imaginatively put yourself in the place of others to genuinely understand them	**Analyticity:** Demanding the application of reason and evidence, alert to problematic situations, inclined to anticipate consequences	**Creativity:** Intellectual inventiveness used to generate, discover, or restructure ideas. Imagining alternatives
Intellectual autonomy: Having control over your beliefs, values, and inferences; being an independent thinker	**Systematicity:** Valuing organization, focusing, and being diligent about problems of all levels of complexity	**Flexibility:** Capacity to adapt, accomodate, modify, or change thoughts, ideas, and behaviors
Intellectual integrity: Being true to your own thinking; applying intellectual standards to thinking; holding yourself to the same standards you hold others; willingness to admit when your thinking may be flawed	**CT self-confidence:** Trusting of one's own reasoning skills and seeing oneself as a good thinker	**Inquisitiveness:** An eagerness to know by seeking knowledge and understanding through observation, and thoughtful questioning in order to explore possibilities and alternatives
Confidence in reason: Confidence that, in the long run, using your own thinking and encouraging others to do the same, gets the best results	**Inquisitiveness:** Curious and eager to acquire knowledge and learn explanations even when the applications of the knowledge are not immediately apparent	**Intellectual integrity:** Seeking the truth through sincere, honest processes, even if the results are contrary to one's assumptions and beliefs
	Maturity: Prudence in making, suspending or revising judgment; awareness that multiple solutions can be acceptable; appreciation of the need to	**Intuition:** Insightful sense of knowing without conscious use of reason
		Open-mindedness: A viewpoint characterized by being receptive to divergent views and sensitive to one's biases

Continued

Table 1-1 HOW OTHER AUTHORS DESCRIBE CRITICAL THINKING TRAITS–cont'd

Paul and Elder's Intellectual Traits*	Facione and Facione's Critical Thinking Dispositions†	Scheffer and Rubenfeld's Habits of the Mind‡
Fairmindedness: Awareness of the need to treat all viewpoints alike, with awareness of vested interests	reach closure even in the absence of complete knowledge	**Perseverance:** Pursuit of a course with determination to overcome obstacles
		Reflection: Contemplation upon a subject, especially one's assumptions and thinking for the purposes of deeper understanding and self-evaluation

*Descriptions summarized from the glossary of Paul, R., & Elder, L. (2001). *Critical thinking: Tools for taking charge of your learning and your life.* Upper Saddle River, NJ: Prentice-Hall.
†Descriptions quoted from Facione, N, Facione, P., & Sanchez, P. (1994). Critical thinking disposition as a measure of competent clinical judgment: The development of the California critical thinking disposition inventory. *Journal of Nursing Education,* 33(8), 346.
‡Descriptions quoted from Scheffer, B., & Rubenfeld, M. (2000). A consensus statement on critical thinking in nursing. *Journal of Nursing Education,* 39(8), 353.

WHAT'S FAMILIAR AND WHAT'S NEW?

We understand something best by comparing it with something we already know: How is it the same and how is it different? This section first addresses critical thinking concepts you're likely to find familiar; then it addresses concepts that are likely to be new.

What's Familiar

PROBLEM SOLVING. Knowing how to solve problems with very specific, carefully reasoned, strategies is the key to thinking critically. Be aware, however, that using *problem solving* interchangeably with *critical thinking* can be a "sore subject." If you have only a "problem-solving mentality"–if all you're doing is solving problems, without making improvements, you're not thinking critically. *Problem solving* is missing the important concepts of *creativity and improvement.* Even if no problems exist, you should be thinking creatively, asking, "What could we be doing better?" and "How can we *prevent* problems before they happen?"

DECISION MAKING. Many nurses use decision making interchangeably with critical thinking. Critical thinking includes decision making, but also includes other concepts like how to do a focused assessment and how to make a diagnosis.

ANALYZING. Critical thinking requires more than analyzing. It also requires coming up with new ideas (right-brain thinking) and analyzing and judging the worth of those ideas (left-brain thinking).

Table 1-2   CRITICAL THINKING: WHAT IT IS AND WHAT IT'S NOT

Critical Thinking	Not Critical Thinking	Example of Critical Thinking
Organized and clearly explained by using words, examples, pictures or graphics	Disorganized and vague	Persisting until you find a way to make your ideas easy to understand; using examples and illustrations to facilitate understanding
Critical for the sake of improvement, new ideas, and doing things in the best interest of the key players involved	Critical for the sake of attacking without being able to suggest new ideas and alternatives; critical for the sake of having it your way	Determining key players affected, then looking for flaws in the way something is done and figuring out ways to achieve the same outcomes easier or better
Inquisitive about intent, facts, and reasons behind an idea or action; thought- and knowledge-oriented	Unconcerned about motives, facts, and reasons behind an idea or action; task-oriented, rather than thought-oriented	Raising questions to deeply understand what happened, why it happened, and what was trying to be accomplished when it happened
Sensitive to the powerful influence of emotions, but focused on making decisions based on what's morally and ethically the right thing to do	Emotion-driven	Finding out how someone feels about something, then moving on to discuss what's morally and ethically right
Communicative and collaborative with others when dealing with complex issues	Isolated, competitive, or unable to communicate with others when dealing with complex issues	Seeking multidisciplinary approaches to planning care as indicated by client needs

THE SCIENTIFIC METHOD AND NURSING PROCESS. There's a lot about critical thinking that's similar to principles of science, the scientific method, and nursing process. For example, critical thinking requires all of the following:
- ◆ **Observing:** Continuously observing and examining to collect data, check for changes, and gain understanding.
- ◆ **Classifying data:** Grouping related information in order to reveal relationships among the observed facts.
- ◆ **Drawing conclusions** that follow logically. If this is so, then …
- ◆ **Conducting experiments:** Performing studies to examine hypotheses (hunches or suspicions) and identify ways to improve.

◆ **Testing hypotheses (hunches):** Determining whether we have factual evidence to support our hunches, assumptions, or suspicions.
CLINICAL REASONING. Often *clinical reasoning* is used interchangeably with critical thinking and clinical judgment. *Clinical reasoning* and *clinical judgment* both refer to critical thinking in the clinical setting.

What's New

STRATEGIES FOR MAXIMIZING HUMAN POTENTIAL. We're only just beginning to learn how to maximize the human potential to think critically. For example, as youngsters most of us were encouraged to memorize. Yet few of us learned *how to memorize* in ways that promote comprehension and retention. We now know that memorizing a list of facts can be a dead end for our minds. It doesn't help us *understand* information, and it doesn't help us *retain it in the long term.* We're beginning to identify strategies like using visual centers of the brain and using preferred learning styles to maximize understanding and retention (see page 24).

MORE IMPORTANCE GIVEN TO THE NEED TO DEVELOP WHAT-IF STRATEGIES. We pay more attention to developing detailed approaches, policies, and procedures to cover what-if scenarios. For example, you have planned policies and procedures to follow if a mistake happens.

INTERPERSONAL SKILLS AND PROMOTING COLLABORATIVE THINKING. We continue to work on developing interpersonal skills and identifying approaches that bring diverse thinkers together. Only then can we facilitate "meetings of the minds" to get the collaborative approaches that are so important to giving quality care.

MORE EMPHASIS ON BEING *VERY SPECIFIC* ABOUT HOW TO MEASURE OUTCOMES (RESULTS). To think critically, you must determine ways you can be clear about whether you really are getting results. For example, in the case of pain management, you don't ask a general question like, "Are you more comfortable?" You ask, "Can you rate your pain on a scale of 0 to 10, with 0 meaning *pain-free*, and 10 meaning *the worst possible pain?*"

NEED FOR EVIDENCE STRESSED. As we have more data, we expect people to provide evidence that supports opinions and solutions. We must be confident in answering questions like, "What evidence do you have that this will work?" and "How do you know this is the problem?"

Box 1-3 gives an overview of additional things that are new about critical thinking. Figure 1-1 is a visual summary of questions that can help you evaluate your potential to think critically.

Box 1-3 WHAT'S NEW ABOUT CRITICAL THINKING

❏ Research findings suggesting that intelligence quotient (IQ) tests may not really measure IQ and that there are other focuses of intelligence (e.g., interpersonal intelligence) that influence our ability to think critically.

❏ The idea that thinking can and must be taught, that practicing thinking skills helps us be better thinkers.

❏ Studies suggesting that the brain is like a muscle: The more you use it, the more capable it becomes.

❏ The belief that personal interests, passions, and commitments, as well as a sense of aesthetics (beauty), mystery, and wonder, play a crucial role in developing attitudes necessary for thinking.

❏ Increased concern about the reasoning process: It's often as important to know how a conclusion or decision is made as it is to know what the conclusion or decision is.

❏ Greater emphasis on understanding other perspectives and using several different perspectives (collaboration) to come to better conclusions. Great minds don't always think alike: Different viewpoints enhance our thinking.

❏ More acceptance of "There's more than one way" and "Sometimes there are no right answers" (each answer is correct in its own way).

❏ Acknowledgment that there are useful mistakes (occasional failure is the price of improvement) and that sharing mistakes is a responsible action that helps others avoid the same errors.

❏ More research on finding ways to "measure" how someone thinks.

❏ The identification of strategies that help us take advantage of how our brains work, including how to:
   • Get information into long-term memory.
   • Form good habits of inquiry.
   • Use both sides of our brains.
   • Enhance creativity.

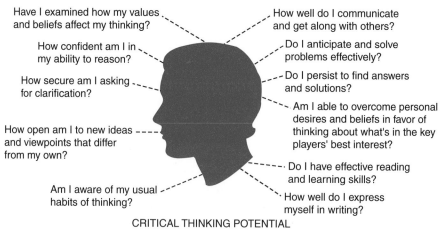

CRITICAL THINKING POTENTIAL

Have I examined how my values and beliefs affect my thinking?

How confident am I in my ability to reason?

How secure am I asking for clarification?

How open am I to new ideas and viewpoints that differ from my own?

Am I aware of my usual habits of thinking?

How well do I communicate and get along with others?

Do I anticipate and solve problems effectively?

Do I persist to find answers and solutions?

Am I able to overcome personal desires and beliefs in favor of thinking about what's in the key players' best interest?

Do I have effective reading and learning skills?

How well do I express myself in writing?

Figure 1-1 ◆ Questions to evaluate your potential to think critically.

Other Perspectives

CRITICAL THINKING MAY BE TRIGGERED BY POSITIVE EVENTS

Here's an example of critical thinking triggered by positive events.

When a baby is born in some hospitals, everyone shares in the celebration. With each birth the public address system plays Brahms' Lullaby. Patients love it—even oncology patients, who say it lifts their spirits and allows them to share someone else's joy. Parents who have just lost their baby are given the option of playing the lullaby or not. Many of them choose to have it played for their baby. "Playing the music is a simple thing that can be done for patients and families that costs virtually nothing and brings a great deal of pleasure."

—Jean Young, ICU Patient Care Manager

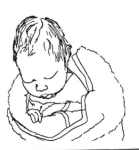

KEY POINTS

Because critical thinking is a complex activity that can be described in more than one way, there's no one right definition—there are several that complement and clarify one another. *Critical thinking* refers to purposeful, results-oriented thinking in any situation. Clinical judgment refers to critical thinking in the clinical setting. Box 1-2, page 8, shows critical thinking indicators (CTIs)—behaviors that demonstrate characteristics that promote critical thinking. There's a lot about critical thinking that's similar to principles of science and the scientific method. Critical thinking requires right-brain thinking (generating new ideas) and left-brain thinking (analyzing and judging the worth of those ideas). Critical thinking is like any skill (e.g., music, art, athletics). We each have our own styles and innate or learned capabilities. And we can all improve by gaining awareness, acquiring instruction, and consciously practicing to improve.

Recommendations for Completing Critical Thinking Exercises

1. Don't let your own thinking be the *weakest link!* Remember the benefits of connecting with your own way of thinking. Use strategies like drawing mind maps—link key concepts, and use your own thinking to decide where things fit in. If you don't know about the benefits of mind mapping or how to draw a mind map, read "Mind Mapping: Getting in the 'Right' State of Mind" beginning on pages 260-262.
2. When writing responses, at first, be more concerned with substance than grammar (as you would if you were writing a diary). However, as you progress, work to make your responses *clear to others*. Making your responses clear to others will help you clarify your thoughts.
3. If you have trouble *writing* and do better *verbally*, tape your response; then play it and write it down. This will save you time in the long run. Or use a voice-activated software program, such as *Naturally Speaking*.
4. Don't be afraid to paraphrase: Paraphrasing helps you gain understanding because you explain what you read using familiar language (your own). To avoid concerns of plagiarism, cite the page numbers that you've chosen to paraphrase.

CRITICAL THINKING EXERCISES

Note: Exercises followed by asterisks have example responses listed in the Response Key at the back of the book beginning on page 246.

1. What is the relationship between outcome achievement and identifying problems, issues, or risks involved?*
2. Personalize the information in this chapter by answering the following:
   ◆ What information did you find to be most relevant or helpful?
   ◆ What information did you find least relevant or helpful?
   ◆ Think of at least two questions the information in this chapter raises for you.
   ◆ How do your responses compare with those of others who read this chapter?
3. Complete the following sentences and then compare your responses with those of others:
   ◆ If I were to tell someone how I think, I would say that I …
   ◆ I do my best thinking when …
   ◆ I do my worst thinking when …
4. Compare and contrast the traits of confidence in reason, critical thinking self-confidence, and confidence, listed in Table 1-1 on page 10.*
5. When you form an opinion, you draw a conclusion from facts or evidence.
   a. What's the difference between facts and opinions?*
   b. How can you determine if an opinion is valid?*

CRITICAL THINKING EXERCISES—cont'd

Note: Exercises followed by asterisks have example responses listed in the Response Key at the back of the book beginning on page 246.

6. Think about the Other Perspectives below. Discuss with a peer (or peers) the effect "mind games" (worrying too much or focusing on the negatives) can have on thinking and performance.

Other Perspectives

YOU ARE YOUR OWN COACH ...

"If you don't talk to yourself and give yourself pep talks, start now. Time was, only crazies talked to themselves; now, you miss the boat if you don't. Our minds are tricky things. We know now that attitude is the base on which knowledge and ability stand."[8]

—Jean T. Penny, PhD, ARNP. www.jtpennys.com

7. Explain how the following Other Perspectives relate to your life today.

Other Perspectives

HOW LITERATE ARE YOU?

"The illiterate of the twenty-first century will not be those who cannot read and write, but those who cannot learn, unlearn, and relearn."

—Alvin Toffler, author of Future Shock

HOW TO THINK LIKE EINSTEIN

"It's not that I'm smart, it's just that I stick with problems longer."

—Albert Einstein

8. Consider Box 1-1 (page 2), addressing workplace skills. Identify three skills you'd like to improve, and then think of some ways you can acquire the three skills you identified.

9. Complete the prechapter self-test, which has been reproduced below:
   a. Describe critical thinking using your own words, based on the definitions in this chapter.*
   b. Explain the difference between thinking and critical thinking.*
   c. Give three reasons why critical thinking is essential for nurses.*
   d. Explain the relationship between outcomes (results) and critical thinking.*
   e. Clarify the term *critical thinking indicator* (CTI™).*
   f. Describe five critical thinking characteristics you'd like to develop or improve.
   g. Address how critical thinking is similar to and different from problem solving.*
   h. Identify four principles of the scientific method that are evident in critical thinking.*

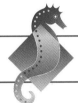

Critical Moments

Connect with people by letting them know your human side and imagining what it would be like to be in their shoes.

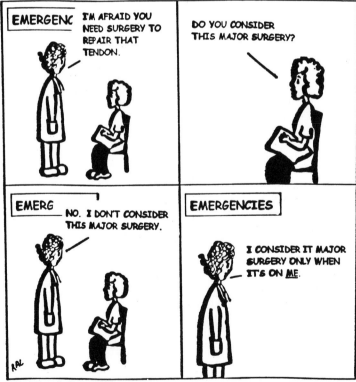

© R. Alfaro-LeFevre 1998.

References

1. The Secretary's Commission on Achieving Necessary Skills [SCANS], The U.S. Department of Labor. (1992). *Learning a living: A blueprint for high performance, a SCANS report for America 2000*. Washington, D.C.: Author.
2. Ennis, R., & Milman, J. (1985). *Cornell tests of critical thinking: Theory and practice*. Pacific Grove, CA: Midwest Publications.
3. Halpern, D. (1984). *Thought and knowledge*. Hillsdale, NJ: Lawrence Erlbaum Associates.
4. Snyder, M. (1993). Critical thinking: A foundation for consumer-focused care. *The Journal of Continuing Education in Nursing, 24*(5), 206–210.
5. Paul, R. (1995). *Critical thinking: How to prepare students for a rapidly changing world*. Santa Rosa, CA: Foundation for Critical Thinking.
6. Colucciello, M. (1997). Critical thinking skills and dispositions of baccalaureate nursing students—A conceptual model for evaluation. *Journal of Professional Nursing, 13*(4), 236–245.
7. Table I, Critical thinking: A statement of expert consensus for purposes of educational assessment and instruction, "The APA Delphi Report" (1990). ERIC Document Number, 315–423.
8. E-mail communication. (May 2002).

See comprehensive bibliography beginning on page 286.

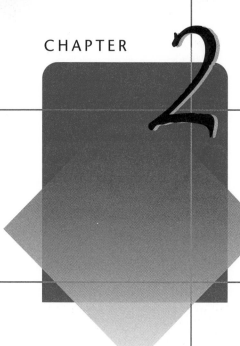

CHAPTER

2 How to Think Critically

THIS CHAPTER at a Glance ...

◆ Gaining Insight and Self-Awareness
◆ What's Your Personal Style and Why Does It Matter?
    Understanding Learning Style Preferences
    How Your Personality Affects Thinking
    Effects of Upbringing and Culture
◆ Mentoring and Building Empowered Partnerships
◆ Factors Influencing Critical Thinking Ability
    Personal Factors
    Situational Factors
    Habits Causing Barriers to Critical Thinking
    Covey's 7 Habits of Highly Effective People®
◆ Outcome-Focused (Results-Oriented) Thinking
    Goals (Intent) versus Outcomes (Results)
    Focusing on End Results
◆ Critical Thinking Strategies
    10 Key Questions
    Using Logic, Intuition, and Trial and Error
    Focusing on the Big and Small Pictures
    Specific Strategies
◆ Knowledge and Intellectual Skill Indicators
◆ How to Read Minds
◆ Developing Character, Acquiring Knowledge, and
  Practicing Skills
◆ Key Points

Read the following Learning Outcomes and decide whether you can readily achieve each one. If you can, you don't need to read this chapter and can go on to Chapter 3. Don't be concerned if you can't achieve any of the outcomes at this time. We come back to these outcomes later in the chapter, in Critical Thinking Exercises.

Learning Outcomes

After completing this chapter, you should be able to:

◆ Explain three key steps to improving thinking.

◆ Describe how your personality and learning style affect your ability to think critically.

◆ Discuss how human habits influence critical thinking ability.

◆ Address how asking the 10 key questions listed on the inside front cover helps you decide your approach to critical thinking.

◆ Describe five strategies that enhance critical thinking, giving reasons why the strategies work.

◆ Identify the roles of logic, intuition, and trial and error in critical thinking.

◆ Decide where you stand in relation to being able to demonstrate Critical Thinking Indicators™ (CTIs)™ for knowledge and intellectual skills.

◆ Explain the relationship between your ability to think critically and developing character, knowledge, and skills.

GAINING INSIGHT AND SELF-AWARENESS

Now that you have an idea of what critical thinking is, let's examine how you can make the most of your potential to think critically. Whether you want to improve your ability to handle personal or professional matters, this chapter helps you learn how to focus your approach to get the results you need in your own way.

As you read this chapter, keep the following in mind:

◆ Thinking is a skill like any other (e.g., music, art, athletics).
◆ As with any skill, we each have our own styles and innate and learned capabilities.
◆ We can all improve by (1) gaining insight and self-awareness, (2) acquiring instruction and feedback, and (3) consciously working to improve.

WHAT'S YOUR PERSONAL STYLE AND WHY DOES IT MATTER?

Developing an awareness of your personal style—how and why you think and learn the way you do—is a key starting point for improving thinking. Research on thinking and learning styles is growing. We now know that many people who consider themselves to be poor thinkers and learners are not so at all. They simply haven't learned to use their own natural abilities.

Two important factors determine whether you can improve your ability to think and learn. You must:

1. Believe in your ability to be a good thinker and learner.
2. Be willing to work at strategies that can help you think and learn more efficiently *in your own way*.

Understanding Learning Style Preferences

If you're one of the millions of people who believe that they aren't good learners, it may just be that you haven't been able to learn in ways that are best for *you*. For example, I have a friend who considered himself to be a poor learner. One day he said, "What I like best about computers is that I never was a good learner ... but with computers, it doesn't matter because you just have to figure things out for yourself ... and I'm good at that." I then pointed out that learning *is* "figuring things out for yourself"—it's 'learning at its *best*' because when you figure things out for yourself, you understand more deeply and retain better. Now *that's* critical thinking! Remember the following:

Rule: **THERE ARE NO RIGHT OR WRONG WAYS TO LEARN—THERE ARE ONLY DIFFERENCES.**

You are responsible for connecting with your preferred style and mastering strategies that can help you learn efficiently in your *own* way. When you figure things out in your own way, you're thinking critically.

If you aren't aware of how you learn best—whether you're a doer, observer, or whatever—review Table 2-1 on page 24, which gives an overview of various learning styles and corresponding strategies to promote learning.

 Other Perspectives

RESPECT YOUR BRAIN
"I have a very weird brain. But I like it; it is the only one I have."[1]

–*Ruth Hansten, FACHE, PhD, MBA, BSN*

CHINESE PROVERB ON LEARNING
"I hear, I forget. I see, I remember. I do, I understand."

–*Quoted by Astronaut John Glenn*

How Your Personality Affects Thinking

Personality plays a major role in how we think and learn. Your personality determines what information you notice and recall, the way you make decisions, and how much structure and control you like. Connecting with your own particular personality's needs helps you understand how and why you think the way you do. It helps you get in touch with your talents and blind spots and find ways to improve. Understanding personality types *different* from your own helps you realize how and why *others* think the way *they* do. Armed with this information, you can facilitate "meetings of the minds."

Study Boxes 2-1 and 2-2, which address personality and thinking styles. Keep in mind that no one style is better than another. They are all good styles with specific strengths and limitations. What's important

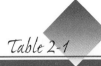

Table 2-1 STRATEGIES FOR LEARNING PREFERENCES

Learning Preference	Strategies To Maximize Learning
Observers (visual learners) Learn best by watching. For example, you'd rather watch someone give an injection before reading the procedure.	Sit in the front of the room, so you stay focused on the teacher, not on what's going on around you. Visualize procedures in your mind's eye, rather than trying to follow individual steps. In skills labs, don't go first. Rather, watch your classmates and take a later turn. Ask for observational experiences. Take lots of notes and use a highlighter. Recopy your notes when you're studying. When learning new terms or concepts or trying to remember something, write them on "sticky notes" and put them where you'll see them frequently (e.g., the bathroom mirror, the computer). Preview chapters by scanning headings and illustrations.
Doers (kinesthetic learners) Learn best by moving, doing, experiencing, or experimenting. For example, you'd rather play with a syringe and inject a dummy before reading the procedure.	Start by doing (e.g., play with equipment before reading about how to use it) because it will make observing, reading, and listening more meaningful. Be sure you know the risks of doing without much knowledge and find ways to minimize them (e.g., if you're playing on the computer, make sure you can't inadvertently erase a file). When taking notes, use arrows to show relationships. Draw boxes and circles around key concepts; make diagrams. Pace up and down while reciting information to yourself; ride a bicycle while listening to an instructional tape. Make tapes with the information you're trying to learn and play them while exercising (e.g., riding a bike), or read while riding a stationary bike. Write key words in the air; use your fingers to help you remember (bend the forefinger as you memorize a concept, then bend the next for the next concept, and so on). Change positions frequently while studying; take frequent short breaks involving activity. Study in a rocking chair; play background music. Ask if you can do assignments in an active way (e.g., create a poster, be part of a discussion group).
Listeners (auditory learners) Learn best by hearing. For example, you learn best when you can listen without worrying about taking notes.	Whisper as you read, listening to your words (especially important when reading test questions). Listen in class without taking notes, focusing on understanding what the teacher says, and then copy someone else's notes. Tape classes and listen to the tapes two or three times before exams. Ask if you can give an oral report or hand in an audiotape for extra credit. Memorize by making up songs or rhymes. Study with a friend, so you talk about the information. Tape yourself as you read key information out loud, and then listen to the tapes.

Box 2-1 WHAT'S YOUR THINKING STYLE?* (MYERS-BRIGGS TYPE INDICATOR)

EXTROVERT	INTROVERT
Thinks out loud	Thinks inside
Draws energy from being with people	Draws energy from being quiet
SENSATE	**INTUITIVE**
Perceives the world discreetly through the five senses	Perceives the world overall
Looks for facts	Looks for meaning
THINKING	**FEELING**
Uses objective data	Uses subjective data
Seeks just decisions	Seeks fair decisions
JUDGING	**PERCEIVING**
Orders the environment	Keeps things flexible and open
Likes to plan	Likes to be spontaneous

From Schoessler, M., Conedera, F., Bell, L., et al. (1993). Use of the Myers-Briggs type indicator to develop a continuing education department. *Journal of Nursing Staff Development, 9(1),9.*

is that you know that there are distinct style differences and that you (1) connect with your own style, celebrating your strengths, and working to overcome limitations, and (2) learn to understand people with styles different from your own, respecting their need to approach things in their own way. Box 2-3 shows the benefits of being sensitive to personality differences.

Effects of Upbringing and Culture

How you were raised and the culture you embrace has a great impact on how you think. For example, if you were raised by strict authoritarian parents who insisted that you "do as you are told, without asking questions," it's likely that you'll find it difficult to approach teachers or leaders to discuss a problem, ask for feedback, or offer suggestions. You'll need to muster courage and work to understand and overcome these deep-seated insecurities.

The more I talk with my international colleagues, the more I realize the impact of cultural beliefs on thinking. For example, in some countries, questioning teachers is considered rude. Teachers are to be respected, and in charge of learning. Yet in the United States we encourage students to question teachers when they don't understand. When students ask questions, everyone benefits, because everyone learns.

Box 2-2   **DO YOU KNOW WHAT TO DO WHEN SOMEONE TURNS BLUE?***

Here's a theory that gives new meaning to turning blue, red, white, or yellow (no, it doesn't mean becoming cyanotic, inflamed, shocky, or jaundiced). Psychologist Taylor Hartman uses colors to represent personality types (by the way, he says you can't really *turn* one personality color or another, you *are* what you are born). Hartman believes that each of us, from birth, is blessed with a core motive—a drive to approach life from a certain perspective. Using colors as labels, here's how he describes four distinct personality types:[†]

Reds have a drive for power. They know how to take charge and make things happen. *Reds'* strengths are that they are confident, determined, logical, productive, and visionary. However, they can be bossy, impatient, arrogant, argumentative, and self-focused.

Blues are driven to achieve intimacy. They love getting to know people well, have strong feelings, and like talking about the daily details of life. *Blues* are creative, caring, reliable, loyal, sincere, and committed to serving others. On the flip side, they can be judgmental, worry-prone, doubtful, and moody. They often have unrealistic expectations.

Whites strive for peace. They're independent, contented people who ask little of those around them. *Whites* are insightful, flexible, tolerant, easygoing, patient, and kind. But *Whites* tend to avoid conflict at all costs, are indecisive, silently stubborn, and may "explode" because they hold things in until there are so many things bothering them that just one more problem pushes them over the edge.

Yellows are driven to have fun. They wake up happy, know how to enjoy life in the present moment, and are simply fun to be around. *Yellows* are outgoing, enthusiastic, optimistic, popular, and trusting. However, they tend to avoid facing facts and can be impulsive, undisciplined, disorganized, and uncommitted.

The Color Code® has a 45-question profile you can take to determine your true color. While you may be a blend of two or more of the above colors, Hartman stresses that you're *dominant in only one*. He also points out that since you're born a particular type, it's useless to wish you were different (it would be like trying to be a different height). Rather, he encourages you to embrace your strengths and to work to overcome limitations by acquiring some of the other colors' strengths.

Applying the *Color Code*® helps you connect with inner drives that often lie dormant, waiting to be harnessed in positive ways. Armed with this knowledge, you can make better "people decisions," like how to nurture a team or get along with difficult people. Imagine how you could apply this theory to help a group come together to give a presentation. You might get a productive, visionary *Red* to coordinate and lead the project; a caring, detail-oriented *Blue* to do the handouts; a peace-loving, insightful *White* to be a "human suggestion box" (no one's afraid to approach a *White*); and a fun-loving *Yellow* to make sure that the class is more than serious stuff (a little fun, humor, and refreshment make it an enjoyable, and therefore, memorable, learning experience).

Box 2-2 **DO YOU KNOW WHAT TO DO WHEN SOMEONE TURNS BLUE?*—cont'd**

Think about what could happen in the previous situation if you switched some of those personalities and tasks around! *The Color Code®* facilitates a crucial first step to improving thinking—understanding how and why we think the way we do (and how and why *others* think they way *they* do). These are challenging times that require us to think and work in teams. Applying these principles helps us spend less time spinning wheels and more time "in gear," fully engaged in progress.

*Adapted from R. Alfaro-LeFevre, *Do you know what to do when someone turns blue?* ©1998. Nursing Spectrum Nurse Wire (www.nursingspectrum.com). All rights reserved. Used with permission.
†Summarized with permission from: Hartman, T. (1998). *The color code.®* New York: Scribner. www.hartmancommunications.com

Box 2-3 **BENEFITS OF PERSONALITY SENSITIVITY**

Partnering and Team Building
♦ Helps diverse personalities come together with understanding and respect, promoting solid relationships
♦ Keeps the focus on common goals, improving quality and efficiency
♦ Helps identify strategies to reduce and resolve conflicts
♦ Facilitates collaboration and makes the most of individual and team talents

Performance and Retention
♦ Promotes critical thinking (people think better when they understand and trust one another)
♦ Reduces stress, allowing more brainpower for finding solutions
♦ Increases self-confidence by providing style-specific strategies
♦ Promotes an environment that nurtures professional and personal growth

Customer Satisfaction
♦ Facilitates communication with "difficult" patients and families
♦ Improves outcomes by helping you tailor approaches to consider different personalities' wants and needs
♦ Patients and families feel understood, empowered, and motivated by receiving care that's "in synch" with their own specific styles

Want to know more about personality sensitivity? Access Alfaro-LeFevre, R. *Don't Worry! Be Happy! Harmonize diversity and improve outcomes* at http://nsweb.nursingspectrum.com/ce/ce236.htm.
Read Hartman, T. (1998). *The Color Code.®* New York: Scribner, or visit Hartman's web site at www.hartmancommunications.com

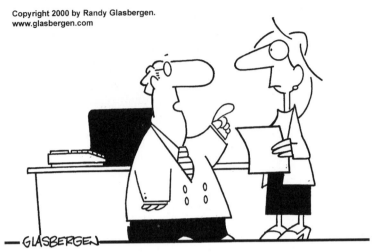

— GLASBERGEN —

**"We need to focus on diversity. Your goal is to hire
people who all look different, but think just like me."**

Other Perspectives

IN SOME CULTURES, QUESTIONING SHOWS WEAKNESS

*"I have trouble asking questions because in my culture, asking questions
is discouraged and a sign of weakness and embarrassment. What I'm
working on and want to know is how to become more confident and
capable in asking questions, for I realize it's essential to critical thinking."*

—*One of My Workshop Participants*

MENTORING AND BUILDING EMPOWERED PARTNERSHIPS

All successful people can identify people in their lives who have made
significant impacts on their thinking. These people are often parents,
teachers, co-workers, or trusted friends. Today, because we know the
value of improving thinking and performance through on-the-job partnerships, many organizations have mentors (also called preceptors).
Mentors are nurses with exemplary skills whose role it is to teach, nurture, and empower new nurses on a one-to-one basis. Learning how to
be a mentor and how to be a "mentee" (knowing how to learn and grow
from a more experienced person) is an important step in critical
thinking. Yet, it's important to have nurses who are well-matched for

this purpose. When matched well, mentors experience the reward of making a difference in someone else's life, and mentees have the benefit of "spreading their wings" under competent, caring guidance. When matched poorly, for example, if the two nurses are very different thinkers or personalities, the end result is frustration, disappointment, and damaged spirits on both sides. Remember that mentoring isn't a "one size fits all" situation. Build empowered partnerships (see page 199 in Chapter 6), pay attention to personal style differences, and address these early. Above all, remember the following:

Rule: **People think best when they like and trust one another. Work to build trust through empowered partnerships. (See page 199 for how to build empowered partnerships.)**

 Other Perspectives

GOOD MENTORS NURTURE POTENTIAL

"… Early in my career, I was powerfully influenced by a nursing instructor who saw potential in me that I did not recognize. Under the watchful, yet caring, tutelage of this person, I began to find my professional self."[2]

–*Patricia Thompson, RN, EdD, President, Sigma Theta Tau International*

"… Expert nurses are made, not born. Remember your first code, your first day in charge, the sadness with the death of your primary patient, or feeling alone? These experiences are all common to the novice nurse. The perception of the experience, as well as what is brought forward to future career events, can be shaped by an experience with a mentor."[3]

–*Margaret M. Ecklund, RN, MS, CCRN*

FACTORS INFLUENCING CRITICAL THINKING ABILITY

Have you ever found yourself saying, "I just wasn't thinking right" or, better yet, "Boy, that really got me thinking–I came up with some great ideas"? We all feel this way at one time or another. Our ability to think well varies, depending on personal factors and circumstances that are present at the time. For example, look at Table 2-2, which lists factors influencing thinking. Then read on for an explanation of *how and why* these factors are so influential.

Table 2-2   FACTORS INFLUENCING CRITICAL THINKING ABILITY

Factors Usually Enhancing Critical Thinking	Factors Usually Impeding Critical Thinking
Personal factors	**Personal factors**
Moral development and fair-mindedness	Dislikes, prejudices, biases
Age (older you are)	Lack of self-confidence
Culture, upbringing*	Limited knowledge of problem solving, decision
Self-confidence*	making, and research principles
Emotional intelligence	Poor communication skills
Knowledge of problem solving, decision making,	Poor writing skills
and research principles	Poor reading and learning skills
Effective communication and interpersonal skills	Unhealthy lifestyles
Habitual evaluation	
Past experience*	**Situational factors**
Effective writing skills	Anxiety, stress, or fatigue
Effective reading and learning skills	Lack of motivation
	Limited knowledge of related factors
Situational factors	Lack of awareness of resources
Knowledge of related factors	Time limitations‡
Awareness of resources	Environmental distractions
Awareness of risks†	
Positive reinforcement	
Presence of motivating factors	

*May impede or enhance thinking (addressed earlier in chapter).
†Sometimes impedes critical thinking.
‡Sometimes enhances critical thinking.

Personal Factors

MORAL DEVELOPMENT AND FAIR-MINDEDNESS. It's likely that there's a positive correlation among moral development, fair-mindedness, and critical thinking: People with a mature level of moral development—those with a clear, carefully reasoned sense of *what's right, wrong, and fair*—are more likely to think critically. It makes sense that those who are keenly aware of their values and beliefs, and approach situations with an attitude of "I must consider all viewpoints and make decisions *in the key players' best interests,*" already are critical thinkers.

AGE. Most authors agree that age tends to correlate with critical thinking ability: The older you get, the better thinker you become. There are two logical reasons for this: (1) Moral development usually comes with maturity. (2) Most older people have had more opportunities to practice reasoning in different situations. (Sometimes older nurses are rigid and set in their ways. In this case, age deters critical thinking).

DISLIKES, PREJUDICES, AND BIASES. These can be subtle but powerful factors that hinder critical thinking. If you don't recognize these factors—put them out on the table, so to speak—and overcome them, you're unlikely to think critically in situations where you have to function in spite of your dislikes, prejudices, and biases.

EMOTIONAL INTELLIGENCE. This is the ability to make emotions work in positive ways, and it enhances critical thinking. *How* you feel about something greatly influences how you think. Yet too often many of us aren't aware of deep, strong feelings. Clarifying emotions and giving them the attention they deserve—making them clear, accepting them, and recognizing how they're influencing thinking—helps us adjust our behavior and get better results. Box 2-4 gives strategies for using emotional intelligence to promote critical thinking.

SELF-CONFIDENCE. For the most part, self-confidence aids thinking. If you aren't confident, you use much of your brainpower worrying about failure, reducing the energy available for *productive thinking*. Occasionally self-confidence is an *impeding* factor: Some people become *overly confident* and believe they can't be wrong or have little to learn from others.

KNOWLEDGE OF PROBLEM SOLVING, DECISION MAKING, NURSING PROCESS, AND RESEARCH PRINCIPLES. Because critical thinking is based on many of these same principles, familiarity with the methods *enhances* critical thinking.

Box 2-4 USING EMOTIONAL INTELLIGENCE TO PROMOTE CRITICAL THINKING

1. **Connect with emotions.** Put your feelings into words and, through dialogue, help others to do the same ("I feel ... because ... "). Never assume you know what someone else is feeling or expect others to know what you're feeling.
2. **Accept true feelings for what they are.** No one's to blame for what he feels.
3. **Master mood management.** Recognize the importance of connecting with how emotions are affecting thinking. Learn to manage feelings like anger, anxiety, fear, and discouragement.
4. **Don't be too concerned with isolated events.** Patterns of behavior are what matter. (Don't sweat the small stuff.)
5. **Keep in mind that emotions are "catching."** If you're depressed, you may trigger depression in someone else. If you're enthusiastic, you may trigger enthusiasm.
6. **Do something to reduce stress.** Take time out, use humor, play a game, take a walk, learn to use yoga or guided imagery.

Recommended reading: Weisinger, H. (1998). *Emotional intelligence at work.* San Francisco, CA: Jossey-Bass.

EFFECTIVE COMMUNICATION AND INTERPERSONAL SKILLS. These are essential to critical thinking. You must be able to understand others, be understood by others, and gain others' trust to get the facts required for sound reasoning. Keep in mind that communication is more than talking and listening: You need to consider the messages you send by your *behavior* over time. For example, if you say that you're committed to giving good care, but consistently arrive late for work with excuses, the message is quite different. Box 2-5 gives communication strategies for enhancing critical thinking.

Box 2-5 COMMUNICATION STRATEGIES FOR ENHANCING CRITICAL THINKING

1. Work to understand what *other people* are trying to say before trying to get *them* to understand you.
2. Clearly state that your intent is not to judge but to understand (e.g., "I'm not here to judge. I just want to understand what's going on").
3. Use strategies that help you see other points of view.
   - Ask for clarification. For example, "I don't mean to be difficult, but I still don't understand. Can you clarify further?"
   - Use phrases like, "From your way of looking at it … or from your perspective." For example, "From your perspective, how do you see this situation?" or "Help me understand what you're trying to do."
   - Paraphrase in your own words. For example, "It seems to me that you're saying … Is that correct?"
4. Listen empathetically (with the intent of understanding the other person's way of looking at the situation). This is often called trying to imagine what it would be like to "walk in someone else's shoes." Listening empathetically requires four steps:
   (1.) Clear your mind of thoughts about how you view the situation or concerns about how you're going to respond.
   (2.) Focus on listening to the person's feelings and perceptions.
   (3.) Rephrase the feelings and perceptions as you understand them to be.
   (4.) Detach and come back to your own frame of reference.
5. Apply strategies that help you get accurate and comprehensive information.
   - Use open-ended questions (those requiring more than a one-word answer). For example, "How do you feel about leaving tomorrow?"
   - Avoid closed-ended questions (those requiring only a one-word answer). For example, "Are you ready to leave tomorrow?"
   - Use exploratory statements that lead the person to expand on certain issues. For example, "Tell me more about … "
   - Don't use leading questions (those that lead someone to a desired answer). For example, "You don't smoke, do you?"
   - Put body language into words. For example, "You looked a little sad… . "
   - Use silence. Allow the person time to gather his thoughts.

Box 2-5 **COMMUNICATION STRATEGIES FOR ENHANCING CRITICAL THINKING**–cont'd

♦ Remember the value of using written communication (letters and diaries really help).
  – Record the information you gathered, and then look to see what's missing and check for inconsistencies.
  – Ask the person to keep a log or diary or keep one yourself.
6. Use strategies that help you get your point across.
  ♦ Make sure the time and place are appropriate.
  ♦ Wait until the person is ready to listen.
  ♦ When voicing an opinion, use phrases that convey you're *voicing an opinion*, rather than dictating what is so (e.g., "From my way of looking at it … From my perspective … ").
  ♦ Ask the person to paraphrase what you've said (e.g., "I need to know you understand. Explain to me what I just said.")
7. Be cognizant of others' communication styles rather than trying to force them to use yours (e.g., don't use touch, even if you like to, if the other person seems to recoil from touch; if someone is formal and reserved, respect his style).
8. Exhibit behaviors that send messages like, I'm responsible, I can be trusted, and I want to do a good job. For example, keep promises, be punctual, accept responsibility, and respect others' time.
9. Acknowledge and apologize when you've caused inconvenience, been careless, made a mistake, or offended someone.
10. Respect others' territory; ask permission (e.g., "May I listen to your chest?" rather than, "Sit up and let me listen to your chest.").

See also Communicating Bad News (pages 194-196).

EARLY EVALUATION. When you make it a habit to evaluate early, for example, reflecting on your thinking and checking whether your information is accurate, complete, and up-to-date, you can make corrections *early*. You avoid making decisions based on outdated, inaccurate, or incomplete information.

PAST EXPERIENCE. Most authors view experience as an enhancing factor. You remember best what you experience. If, however, your past experience isn't congruent with the current situation, experience may be an inhibiting factor. For example, if a mother has had a bad experience breast-feeding her firstborn child, it may be difficult for her to think clearly about breast-feeding subsequent children.

EFFECTIVE WRITING SKILLS. These promote critical thinking. When you learn how to make yourself clear in writing, you learn to apply critical thinking principles like identifying an organized approach, deciding what's relevant, and focusing on others' perspectives.

EFFECTIVE READING AND LEARNING SKILLS. These are enhancing factors. Because critical thinking often requires that you use resources independently, you must know how to read and learn well. Having effective reading skills doesn't mean knowing how to read rapidly. It means knowing how to read efficiently, identifying what's important, and drawing conclusions about what the material implies.

Situational Factors

ANXIETY, STRESS, FATIGUE. For the most part, these *impede* thinking. High levels of anxiety and stress, often the first to tap your brain energy, make concentration difficult. When you're fatigued, you're already operating on a "low battery." A *low* anxiety level, however, like being a little nervous about a test, can *promote* critical thinking by motivating you to prepare.

AWARENESS OF RISKS. Usually this is an *enhancing* factor. When you know the risks, you think more carefully, making sure you've made a prudent decision before acting. Sometimes awareness of the risks can increase anxiety to a level that *impedes* critical thinking. For example, most of us remember how hard it was to think critically when we gave our first injection.

KNOWLEDGE OF RELATED FACTORS. The more you know about a situation, the better you'll be able to reason. For example, you might know about diabetes, but if you don't know the *person* you're going to teach–know the person's lifestyle, desires, and motivations–you'll be unlikely to design a plan that the person will follow.

AWARENESS OF RESOURCES. Awareness of *resources* allows us to think critically, even with limited knowledge. For example, nurses frequently think critically about drug administration with limited drug-specific knowledge. They check with resources like pharmacists and drug manuals before giving unfamiliar drugs (e.g., they find out usual dose range, contraindications, and possible side effects).

POSITIVE REINFORCEMENT. Positive reinforcement *promotes* critical thinking by building self-confidence and focusing on what's being done *right*.

EVALUATIVE OR JUDGMENTAL STYLES. Conveying an evaluative or judgmental style usually *impedes* critical thinking. People who feel they're being evaluated or judged often spend more energy worrying about what *others* are thinking than what *they're* thinking.

PRESENCE OF MOTIVATING FACTORS. Things that motivate you to think critically aid thinking because they connect with your desires, enticing you to get your brain "in gear." An example of a common motivating factor for critical thinking is knowing why you're asked to do something. Think how much more motivated you are to learn when someone says, "You must know this because you run into it a lot, and you must be able to handle it."

TIME LIMITATIONS. This can be an *enhancing* or *impeding* factor. Time limitations can be motivating factors—deadlines stimulate us to get things done. If there's *too little time*, however, you may make decisions quicker than you'd like and come up with less than satisfactory answers. It's interesting to note that the courts give more leeway to decisions that were made in emergency situations than to those made with plenty of time for thinking.

ENVIRONMENTAL DISTRACTIONS. These impede critical thinking for obvious reasons—the more distractions, the more difficult it is to stay focused. For example, it's best to chart in a quiet place, where there are few interruptions and distractions.

Habits Causing Barriers to Critical Thinking

As humans, we instinctually develop habits that can cause barriers to critical thinking. These habits, summarized in Box 2-6, are addressed in the section that follows. Keep in mind that these habits are simply a result of human nature. Whether we realize it or not, we're all victims of these behaviors to some extent at one time or another.

SELF-FOCUSING. Focusing on ourselves is a carry-over from primitive survival instincts—in the early days of man, humans had to be keenly centered on their own needs to survive. We still have this instinct. To think critically, we must overcome the natural tendency to focus on how things affect *us*, and what *we* must do more than how things affect *others* and what *they* must do. We must ask questions like, "Am I doing this more for me than them?" "How are others likely to see this?" and "What's in the best interest of others involved?"

Box 2-6 **BARRIERS TO CRITICAL THINKING**

> Self-focusing
> Mine-Is-Better
> Tunnel Vision
> Choosing-Only-One
> Face-saving
> Resistance to Change
> Conformity
> Stereotyping
> Self-deception

MINE-IS-BETTER. We all tend to regard our ideas, values, religions, cultures, and points of view as being superior to others. To enhance your critical thinking potential, you need to consciously work to control this habit as you search for truth.

TUNNEL VISION. Tunnel vision is a universal problem. We see what we expect to see, often misinterpreting what's before us. A classic example of tunnel vision is when a psychiatric nurse fails to consider whether someone's confusion is related to a *medical problem*, and vice versa (a medical-surgical nurse fails to consider whether someone's confusion is related to a *psychiatric problem*).

CHOOSING-ONLY-ONE. When faced with two choices, we tend to choose *only one* of the two. We forget to think about things like, Are there other, better choices? Can we do both? Do we have to do either? Beginners are most vulnerable to the choosing-only-one habit. They tend to blindly accept that if they've chosen one of two options, they've made a good decision. They also tend to make the assumption that there must be one best way to do something, rather than thinking that there probably are several good ways of getting something done, and each has advantages and disadvantages, depending on circumstances. We can overcome this tendency by remembering to ask ourselves, Must I choose only one? or Is this the only way? What approaches can we combine?

FACE-SAVING. When we feel we said or did something wrong, we have a strong instinct to protect our image—we try to save face. Critical thinking requires that we learn and grow. As we learn and grow, we'll make mistakes or realize our old ways of thinking or doing things can be improved. To be a critical thinker, we must be comfortable saying things like, I'm not sure, I was wrong, or I have to think about that.

RESISTANCE TO CHANGE. We all tend to resist change. Too often change is considered "guilty until proven innocent." Overcoming this barrier doesn't mean embracing every new idea uncritically. It means being willing to suspend judgment long enough to make an informed decision on whether the change is worthwhile. (See more on facilitating and navigating change on pages 190–193.)

CONFORMITY. While some conformity, like following policies and procedures, is good, we sometimes engage in *harmful conformity*. Harmful conformity is when we conform to group thinking just to avoid being viewed as "different." Conforming without thought stifles the ability to be creative and improve. An example of conformity that *may* be harmful is supporting a political leader simply because of peer pressure rather than seeking to understand the policies supported by the leader.

STEREOTYPING. We stereotype when we make fixed and unbending overgeneralizations about others (e.g., homeless people aren't very bright).

When our minds are fixed and unbending, we're unlikely to see what's really before us. By recognizing our tendency to stereotype, we can make a conscious effort to overcome this habit.

SELF-DECEPTION. This is the subconscious forgetting of things about ourselves we don't particularly feel good about. An example of this is experienced nurses who deceive themselves into believing they were never as shy, nervous, or insecure as the students they encounter today.

Critical Moments

MOTIVATION: WHAT'S IN IT FOR THEM?
Connecting with others' motivations can spark them to think critically. When trying to motivate others, use the human instinct to self-focus to your advantage. Ask yourself questions like: What's in it for them? and How can I make this relevant and worth their while?

Covey's 7 Habits of Highly Effective People®*

Stephen Covey, author of the highly successful book *The 7 Habits of Highly Effective People*®, addresses the importance of replacing old patterns with new habits. These habits, listed below, enhance critical thinking.*

1. **Be Proactive.**® Choose to be responsible for your own life, anticipate responses, and act before things happen.
2. **Begin With the End in Mind.**® Develop goals and make your expectations explicit.
3. **Put First Things First.**® Decide what's important and stick to priorities moment by moment, day by day.
4. **Think Win-Win.**® Seek mutual benefit in all human interactions.
5. **Seek First to Understand, Then to Be Understood.**® Communicate effectively.
6. **Synergize.**® Recognize that the whole is greater than the sum of its parts: Collaborate, bringing diverse ideas and talents together to create new and better ideas.
7. **Sharpen the Saw.**® Look after yourself physically, emotionally, and spiritually. (Covey explains Sharpening the Saw by telling a story about a man who is sawing a tree trunk for hours: The saw is dull, and the man is exhausted. Someone suggests that he might do better if he sharpens the saw. The man responds, "I don't have time" and continues to work ineffectively.)

---

*Summarized from Covey, S. (1989). *The 7 habits of highly effective people.*® New York: Simon & Schuster, © 1989 Stephen R. Covey. Used with permission of Franklin Covey Co. All trademarks of Franklin Covey are used with permission. All rights reserved. www.FranklinCovey.com

CRITICAL THINKING EXERCISES

Note: Exercises followed by asterisks have example responses listed in the Response Key at the back of the book beginning on page 246.

1. Study Boxes 2-1 (What's Your Thinking Style?) and 2-2 (Do You Know What to Do When Someone Turns Blue?). In a group or in a personal journal, discuss:
   a. Your thoughts about your thinking style and main motive according to Myers-Briggs and Hartman.
   b. How your style and innate motives affect your ability to think clearly.
   c. How working with people with styles different than your own affects your thinking.
   d. How you would feel about taking one of the personality tests for your own personal knowledge versus for use at school or work.
2. a. Emotive thinking is thinking that's driven by feelings: How does this relate to critical thinking?*
   b. Write a paragraph explaining how intelligent use of emotions facilitates better thinking.*
   c. In a personal journal, write about the influence of feelings on your thinking. For example, are you ruled more by your heart than your head, or vice versa, and what difference does that make? Identify at least one thing you can do to improve your ability to have more balanced thinking (thinking that considers both "heart" and "head").
3. Respond to the following from the prechapter self-test:
   a. Explain three key steps to improving thinking.
   b. Describe how your personality and learning style affects your ability to think critically.*
   c. Discuss how human habits influence critical thinking ability.*

OUTCOME-FOCUSED (RESULTS-ORIENTED) THINKING

As addressed in Chapter 1, critical thinking is outcome-focused (results-oriented) thinking. This section clarifies the relationship between goals (your intent) and outcomes (the actual results you get). It also explains why focusing on outcomes promotes better thinking.

Goals (Intent) versus Outcomes (Results)

The terms goal and outcome are often used interchangeably. While these two terms have similar meanings, there's a significant difference. Remember the following rule:

Rule: ◆ Use *goal* to state general intent (your purpose, what you aim to do). *Example:* My goal is to teach Steve about diabetes by the time he is discharged.

Continued

> *Rule:* cont'd
>
> ◆ Use ***outcome*** to describe *specific results* that others can observe at a certain time when the goal is achieved. *Example:* By the time he is discharged, Steve will be able to tell us how he will manage his diet and insulin injections to maintain his blood sugars within normal range.

Understanding the above relationship between goals and outcomes is important. Goals are often quite vague, and can be somewhat idealistic. Outcomes, because they center on *clearly observable results*, force you to think things through, helping you be realistic and focused from the start. Use the following memory jog to help you remember these two terms

G=G (**G**oals = **G**eneral intent)

O=O (**O**utcomes = **O**bservable results)

Focusing on End Results

To some people, outcome-focused thinking is just a buzzword that gets too much attention—it seems obvious that you need to focus on end results to reason well. But think about the following scenario that shows determining the end results isn't always obvious.

Case scenario
FOCUSING ON OUTCOMES (END RESULTS)

A group gathers to discuss building a bridge in a rural town. Someone says, "Let's first be sure that we all agree on the end result." Several members consider this a dumb statement because the end result, obviously, is that the town will have a bridge. It seems like a clear and observable outcome, right? How about if I tell you this is very limited thinking? The *real* end result they must focus on is that whoever wants to get across that bridge is able to do so. To think critically, they have to pay attention to the end users, the people who will use the bridge. They must begin by asking questions like, "Who will use this bridge?" "How much room will they need to get their vehicles across?" When will there be the most traffic, and how much will that traffic weigh?" "Where is the best place for this bridge?" If these questions aren't raised *in the beginning* it's likely that they'll end up with a costly, useless, inconvenient, or even dangerous bridge.◆

Remember the following rule:

Rule: **Determining outcomes requires you to be clearly centered on the *key people* who will demonstrate that your desired end result has been achieved. In the previous scenario, the key people are those *who travel the bridge.* In health care, it's your *patients or clients.***

Determining client-centered outcomes, a key critical thinking skill for nursing, is addressed in depth in Chapter 5 (pages 171-174), where there are opportunities to practice determining outcomes in nursing situations. For now, just remember that if you haven't given enough thought to exactly what end results you need, you aren't thinking critically.

Critical Moments

FOCUSING ON OUTCOMES: IMAGINE THE FUTURE
Focusing on outcomes—the end products or results—helps you think things through and avoid what I call "best laid plans" problems. To think critically, put your mind in the future and imagine what things will be like on the day you reach the outcomes. For example, once I was on a planning committee for a conference. One of our goals was to keep costs down, so we decided to skip refreshments for the afternoon break. This seemed to make sense until someone put her mind in the future, focused on the end results, and said, "I don't want to be the one who has to stand up in front of 100 tired, thirsty people and announce, 'there will be no refreshments during this break.'" After that comment, we changed our minds. When determining outcomes, "think future." Imagine consequences: exactly how things will be on the day you reach your outcome.

CRITICAL THINKING STRATEGIES

This section first summarizes 10 key questions that promote critical thinking, and then goes on to other strategies.

10 Key Questions

Ask 10 key questions to determine your approach to critical thinking in different situations.

1. **What major outcomes (observable results) will drive our thinking**? Critical thinking is purposeful. Before you start, clarify exactly what results you need, and what it will "look like" when

results are achieved. For example, compare the vague outcome in situation *a* below, with the more specific outcome in situation *b*.
   a. Jody will be discharged home in two days.
   b. Jody will be discharged home in two days in the care of her mother, who will be able to demonstrate sterile dressing change by then.

2. **Exactly what are the problems, issues, or risks that must be addressed to achieve the major outcomes?** Clearly identifying the problems, issues, and risks that may impede progress is at least 80% of the critical thinking challenge. Asking this question helps you prioritize—you have only so much time, and you must assign top priority to addressing problems, issues, or risks that may impede getting results. Using the above example, Jody's mother tells you that she knows nothing about changing sterile dressings and also wants to know how she can improve her parenting skills. If time is short, you must give top priority to teaching her about dressing changes, and handle the issue of how to be a better parent by giving her information on reference materials and support groups.

3. **What are the circumstances (what is the context)?** The approach to critical thinking varies, depending on the circumstances (context). For example, you're in class and you're asked how to manage a patient in shock. You aren't sure, but you think you know, so it's appropriate for you to answer. If you're in the clinical setting, however, trying to manage shock based on uncertain knowledge is inappropriate.

4. **What knowledge is required?** Discipline-specific theoretical and experiential knowledge is essential to being able to think critically. For example, how can you think critically about managing cardiac pain if you don't know the causes and common treatments of cardiac pain? If you don't know what knowledge is required, you probably don't know enough to get involved—you must get help.

5. **How much room is there for error?** When there's less room for error, we must carefully assess the situation, examine all possible solutions, and make every effort to make prudent decisions. For example, which situation below has less room for error, and how might your approach to decision making differ in each situation?
   a. You're trying to decide whether to give an over-the-counter antihistamine to someone who's been in excellent health but who's been having trouble sleeping.
   b. You're trying to decide whether to give an over-the-counter antihistamine to someone with multiple health problems.
   Obviously, situation *a* has more room for error because the person is less likely to have preexisting conditions that might be aggravated by an antihistamine. In situation *b*, you need to consult the person's attending physician.

If there is plenty of room for error—if there are few or no risks involved—you can be more creative and spontaneous (for example, in a brainstorming session).

6. **How much time do I/we have?** If we have plenty of time to make a decision, we can take time to think independently, using resources such as textbooks to guide our thinking. If we don't have much time, we may be required to refer the problem to an expert immediately to ensure timely attention.

7. **What resources can help?** Identifying resources (for example, textbooks, computers, or experts) is essential to getting the information you need to think critically. For example, most nurses don't know every hospital policy by heart. Rather, they know what situations are covered by policies and refer to the policy manual as needed.

8. **Whose perspectives must be considered?** Critical thinking requires you to consider the perspectives of all of the key players involved or you risk having conflicting purposes. For example, to develop an effective plan for home care, you must consider the perspectives of the patient, other household members, and other key members of the health care team. Imagine what could happen if you sent a grandmother home with many brightly colored medications and everyone forgot to consider the perspective of a toddler in the home!

9. **What's influencing thinking?** Recognizing influencing factors such as personal biases helps us identify vested interests, an important step in making fair-minded choices. For example, a nurse who is strongly against abortion would be wise to avoid working in gynecology, where women's decisions might make it difficult to give objective nursing care.

10. **What must we do to prevent, control, or eliminate the problems or issues identified in question *2* above?** Getting results depends on your ability to identify specific strategies to prevent or manage problems that are likely to be barriers to outcome achievement. For example, if you have a bedridden patient who has surgery, preventing skin breakdown is a problem that must be managed to ensure timely discharge.

The inside front cover summarizes these 10 key critical thinking questions.

Critical Moments

CONSIDERING ALTERNATIVES GETS RESULTS
People aren't successful because they come up with one right answer or explanation. Rather, it's because they come up with many *answers or explanations. To get results, make it a habit to look for alternative explanations, problems, or solutions.*

Using Logic, Intuition, and Trial and Error

Let's consider when and how to use *logic, intuition,* and *trial and error.*

Logic, or sound reasoning that's based on facts (evidence), is the foundation for critical thinking. It's the safest, most reliable strategy. For all important decisions and opinions, make sure you can explain the logic of your FINAL ANSWER (pardon the cliché).

Intuition, a valuable part of thinking that we should nurture, is best described as knowing something without evidence. Intuitive hunches often speed up problem solving, especially for experts, who have large mental banks of previous experience to draw upon. If you get a sense that something requires more investigation, monitoring, or preparedness, pay attention. Bring logic to your thinking and continue to look for evidence, as you act with caution. If you have no evidence to support intuitive feelings, consider the risks of acting on intuition alone (e.g., what are the risks of harm?). Pages 84-85 address the use of logic and intuition in clinical judgment and provide examples of how these two ways of thinking complement one another.

Trial and error, or trying several solutions until you find one that works, can be *risky* but necessary. Use trial and error *only* when there's plenty of room for mistakes, when the problem can be monitored closely, and when the solutions have been logically thought through. A common example of useful trial and error in nursing is determining the best way for a dressing to be applied to an awkward wound–it may take several tries before determining the best way.

 Other Perspectives

TRIAL AND ERROR: A CONTINUOUS PROCESS
"Trial and error, the process of trying one thing and observing the outcome, and then analyzing the outcome and making changes, is an important learning experience. It requires a great deal of critical thinking. Getting input from trying to do something in the real world is one of the most important experiences that can improve outcomes. Call it what you want, but it's important for individuals and health care organizations to be able to interact with the world, learn from experience, and then use that experience to improve the next attempt. However, trial and error is a continuous cycle. You must constantly try to improve care quality based on what you learn from experience–it isn't just a one-time thing."

–One of My Workshop Participants, a Quality Improvement Expert

Focusing on the Big and Small Pictures

Whether you think you're a "big picture" person or a "details" person, it's important not to become a victim of the *choosing-only-one* habit addressed earlier. Critical thinking requires you to focus on *both* the big picture and the details—the whole and the parts. Think about the following examples.

◆ Mr. Martinez, who has cardiac problems, tells you he has chest pain and is afraid he might die. Treating both "the whole" (Mr. Martinez's pain and anxiety) and "the parts" (Mr. Martinez's oxygen-deprived heart) is essential to resolving the chest pain (and, perhaps, to saving his life).

◆ You're trying to teach Tonya how to care for her newborn. You're well-prepared with lots of nice pamphlets. She seems interested, but she keeps yawning and doesn't seem to retain information very long. Finally you say, "Is there a better time we could do this?" She admits that she hasn't slept all night and is too tired. You come back later after Tonya's had a good rest. She learns readily. In this case, paying attention to an important detail (fatigue) helped you be a more effective teacher.

Remember to ask questions like, "What's the big picture here?" "Am I considering both the parts and the whole?" and "Am I paying attention to key details?"

Specific Strategies

Part of learning to think critically is learning specific strategies that help promote critical thought. Consider how using the following strategies expands your thinking.

◆ **Anticipate the questions others might ask** (e.g., What will my instructor want to know? or What will the doctor want to know?). This helps identify a wider scope of questions that need to be answered to gain relevant information.

◆ **Ask what-else questions**. For example, change Have we done everything? to What else do we need to do? Asking what-else questions pushes you to look further and be more complete.

◆ **Think out loud or write your thoughts down.** When you put your thinking into words, you make your ideas, reasons, and logic explicit, making it easier to evaluate and correct yourself.

◆ **Ask an expert to think out loud.** When you ask experts to think out loud, you often learn organized systematic approaches to solving problems and making decisions.

◆ **Ask what-if questions** like, What if the worst happens? or What if we try another way? This helps you be proactive instead of reactive. It enhances your creativity and helps you put things in perspective.

◆ **Ask why** (determine underlying purpose or reasons). To fully understand something, you must know *what* it is and *why* it's so. There's a saying, "She who knows *what and how* is likely to get a good job. She who knows *why* is likely to be her boss."

◆ **Paraphrase in your own words.** Paraphrasing helps you understand information using a familiar language (your own).

◆ **Compare and contrast.** This forces you to look closely at the parts of something as well as the *whole*, helping you get more familiar with both things you're comparing. For example, if I asked you to compare two different kinds of apples, you'd have to look closely at both of them. As a result of comparing them, you'd also be more likely to know and *remember* each type of apple better.

◆ **Organize and reorganize information.** Organizing information helps you see certain patterns, but it may make you *miss* others. Reorganizing it helps you see some of those *other* patterns. For example, compare the following groups of numbers (each group contains the same numbers, organized differently). What patterns do you see and which is easier to remember?

    36345643   34343 656   333 44 566

◆ **Look for flaws in your thinking.** Ask questions like, What's missing? and How could this be made better? If you don't go looking for flaws, you'll be unlikely to find them. Once you've found them, you can make corrections early.

◆ **Ask someone else to look for flaws in your thinking.** This offers a "fresh eye" for evaluation and may bring new ideas and perspectives.

◆ **Develop good habits of inquiry** (habits that aid in the search for the truth, such as keeping an open mind, verifying information, and taking enough time).

◆ **Revisit information.** When you come back and look at something after a period of time, you'll probably view it differently.

◆ **Replace the phrases "I don't know" or "I'm not sure" with "I need to find out" or "Let's find out."** This shows you have the confidence and ability to find answers and mobilizes you to locate resources.

◆ **Turn errors into learning opportunities.** We all make mistakes. They're stepping-stones to maturity and new ideas. If you aren't making any mistakes, maybe you aren't trying enough new things.

◆ **Share your mistakes–they're valuable.** Sharing your mistakes helps others avoid making the same mistake and may identify common misconceptions or problems that need to be rectified.

Critical Moments

MENDING FENCES: SOMETIMES ESSENTIAL TO CRITICAL THINKING
Critical thinking often requires collaboration. When you and someone else have begun a pattern of arguing and obstruction, work to mend fences. Point out that you have gotten into a bad pattern (or off to a bad start). Ask for agreement to wipe the slate clean and promise to focus on common goals. You can change the pattern.

KNOWLEDGE AND INTELLECTUAL SKILL INDICATORS

In Chapter 1 we addressed critical thinking indicators (CTIs)™—behaviors that demonstrate attitudes (characteristics) that promote critical thinking (pages 7 to 8). Now let's look at two other types of CTIs: *knowledge* and *intellectual skill* indicators. Study Table 2-3, showing CTIs for knowledge and intellectual skills. Notice that the second column (intellectual skills) requires you to be able to *apply* the knowledge listed in the first column. Once you recognize this relationship between the two columns, assess your abilities as you did with the CTIs in Chapter 1: Think about each indicator and rate your ability to demonstrate the behavior using a scale of 0–10 (0 = I often have trouble demonstrating this indicator and 10 = I usually demonstrate this

Table 2-3   CRITICAL THINKING INDICATORS™

Behaviors Demonstrating Knowledge

Requirements vary, depending on context (for example, specialty practice):

Clarifies:
- ❏ nursing and medical terminology
- ❏ nursing vs. medical and other models, roles, and responsibilities
- ❏ signs and symptoms of common problems and complications
- ❏ related anatomy, physiology, pathophysiology
- ❏ normal and abnormal function (bio-psycho-social-cultural-spiritual)
- ❏ factors that promote or inhibit normal function (bio-psycho-social-cultural-spiritual)
- ❏ related pharmacology (actions, indications, side effects, nursing implications)
- ❏ reasons behind interventions and diagnostic studies
- ❏ normal and abnormal growth and development
- ❏ nursing process, nursing theories, and research principles
- ❏ applicable standards, laws, practice acts
- ❏ policies and procedures and the reasons behind them

- ❏ ethical and legal principles
- ❏ spiritual, social, and cultural concepts
- ❏ where information resources can be found

Demonstrates:
- ❏ focused nursing assessment skills (e.g. breath-sounds or IV site assessment)
- ❏ related technical skills (e.g. n/g tube or other equipment management)

Clarifies:
- ❏ personal values, beliefs, needs
- ❏ how own thinking, personality, and learning style preferences may differ from others' preferences
- ❏ organizational mission and values

Table 2-3   CRITICAL THINKING INDICATORS™–cont'd

Behaviors Demonstrating Intellectual Skills/Competencies

Nursing process and decision-making skills:

❑ Applies standards and principles when planning, giving, and adapting care

❑ Assesses systematically and comprehensively; uses a nursing framework to identify nursing concerns, uses a body systems framework to identify medical concerns

❑ Detects bias; determines credibility of information sources

❑ Distinguishes normal from abnormal; identifies risks for abnormal

❑ Determines significance of data; distinguishes relevant from irrelevant; clusters relevant data together

❑ Identifies assumptions and inconsistencies; checks accuracy and reliability; recognizes missing information; focuses assessment as indicated

❑ Concludes what's known and unknown; makes reasonable inferences (conclusions) and judgments—gives evidence to support them

❑ Considers multiple explanations and solutions

❑ Identifies both problems and their underlying cause(s) and related factors; includes patient and family perspectives

❑ Determines individualized outcomes; focuses on results

❑ Manages risks, predicts complications, promotes health, function, and well-being; anticipates consequences and implications—plans ahead accordingly

❑ Sets priorities and makes decisions in a timely way; includes key stakeholders in making decisions

❑ Weighs risks and benefits; individualizes interventions

❑ Reassesses to check responses and monitor results (outcomes)

❑ Communicates effectively orally and in writing

❑ Identifies ethical issues and takes appropriate action

❑ Identifies and uses technologic, information, and human resources

Additional Related Skills:

❑ Establishes empowered partnerships with patients, families, peers, and coworkers

❑ Teaches patients, self, and others

❑ Addresses conflicts fairly; fosters positive interpersonal relationships

❑ Facilitates and navigates change

❑ Manages time and environment

❑ Gives and takes constructive criticism

❑ Facilitates teamwork (focuses on common goals; helps and encourages others to contribute in their own way)

❑ Delegates appropriately; leads, inspires, and motivates others

❑ Demonstrates systems thinking (shows awareness of the interrelationships existing within and across healthcare systems)

indicator). If you're a beginning student, don't be concerned about low scores. As you get repeated practice in real situations, consciously working to improve, you'll soon find that many of these behaviors become habit. You'll also have many opportunities to practice and develop these skills as you read on and complete the exercises throughout the book. What's important is that you start to get a picture of what behaviors promote critical thinking.

Box 2-7 RESULTS OF TWO STUDIES DESCRIBING CRITICAL
THINKING SKILLS

The skills below were incorporated into critical thinking indicators (CTIs).

SCHEFFER AND RUBENFELD*

Analyzing: Separating or breaking down a whole into parts to discover their nature, function, and relationships

Applying standards: Judging according to established personal, professional, or social rules or criteria

Discriminating: Recognizing differences and similarities among things or situations and distinguishing carefully as to category or rank

Information seeking: Searching for evidence, facts or knowledge by identifying relevant sources and gathering objective, subjective, historical, and current data from those sources

Logical reasoning: Drawing inferences or conclusions that are supported in or justified by evidence

Predicting: Envisioning a plan and its consequences

Transforming knowledge: changing or converting the condition, nature, form or function of concepts and contexts

THE APA DELPHI REPORT[†]

Interpretation: Categorizing, decoding sentences, clarifying meaning

Analysis: Examining ideas, identifying arguments, analyzing arguments

Evaluation: Assessing claims, assessing arguments

Inference: Querying evidence, conjecturing alternatives, drawing conclusions

Explanation: Stating results, justifying procedures, presenting arguments

Self-Regulation: Self examination, self correction

*Scheffer, B. & Rubenfeld, M. (2000). A consensus statement on critical thinking in nursing. *Journal of Nursing Education, 39(8)*,353.
[†]*Table I, Critical thinking: A statement of expert consensus for purposes of educational assessment and instruction,* "The APA Delphi Report" (1990) ERIC Document Number, 315–423.

Box 2-7 shows the results of two studies that aimed to describe critical thinking skills. These skills were incorporated into the CTIs listed in Table 2-3.

HOW TO READ MINDS

Unlike *Star Trek*'s Dr. Spock, we humans can't read minds—we have to look at behavior and seek explanations to understand someone else's thinking. Looking at *patterns of behavior* over time is important when trying to determine if someone is a critical thinker. For example, does the person usually achieve desired results? Does the person usually seem confident? Understand, however, that motives and intentions often aren't clear in behavior alone. Get explanations by saying things like, *Help me understand what you're trying to do, and why and how you're trying to do it. What do you expect to happen when you do this? What if (fill in the blank) happens—how will you handle it?* and *What alternatives have you thought about?* Only when you get explanations do you have an idea of what's going on in the other person's head.

It takes a knowledgeable, experienced, critical thinker who is cognizant of key elements of performance evaluation to evaluate thinking in the workplace. Remember that differences in personal styles sometimes make understanding others' thinking difficult. For example, someone who is a very logical, step-by-step thinker may have trouble understanding a creative person who's great at multitasking. Consider this tennis analogy in relation to judging someone else's thinking: You may know tennis strokes that work for your own game. But it takes years of instruction, practice, and insight before you're qualified to teach, judge, and formally comment on someone else's game. The same goes for critical thinking.

DEVELOPING CHARACTER, ACQUIRING KNOWLEDGE, AND PRACTICING SKILLS

In summary, learning to think critically requires you to do four things:

1. **Develop a critical thinking character.** Hold yourself to high standards and make a commitment to demonstrating CTIs. Remember, others determine how you think by your behavior over time. You may *want* to be patient and understanding, but if your behavior over time sends different messages, *this* is the reality of what's happening.

2. **Take responsibility and get actively involved.** Seek out learning resources and experiences that help you acquire the theoretical and experiential knowledge you need to think critically. Practice intellectual skills such as assessing systematically and comprehensively. Just as practicing physical skills improves your ability to perform physically, practicing thinking skills improves your ability to perform intellectually.

3. **Gain interpersonal skills like resolving conflicts, getting along with others, and working as a team.** These skills are essential to getting the information you need to think critically. Keep in mind that "being too nice" problems (for example, not giving

constructive criticism because of concerns of offending someone) can be as bad as "not being very nice" problems (for example, demonstrating arrogance, sarcasm, or intolerance to other ways of doing things). Learn how to give and take feedback. To improve, we must get through the negative aspects of criticism.

4. **Practice related technical skills** (e.g., using computers and managing IVs). Until these skills become second nature, they create a "brain drain" that leaves you with little energy for paying attention to other important things, such as monitoring physical and psychological responses to care.

Finally, a picture is worth a thousand words. Study Figure 2-1, which gives a visual graphic of what it takes to think critically.

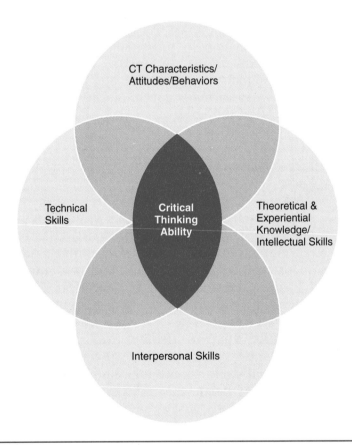

Figure 2-1 ◆ Looking at the illustration clockwise, critical thinking ability depends on demonstrating (1) critical thinking characteristics, (2) theoretical and experiential knowledge, (3) interpersonal skills (e.g., resolving conflicts and working as a team, and (4) related technical skills (e.g., using computers or starting IVs) to prevent the "brain drain" of mastering these types of skills.

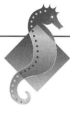

Critical Moments

PICTURE THIS

When you're trying to understand, explain, or remember something, try drawing pictures, diagrams, or graphs. Our brains usually do better with pictures than words. For example, which of the ways of expressing percentages provided below is easiest for you to understand?

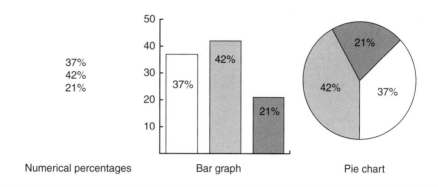

Numerical percentages   Bar graph   Pie chart

KEY POINTS

Learning how to think critically requires gaining insight into what critical thinking entails, acquiring instruction and feedback, and consciously practicing to improve. Becoming aware of your personal style—how and why you think and learn the way you do—is an excellent starting point for improving thinking. Each of us is responsible for connecting with our preferred styles and working at strategies that can help us think and learn effectively in our own way. Connecting with your own particular personality type helps you gain insight into how and why you think the way you do. Understanding personality types different from your own helps you realize how and why *others* think the way they do. Box 2-1 and Box 2-2 summarize two different and complementary ways of describing personality type. Habits creating barriers to critical thinking include self-focusing, tunnel vision, mine-is-better, choosing-only-one, face-saving, resistance to change, conformity, stereotyping, and self-deception. Stephen Covey offers seven habits that can enhance critical thinking (page 37).

Goals, because they focus on intent, may be vague, lofty, and unrealistic. Identifying specific, observable, expected outcomes (results) helps you be realistic and focused from the start. Logic, sound reasoning based on evidence, provides the foundation for critical thinking. Using intuition as a guide to look for evidence is an effective strategy that should be nurtured. Before acting on intuition alone, however, be sure your actions won't cause harm. Trial and error, or trying several solutions until you find one that works, is sometimes risky, but often a necessary and useful approach to problem solving. Table 2-3 describes CTIs™ that demonstrate the knowledge and intellectual skills required to think critically.

CRITICAL THINKING EXERCISES

Note: Exercises followed by asterisks have an example responses listed in the Response Key at the back of the book beginning on page 246.

1. Using your own words and giving an example(s), explain how the terms goal and outcome are related.*
2. Think of an outcome that you'd like to achieve six months from now; then apply the 10 key critical thinking questions listed on the inside front cover to determine your approach to achieving your outcome.
3. How would your approach to critical thinking change in the following two situations?*
   a. You want your committee to produce a number of creative ideas to be evaluated later.
   b. You want your committee to develop a policy for managing postoperative complications.
4. a. Arranging information into related patterns helps you remember better. Rearrange the following numbers into a pattern that helps you remember them: 992887656780898
   b. Using spatial intelligence (e.g., using shading, boxes, and circles to call out information) enhances learning. Draw a circle around the group of numbers listed above. Notice how they stand out from the rest of the page.
5. Identifying assumptions–recognizing things you've taken for granted without realizing–is essential for critical thinking. Answer the following riddle, and then check the response on page 24 to see what assumptions you made. Think of a question you could have asked that may have helped you avoid making the assumptions.*

Riddle: JACK AND JILL WERE FOUND DEAD ON THE FLOOR, SURROUNDED BY WATER AND PIECES OF BROKEN GLASS. THERE WAS NO BLOOD. WHAT HAPPENED?

6. Respond to the following from the prechapter self-test:
   a. Address how asking the 10 key questions listed on the inside front cover helps you decide your approach to critical thinking.
   b. Describe five strategies that enhance critical thinking, giving reasons why the strategies work.

c. Identify the roles of logic, intuition, and trial and error in critical thinking.

d. Decide where you stand in relation to being able to demonstrate CTIs for knowledge and intellectual skills.

e. Explain the relationship between your ability to think critically and developing character, knowledge, and skills.

References

1. E-mail communication. November 2001.
2. Thompson, E. (2000). Mentoring power. *Reflections on Nursing LEADERSHIP, 26 (1)*, 7.
3. Ecklund, M. (January 2001). Reach Out and Touch: Making the Mentoring Connection. Retrieved June 29, 2002 from http://www.aacn.org/AACN/freece.nsf/ ff1487bfe89b77df882565a6006cfc3f/9af5547588f2cc52882569e0006b38ba?OpenDocument.

See comprehensive bibliography beginning on page 286.

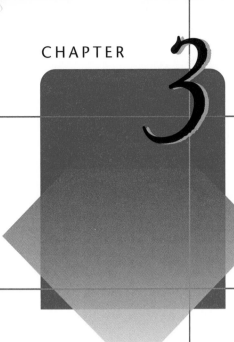

Critical Thinking and Clinical Judgment

THIS CHAPTER at a Glance ...

◆ Critical Thinking and Clinical Judgment
    Applied Definition
    Other Ways Nurses Describe Critical Thinking
    What about Critical Thinking Indicators™ (CTIs™)?
◆ Goals and Outcomes of Nursing
    Major Goals of Nursing
    Major Outcomes of Nursing
    What Are the Implications?
◆ Novice Versus Expert Thinking
◆ A New Mindset
    From "Diagnose and Treat" to a Predictive Approach
        Predict, Prevent, Manage, Promote (PPMP)
        Treating versus Managing
    Outcome-Focused, Data-Driven, Evidence-Based Care
    Clinical, Functional, and Other Outcomes
◆ A Changing Nursing Process
    More Proactive and Dynamic
    Is the Care Plan Dead?
    What Do Nurses Diagnose?
    Nursing Responsibilities Related to Diagnosis
◆ Developing Clinical Judgment (Clinical Reasoning Skills)
    Where Do Intuition and Logic Fit In?
    What about Creativity?
    Scope of Practice Decisions
    Decision Making and Nursing Standards and
        Guidelines
    How to Develop Effective Clinical Judgment
    10 Strategies for Developing Clinical Judgment
◆ Making Sure Your Charting Reflects Critical Thinking
◆ Key Points

Read the following Learning Outcomes and decide if you can readily achieve each one. If you can, you don't need to read this chapter and can go on to Chapter 4. Don't be concerned if you can't achieve any of the outcomes at this time. We'll come back to these outcomes later in the chapter, in Critical Thinking Exercises.

Learning Outcomes

After completing this chapter, you should be able to:

♦ Describe what critical thinking and clinical judgment means to you in relation to the descriptions in this chapter.

♦ Address the implications of the major goals and outcomes of nursing.

♦ Explain what outcome-focused, data-driven, evidence-based care means.

♦ Compare and contrast the *Diagnose and Treat (DT)* and the *Predict, Prevent, Manage, Promote (PPMP)* approaches to health care delivery.

♦ Clarify your responsibilities related to diagnosis and management of medical and nursing problems.

♦ Explain the role of ethics codes and national and organizational standards and guidelines in making decisions.

♦ Identify three things you will begin doing immediately to develop your clinical reasoning skills.

Other Perspectives

As you can see from the above Other Perspectives, health care consumers are all too aware that caring and compassion aren't enough—they value having nurses who have the knowledge, confidence, and thinking skills required to deal with the complex problems they face on a daily basis. This chapter and the next one are designed to help you meet the challenges of acquiring the knowledge, confidence, and thinking skills required to succeed in six common nursing situations: reasoning in the clinical setting (clinical judgment), moral and ethical reasoning, nursing research, teaching others, teaching ourselves, and test taking. To keep the length of the chapters manageable—to avoid asking you to do too much at one time—content is divided into two chapters. This chapter focuses on how to use critical thinking to promote clinical reasoning skills (clinical judgment). Chapter 4 focuses on moral and ethical reasoning, nursing research, teaching others, teaching ourselves, and test taking.

CRITICAL THINKING AND CLINICAL JUDGMENT

As explained in Chapter 1, nurses often use *critical thinking, clinical judgment,* and *clinical reasoning* interchangeably, even though they are slightly different terms (see page 5). This section first looks broadly at critical thinking, and then it goes on to address specific principles and strategies for developing clinical reasoning skills (clinical judgment). Chapter 5, Practicing Clinical Judgment Skills: Up Close and Clinical, focuses entirely on giving you opportunities to practice clinical judgment skills in context of case scenarios based on experiences from real clinical situations.

Applied Definition

Let's begin to examine critical thinking and clinical judgment in nursing by reviewing the applied definition from Chapter 1.

CRITICAL THINKING AND CLINICAL JUDGMENT IN NURSING:

◆ Entails purposeful, informed, outcome-focused (results-oriented) thinking that requires careful identification of key problems, issues, and risks involved.

◆ Is driven by patient, family, and community needs.*

◆ Is based on principles of nursing process and scientific method (e.g., making judgments based on evidence rather than guesswork).

◆ Use both intuition and logic, based on knowledge, skills, and experience.

◆ Is guided by professional standards and ethics codes.

◆ Requires strategies that make the most of human potential (e.g., using individual strengths) and compensate for problems created by human nature (e.g., overcoming the powerful influence of personal views).

◆ Is constantly reevaluating, self-correcting, and striving to improve.

Too often, nurses want to focus only on outcomes or only on the problems, which is narrow thinking. Remember the following rule, that was first introduced in Chapter 1:

Rule: To think critically and make reasoned clinical judgments, you must be clear about the outcomes (results) you expect, and also *clearly and specifically* identify the problems, issues, and risks that must be managed to reach the outcomes. For example, if you have an expected outcome that a patient who *will be discharged in three days will be able to manage wound care,* you must identify any problems or risks that may stop you from reaching this outcome (for example, an infection or unmet learning needs).

Other Ways Nurses Describe Critical Thinking

To many nurses, critical thinking simply means good problem solving. While problem-solving skills are required, you need a broader view of critical thinking to succeed in today's competitive health care setting. If you don't have a sincere desire to improve—to find ways to broaden your knowledge and skills and to make current practices more efficient and effective, you aren't thinking critically.

Another way to describe critical thinking is a commitment to look for the best way, based on the most current research and practice findings (e.g., the best way to manage pain in a specific person or for a

---

*To think critically, nurses must be clearly grounded in meeting patient and consumer needs. It's important to point out, however, that meeting nurses' and other disciplines' needs is often essential to meeting patient and consumer needs. For example, meeting nurses' requests for user-friendly, streamlined charting systems results in better communication and more time for patient care.

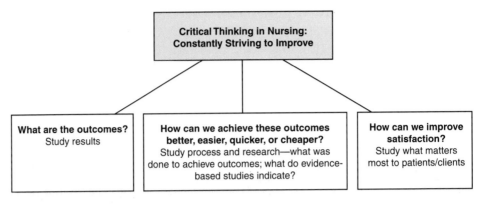

Figure 3-1 ◆

specific health problem. Figure 3-1 shows how critical thinking in nursing constantly strives to improve by focusing on three key questions: (1) What are the outcomes? (2) How can we achieve these outcomes more efficiently? and (3) How can we improve consumer satisfaction? Box 3-1 shows words of wisdom on critical thinking from other nurses.

Box 3-1 WORDS OF WISDOM ON CRITICAL THINKING*

"Fostering, supporting, and rewarding critical thinking is key to recruitment and retention. If we don't encourage nurses to grow in these skills, they become task-oriented and frustrated with the organization ("I'll just do as I'm told, try not to think too much, and not say a word"). Nurses must find ways to promote critical thinking throughout their departments and organizations, for it will ultimately help recruit and retain nurses with exemplary critical thinking skills."

—Donna D. Ignatavicius, MS, RN, Cm, DI Associates, Inc, iggy@diassociates.com

"Improving thinking allows nurses to develop the most important tool they have in their toolbox: themselves ... all designed to better impact patient outcomes. Improving thinking involves being clear about who you are as a person, and how your attitudes, assumptions, frames of reference, and tendencies to stereotype affect problem solving—how your personal choices and behaviors affect communication and interpersonal relationships."

—Ruth Hansten, RN, PhD, FACHE, MBA, BSN, Hansten Healthcare. www.Hansten.com

"To think critically, you must be willing to look at each situation objectively, uncovering each layer to get a deep understanding of what's happening. This often requires playing devil's advocate, looking at the circumstances from all angles, even those you'd rather not consider. You have to overcome human tendencies to be partial and subjective, and to form opinions based on individual preferences, rather than evidence."

—Karen Seyfert, RN, BSN, Coatesville VA Hospital. Kme413@cs.com

Continued

Box 3-1 WORDS OF WISDOM ON CRITICAL THINKING*–cont'd

"Thinking critically involves paying attention to how one is thinking as nursing care is accomplished. Nurses should ask themselves questions like, What are my assumptions in this situation? Are they accurate? What additional information do I need? How can I look at this situation in a different way? This kind of thinking can occur while doing, or it can occur after doing. The important point is that nurses observe how thinking occurs and how effective it is. Critical thinking following doing is called reflective thinking. Thinking while doing is called thinking in action."

–Joan Jenks, RN, PhD

"Critical thinking involves using our brainpower to view and interact with the world and to act in a reflective, discerning way. It includes having intellectual curiosity, being creative, being open to new ideas, examining underlying assumptions, and considering alternative lines of reasoning to make reasoned judgments that are sensitive to context."

–Theresa M. Valiga, EdD, RN, National League for Nursing. http://nln.org/

"What's wrong with this picture? Or, if nothing is wrong, what could be improved? is my all-time favorite critical thinking question. This question works well in all dimensions of professional and personal life. It raises our suspicion and triggers critical thoughts."

–Bette Case, PhD, RN, C, Clinical Care Solutions. bcase13747@aol.com

"There's an interesting paradox when addressing critical thinking. We emphasize the need to be able to respond quickly in the clinical setting. Yet one of the toughest mental disciplines that's fundamental to problem solving is being able to suspend judgment (withhold a response) until we have sufficient quality data."

–Marilyn Jackson, PhD, MA, RN. Intuitive Options. www.IntuitiveOptions.com

*E-mail communications, 2002.

Other Perspectives

CRITICAL THINKING: A SIXTH SENSE?

Here's how my mother, a British World War II nurse, describes critical thinking:

"Critical thinking is a 'sixth sense' that's developed over time from an accumulation of years of knowledge and experience—both personal and what you've learned from others. When you do a job for years, you learn what to look for and what to do. In almost a split second, you evaluate what you see, correlate it with what you've learned, and take appropriate action."

–Doris Alfaro, SRN, Class of 1944, Chesterfield Royal Hospital, Derbyshire, UK

What about Critical Thinking Indicators™ (CTIs™)?

Being familiar with CTIs™—short descriptions of behaviors that demonstrate the knowledge, characteristics, and skills that promote critical thinking—is central to learning to think critically in nursing. If you're not familiar with these, take time now to review pages 8 and 46. Keep in mind that no one is perfect, able to demonstrate all of the behaviors perfectly all the time. But the CTIs™ do provide a picture of what critical thinking in nursing "looks like." If you use the CTIs™ as a checklist, you can compare yourself with the listed indicators and target areas to develop. You can also use the CTIs™ to jog your mind about what you have to do to think critically when you're in a new or complex situation. For example, when you know that a key indicator is assessing systematically and comprehensively, it's likely that one of your first thoughts will be, "I need to figure out a way to assess this patient in a systematic, comprehensive, organized way."

◆ GOALS AND OUTCOMES OF NURSING

To better understand nursing's critical thinking, let's consider the questions, What major goals and outcomes do nurses aim to achieve? and What are the implications of these outcomes? Study the following goals and outcomes, paying attention to the fact that goals state *intent* and outcomes state the *evidence*, or observable results, which show the expected benefits of care.

Major Goals of Nursing

Broadly speaking, nurses aim to achieve the following goals in a humanistic way:
1. To help people avoid illness and its complications.
2. To help people—whether they are ill, injured, disabled, or well—gain optimum function, independence, and a sense of well-being. (In cases of terminal illness the goal of dying peacefully is also appropriate.)
3. To continually improve care practices, finding ways to improve patient outcomes.

Major Outcomes of Nursing

Broadly speaking, the following shows the major outcomes that demonstrate the benefits of nursing care:

After receiving individualized, state of the art, nursing care, people will demonstrate improved physical, mental, and spiritual health, as evidenced by:
◆ Absence of (or reduction in) signs, symptoms, and risk factors of illness, disability, or injury

♦ Use of behaviors and strategies that evidence shows promotes health, function, and quality of life (health promotion behaviors include things like managing therapeutic regimens, reducing risk factors, getting enough rest and exercise, and going for health screening; quality of life indicators include things like ability to do desired, as well as required activities with minimal or no discomfort)

♦ Nursing documentation of individualized, state-of-the-art care

What Are the Implications?

Three major implications of the goals and outcomes of nursing follow:

1. Because the conclusions and decisions we as nurses make affect people's lives, our thinking must be guided by sound reasoning—precise, disciplined thinking that promotes accuracy and depth of data collection and seeks to clearly identify the problems, issues, and risks at hand.

2. Since our ultimate aim is for people to be able to manage their own health care to the best of their ability, we *must* stay focused on patient perceptions, needs, desires, and capabilities.

3. Because we're committed to achieving quality outcomes in a cost-effective, timely way, we must constantly seek to improve both our personal ability to give nursing care and the overall quality of health care delivery. We must continue to work to find answers to questions like, How can we achieve better outcomes? How can we improve satisfaction with our services? How can we contain costs, yet maintain high standards? and How can we ensure competent nursing practice?

◆ NOVICE VERSUS EXPERT THINKING

Consider the following scenario:

Case scenario   A car hits a young man riding his bicycle in the park. Thrown 60 feet, he lies motionless. Within minutes two park rangers arrive. They put on latex gloves and begin to assess his injuries. An ambulance pulls up and one ranger yells, "We'll need intubation equipment!" A woman, out for a walk, looks on from a distance. A second woman, biking, comes upon the scene. Here's how the conversation goes:

First woman: This is terrible. I wish the ambulance had gotten here sooner.

Biking woman: Oh?

First woman: Yes. He was thrown at least 50 feet. If the ambulance had arrived sooner, they could have done more. I can't believe these two rangers didn't start resuscitation right away. They waited for this ambulance … they should have been breathing for him.

Biking woman: These rangers look like they know what they're doing. They would have started resuscitation if he needed it. This young man has been thrown so far, I'm sure they're concerned about spinal cord injuries. If they tilt his head back to start respirations, they risk severing his spinal cord—they don't want to do that unless it's absolutely necessary.◆

The above is a true story. I was the biking woman. As I talked more with the woman, I learned she was a student nurse. She thanked me for pointing out something she hadn't thought about. After it was all over, I realized our conversation demonstrated a common difference between expert and novice thinking: The student nurse felt a need to act immediately. As an experienced nurse, I knew the importance of assessing before acting.

We're all novices at one time or another. We all know what it's like to be new at something and watch an experienced professional and wonder, Will *I* ever know this much? And almost always, with time and commitment, we soon find ourselves helping someone *else* who looks at *us* and thinks, Will I ever know this much?

To help you gain insight into the difference between novice and expert thinking, study Table 3-1, which compares the two: If you're a novice, determine some things you can do to enhance your ability to think critically; if you're an expert, decide how you can help a novice.

 Other Perspectives

THE DIFFERENCE BETWEEN NOVICES AND EXPERTS

"There is an accumulation of evidence that expert problem solving … is dependent on (1) a wealth of prior specific experiences that can be used in routine solution of problems by pattern recognition … and (2) elaborate conceptual knowledge applicable to the occasional problematic

Continued

situation .... The main difference between expert clinicians and students is that experts generate better hypotheses (from the beginning, they have better hunches about what the problems may be)."[2]

—Dr. Geoffrey Norman

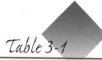

Table 3-1   NOVICE THINKING COMPARED WITH EXPERT THINKING*

Novice Nurses	Expert Nurses
◆ Knowledge is organized as separate facts. Rely heavily on resources (e.g., texts, notes, preceptors). Lack knowledge gained from actually doing (e.g., listening to breath sounds).	◆ Knowledge is highly organized and structured, making recall of information easier. Have a large storehouse of experiential knowledge (e.g., what abnormal breath sounds sound like, what subtle changes look like).
◆ Focus so much on *actions* that they tend to forget to *assess* before acting.	◆ *Assess* and think things through before *acting.*
◆ Need clear-cut rules.	◆ Know when to bend the rules.
◆ Are often hampered by unawareness of resources.	◆ Are aware of resources and how to use them.
◆ Are often hindered by anxiety and lack of self-confidence.	◆ Are usually more self-confident, less anxious, and therefore more focused.
◆ Must be able to rely on step-by-step procedures. Tend to focus more on *procedures* than on the *patient response* to the procedure.	◆ Know when it's safe to skip steps or do two steps together. Are able to focus on both the parts (the procedures) and the whole (the patient response).
◆ Become uncomfortable if patient needs preclude performing procedures exactly as they were learned.	◆ Comfortable with rethinking procedure if patient needs require modification of the procedure.
◆ Have limited knowledge of suspected problems; therefore, they question and collect data more superficially.	◆ Have a better idea of suspected problems, allowing them to question more deeply and collect more relevant and in-depth data.
◆ Tend to follow standards and policies by rote.	◆ Analyze standards and policies, looking for ways to improve them.
◆ Learn more readily when matched with a supportive, knowledgeable preceptor or mentor.	◆ Are challenged by novices' questions, clarifying their own thinking when teaching novices.

*The depth and breadth of expert knowledge, largely gained from opportunities to apply theory in real situations, greatly enhance critical thinking ability.

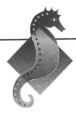

Critical Moments

WHEN AN EXPERT IS A NOVICE

Being an expert means not only having a lot of knowledge and experience, but also being very familiar with the patients and situations at hand. For example, you may be an expert perioperative nurse, and feel like a fish out of water if pulled to work on a medical-surgical floor. Here's another example: Some nurses are experts on clinical care but forget that patients and families are experts about themselves. Don't be a know-it-all. Seek out and acknowledge formal and informal experts. And if you see an expert acting like a fish out of water, lend a hand.

 # A NEW MINDSET

A new "mindset" is almost an oxymoron (a figure of speech with contradictory ideas) when it comes to critical thinking. Being a critical thinker requires us to avoid having a mindset—to keep an open mind that constantly questions the status quo. However, as a whole, we do have a new mindset in health care delivery. And we must understand it to be able to think independently and critically. As you read this section, remember the importance of understanding the mindset while challenging the status quo, looking for better ways. Keep in mind that health care delivery trends have a profound influence on how we think.

Let's start by looking at how care delivery has shifted to a predictive model, a more proactive approach that prevents problems and promotes health and independence.

From "Diagnose and Treat" to a Predictive Approach

Today we have shifted from to a *diagnose and treat* (DT) approach, which implies we wait for evidence of problems before starting treatment, to a predictive model—one that focuses on identifying and managing risk factors *before* problems arise. The predictive model is based on evidence. Thanks to research and efforts to come to clinical consensus, we can often predict who is at risk for certain problems and, if needed, begin an aggressive prevention plan, which may include "treatment." Think about these examples:

◆ We may give an influenza vaccine to someone who has chronic lung disease and also vaccinate his entire family, thus reducing his risk of coming in contact with the influenza virus.

◆ In hip, back, and neck surgery, we routinely "treat to prevent" the potential complication of embolus (clot) formation. We apply pulsating antiemboli stockings and give anticoagulants to high-risk patients.

◆ For those with significant exposure to the AIDS virus, treatment begins before we have evidence of the virus in the blood.

◆ Sometimes taking an antihistamine for a week before allergy season can significantly reduce allergic response.

The predictive model is based on the fact that we now know that recovery from many problems follows an orderly pattern along predictable milestones. We know the importance of recognizing early when patients aren't progressing as expected and intervening to get the patient back on track to recovery. When patients fail to achieve a specific milestone (for example, if someone who has had open-heart surgery isn't off the ventilator and breathing on his own within 24 hours of surgery), a multidisciplinary team evaluates whether there are problems to be solved or resources needed to get him back on track. (The milestone in this case is that the person should be able to breathe on his own within 24 hours of surgery.)

PREDICT, PREVENT, MANAGE, PROMOTE (PPMP). Using a predictive model requires *predicting, preventing,* and *managing* problems and their likely complications. It also requires *promoting* function and well-being. The PPMP approach requires you to do four things:

1. Identify actual problems present, then predict the most likely and most dangerous complications and take immediate action to a) prevent them, and b) be prepared to manage them in case they can't be prevented. *Example:* In cardiac emergencies, after defibrillation, experienced nurses anticipate that IV drugs may be given to prevent more dysrhythmias. They keep emergency drugs and intubation equipment readily available to manage unavoidable complications.

2. Look for evidence of causative or risk factors (things we know cause problems or put people at risk for problems) and control them to prevent the problems themselves. ***Example:*** You're making a home visit to assess an infant. As part of the assessment, look for risks to the infant's safety (check where the baby sleeps, find out if the parents are aware of possible infant hazards). If you identify risks to the baby's safety, you're responsible for making a plan to correct the situation. Failing to make such a plan may be considered negligence.

3. Screen for common health problems, even if risk factors aren't evident. *Example*: Screen for developmental delays in a healthy baby.

4. Encourage behaviors that promote optimum function, independence, and sense of well-being. ***Example:*** Explain to a sedentary asthmatic mother that beginning a walking or exercise program is key to promoting optimum lung function.

The PPMP approach—*predict, prevent, manage, promote*—helps prevent problems, prioritize care, improve satisfaction, and contain costs. Think about the following example: Nursing home residents who

III, Injured, or Disabled People	Healthy People
Focus: Disease, injury, and disability management and prevention; risk management and health promotion	**Focus:** Illness and injury prevention; risk management and health promotion
Approach: ◆ Identify patient problems and their causes (risk/related factors); monitor and manage related signs, symptoms and risk factors	**Approach:** ◆ Identify patient risk factors
◆ Identify risk factors for complications—monitor and manage these as indicated	◆ Predict possible health problems based on risk factors—monitor and manage risk factors
◆ Predict most likely and dangerous complications based on risk factors and problems present—monitor closely and be prepared to manage	◆ Screen for common problems (even if risk factors aren't evident)
◆ Promote optimum independence and function (bio-psycho-social-cultural-spiritual) through teaching and encouraging use of healthy behaviors (e.g., biofeedback; eating and drinking enough, having an exercise regimen if possible, managing stress)	◆ Promote optimum function, independence, and well-being (bio-psycho-social-cultural-spiritual) through teaching and encouraging use of healthy behaviors and resources (e.g., biofeed back, eating and drinking enough, having an exercise regimen, managing stress, getting help from relatives)

Table 3-2   PREDICTIVE MODEL: PREDICT, PREVENT, MANAGE, PROMOTE(PPMP)

From workshop handouts. © 2001, 2002. R. Alfaro-LeFevre.

aren't closely monitored and treated for risk factors for skin breakdown get decubiti, which are costly, care-intensive, painful, and demoralizing. Table 3-2 summarizes the focus and approach of the predictive model.

TREATING VERSUS MANAGING. We hear a lot about treating versus managing. So, what's the difference? *Managing* implies that you do more than treat. For example, in cases of asthma, you don't just keep treating asthma attacks. You monitor the person when healthy and fine-tune medications and inhalers to try to keep the person symptom-free.

The following Critical Moments show the importance of being proactive when managing health problems. For specific strategies to predict, prevent, and manage health problems, see Promoting Health by Identifying and Managing Risk Factors (page 159) and Diagnosing Actual and Potential (Risk) Problems (page 161) in Chapter 5.

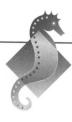

Critical Moments

IMPROVE PERFORMANCE: PREDICT, PREVENT, AND MANAGE DEHYDRATION

Living in Florida where we have heat, humidity, and a lot of elderly people, I've learned the need to manage, rather than treat, dehydration firsthand. Too often, people are told to walk as much as possible to gain or regain strength. Sometimes, these instructions backfire, and people faint from too much effort.

If you or someone else is going to exercise, improve performance by being sensible about pace and ensuring adequate hydration. On hot or humid days, predict the risk of dehydration and heat stroke. Prevent it by monitoring for (and teaching about) risk factors (for example, old or young age, obesity, alcohol or caffeine use, and some medications like diuretics). Look for (and teach) the signs of heatstroke (weakness, nausea, vomiting, chills, confusion, disorientation, hallucinations). Stress the importance of improving exercise performance by drinking water before exercising (so you start out well hydrated), wearing loose-fitting clothes, avoiding the hotter parts of the day, avoiding tea or caffeine (they act as diuretics), and replacing fluids during exercise (water is usually best).

If you suspect heatstroke, manage it by cooling down the person immediately (place him near an air conditioner or place damp towels all over the body, especially to the temples and wrists where blood vessels are near the skin). If the person can tolerate liquids, offer cool fluids. If the person becomes dazed, confused, or has stopped sweating, head for the emergency room because dehydration is severe, requiring immediate medical management.

Want to know more about risk management?

Go online to the Harvard Center For Risk Analysis at http://www.hcra.harvard.edu/. The center is dedicated to promoting reasoned public responses to health, safety, and environmental hazards. It also addresses statistics and approaches for problems like stroke, heart disease, suicide, cancer, and drowning and other accidents. The Centers for Disease Control and Prevention Web page (http://www.cdc.gov/) also has a wealth of information on disease and disability prevention.

Outcome-Focused, Data-Driven, Evidence-Based Care

From professional and economic perspectives, the care we give must be driven by the best available evidence. We must recognize the importance of being able to answer questions like:

◆ Exactly what are the expected outcomes (specifically what benefits will be observed *in this client or group* after nursing care)?

◆ By when do you expect to achieve these outcomes?

◆ What evidence indicates that you're likely to achieve these outcomes? Granted, in some situations, the best available evidence may be "I looked it up in two clinical references and they both say the same thing." But in important situations you need the best scientific evidence to support that you are using the most appropriate approach (see

Box 3-2   CLINICAL PRACTICE GUIDELINES AND EVIDENCE-BASED PRACTICE

What are clinical practice guidelines (CPGs)?*

CPGs are recommendations for how care should be managed in specific diseases, problems, or situations (e.g., how to best manage smoking cessation or neonate umbilical cord care). CPGs must be developed for specific use, and are best designed by a collaborative panel of clinical and scientific experts. When scientific evidence is sufficient, practice guidelines are obvious and clear. When scientific evidence is insufficient, other sources of knowledge (e.g., wisdom gained from clinical experts or specific cases) must be brought to bear on the recommendations to fill in the gaps in the research evidence.

What are the best evidence-based practice (EBP) Web sites for updating practice standards?

The two best EBP resources are the Agency for Healthcare Research and Quality (AHRQ), found at www.ahrq.gov and the Cochrane Library, found at http://www.cochrane.org/cochrane/cc-broch.htm#CC and http://www.update-software.com/cochrane/.

How do you best use the information on these Web sites?

AHRQ offers free access to evidence summaries and reports (on their home page, click on *Evidence-Based Practice*, then see listings under *Evidence Reports*). They also archive their old CPGs developed during 1992–1996. If you access archived CPGs, use the information only after updating them with the latest research on the topic.

The Cochrane Library produces systematic reviews, which give a single statement that summarizes the state of the science and draws on all research on a given topic. A systematic review is the strongest level of evidence for clinical decisions. Evidence summaries can be searched and located through the bibliographic database (such as CINAHL) by limiting results of the search to "publication type: systematic review." Full text summaries are available only through subscription (to subscribe, go to http://www.updatesoftware.com/ccweb/cochrane/cdsr.htm).

Evidence summaries and reports are the essence of EBP and hold promise for improving care, patient outcomes, and efficiency of health care. Moreover, EBP provides mechanisms for fulfilling our social responsibility to provide the *best* care in the most effective and affordable way.

*The term *clinical practice guideline* is sometimes used interchangeably with *practice standard* and *protocol*. All three terms address how care should be managed in certain situations.
(Answers provided by Kathleen R. Stevens, RN, EdD, FAAN, Professor and Director, Academic Center for Evidence-Based Practice (ACE), The University of Texas Health Science Center at San Antonio. Phone: 210-567-3135. Fax: 210-567-5822. E-mail: acestar@uthscsa.edu).

Box 3-2). The following example shows the importance of considering evidence when weighing risks of treatment.

EXAMPLE: ANTHRAX EXPOSURE: WEIGHING THE RISKS. Predicting, preventing, and managing health problems requires knowing the evidence related to treatment risks. You don't treat risk factors in the absence of disease until you weigh the risks of *treatment-related* harm against the probability of *disease-related* harm. For example, in 2001, people potentially infected with anthrax following the terrorist attacks received prolonged courses of antibiotics only after doctors weighed the risks of treatment against getting a deadly respiratory anthrax infection. They made a difficult choice based on the best available evidence at the time.

Clinical, Functional, and Other Outcomes

While how to develop specific, client-centered outcomes is addressed in Chapter 5, this section looks at clinical, functional, and other outcomes to better understand advances in clinical reasoning. Clinical outcomes, at a basic level, are whether a problem is fixed or not. For example, if someone has surgery to repair a fractured hip, did the hip heal? Looking at clinical outcomes only is narrow thinking. Even if you have a clinical outcome of a hip fracture that's healed, you may still have a *functional outcome* of a person who is unable to walk—a very different picture of how beneficial the procedure was. Study the following types of outcomes that use *repair of a fractured hip* as an example. Think about the difference between health care systems that focus only on clinical outcomes compared to those that use a more holistic approach, also considering the others listed.

- ◆ **Clinical Outcomes:** To what degree are the patient's health problems resolved? For example, is the hip healed?
- ◆ **Functional Outcomes:** To what degree is the patient able to function independently, physically, cognitively, and socially? For example, is the person able to do required daily activities without help? Were there complications resulting in cognitive function problems?
- ◆ **Symptom Severity/Quality of Life Outcomes**: To what degree is the patient free of symptoms and able to do desired, as well as required, activities (e.g., is there any hip pain and is the person able to meet physical work requirements and do favorite activities?)?
- ◆ **Risk Reduction Outcomes:** To what degree is the patient able to demonstrate ways to reduce health risks? For example, is he able to explain ways of improving safety, such as using a cane when fatigued? Does he keep his home free from hazards that may cause falls?
- ◆ **Protective Factor Outcomes:** To what degree does the patient's environment protect him from deteriorating health (for example, when bedridden, are bedrails up as needed and skin care protocols followed?)?

◆ **Therapeutic Alliance Outcomes:** To what degree does the patient express a positive relationship between himself and health care professionals (for example, when asked, does he state that he feels free to ask questions?)?

◆ **Satisfaction Outcomes:** To what degree do the patient and family express satisfaction with care given (for example, when asked, do they state that they had competent, efficient treatment? Were services convenient?)?

◆ **Use of Services Outcomes:** To what degree were appropriate nursing services used (for example, was a case manager used, if needed?)?

Box 3-3 summarizes additional health care delivery trends influencing how nurses think.

Box 3-3   TRENDS INFLUENCING THINKING

Nurses Take on More Responsibilities. Nurses continue to take on more responsibilities for both diagnosis and management of health problems. Lifelong learning, focus on mastering essential knowledge and skills, willingness to broaden clinical skills and responsibilities are keys to success.

Nurses Must Prove Value. Regulatory requirements stress that nurses must prove their value to both consumers and their employers, showing how they impact on patient outcomes.

New Threats Emerge. Resistant bacteria, due to antibiotic overuse, threaten us with new infections. Terrorism, including bioterrorism, is a constant threat, requiring new levels of preparedness, responsiveness, and critical thinking.

Partnerships Nurtured, Collaboration Encouraged. Professional, teacher-learner, and nurse-patient relationships are encouraged to be more equal, with an emphasis on developing partnerships that focus on common goals.

Cultural Needs and Patients' Rights. Nursing and health care organizations mandate that we identify and address cultural and spiritual needs. See also Patients' Rights (page 107).

More Concern for Care of the Elderly and Chronically Ill. Many people are living longer with illnesses and disabilities, creating new challenges to keep them as healthy and independent as possible. When these people get sick, the problems are often more complex than usual because of preexisting problems.

New Diagnostic and Treatment Modalities. Researchers study new diagnostic and treatment modalities such as vaccine use and genetic manipulation to prevent illness and find new cures.

Ethical Dilemmas Grow. Ethical issues (e.g., end-of-life care, assisted suicide, fertility issues, cloning, and stem cell research) grow in complexity, requiring thinking that's clearly focused on ethical principles (see next chapter).

Increased Home Care. Nurses must be able to give "high tech" care in homes, and have excellent assessment and interpersonal skills. Being flexible, resourceful, and practical in the home is key.

Continued

Box 3-3 TRENDS INFLUENCING THINKING–cont'd

Case Management. Case management–the use of collaborative approaches to ensure that the best available resources are used to reach outcomes efficiently–promotes quality. This approach is firmly grounded in prevention and early intervention. Today all nurses are expected to be "case managers," closely monitoring progress toward outcomes to detect variances in care (a variance in care is when a patient isn't progressing toward outcomes in the expected time frame–for example, if someone has surgery and is expected to get out of bed on the first day after surgery but is unable to do so, it's considered a variance in care, which needs further evaluation).

Evidence-Based Standards, Practice Guidelines, Protocols, and Best Practices. To reduce useless or harmful practices, federal, state, local, managed care, and private organizations set standards, protocols, guidelines, and best practices (see Box 3-2).

Healthy People 2010. National, state, and local government agencies; nonprofit, voluntary, and professional organizations; and businesses, communities, and individuals come together to achieve two major goals: (1) To help people of all ages improve life expectancy and quality of life, and (2) To eliminate health disparities among different segments of the population. Specific focus areas and objectives are targeted (these can be found on the Web at http://web.health.gov/healthypeople/ prevagenda/focus.htms).

Critical Paths (also known as clinical pathways and CareMaps™) Refined. Critical paths, standard multidisciplinary plans used to predict and determine appropriate care for specific problems, are refined and improved. (Pages 266 shows an example of a critical pathway.)

Computer Use. Computers make it possible to track information in ways that were impossible in the past, giving us specific data on treatments that work. We have instant access to vast knowledge stores, databases, and diagnosis and decision-support systems. More documentation is done directly on the computer, often at patients' bedsides. Computerized patient records (CPR), sometimes called computerized medical records (CMR) or OLPR (On Line Patient Records), are common.

Services Driven by Consumer and Community Needs. Health care organizations aiming to succeed recognize that they must compete for their clients' dollars–services must be driven by consumer needs and customer satisfaction. Insurance companies and consumers alike want to know that they are getting the best value for their dollar.

Managed Care. Managed care organizations aim to furnish services within a group of providers who network to provide quality care in the most cost-effective manner. Nurses, physicians, and therapists working in a managed care environment are challenged to deliver the highest standard of care with the best value.

Wellness Centers and Holistic and Alternative Therapies. More people recognize the value of keeping people healthy and triggering the body's natural healing powers through holistic and alternative therapies (for example, diet, exercise, acupuncture, and stress reduction through meditation and aroma therapy).

Teaching and Counseling Remain Key Responsibility. Nurses are called on to help consumers at both ends of the "knowledge spectrum," from those who are illiterate to those who surf the Internet, becoming experts on the latest information on their problems.

Critical Moments

ELDERLY AND CHRONICALLY ILL: BE CAREFUL OF ASSUMPTIONS

When dealing with aging and chronically ill clients, be especially careful of the human tendency to make assumptions. The complexity of their health status often hides problems that might otherwise be quite obvious. For example, we had a 70-year-old man with chronic back pain. He complained of increasing pain for weeks before someone said, "Maybe it's not his back. Has anyone checked his kidneys?" Only then were kidney stones diagnosed. Getting results requires you to examine alternative explanations, problems, or solutions. The more alternative solutions, explanations, and problems you consider, the more likely it is that you're thinking critically.

CRITICAL THINKING EXERCISES

Note: Exercises followed by asterisks have example responses listed in the Response Key at the back of the book beginning on page 246.

1. Get a piece of paper and make two columns. On the left, list the key points of the applied critical thinking definition on page 57. On the right, write your own interpretation of what each key point implies about what you need to do to think critically in nursing.
2. Write a few statements that address the implications of the following Critical Moments in relation to developing critical thinking skills.*

Critical Moments

ACQUIRING KNOWLEDGE AND SKILLS

Clinical expertise comes from applying knowledge in practice, not from memorizing facts in a book. Seek out simulated observation and real experiences that can help you apply your knowledge and also identify things you may not find in a textbook.

3. Study Table 3-1, page 63 (Novice Thinking Compared with Expert Thinking). Write a paragraph or two about where you stand in relation to the descriptions in this table.
4. What's wrong with this "picture" (the following scenario)?*

> **CASE SCENARIO.** Mr. Vina, an elderly diabetic, is seen at home every other day by a nurse, who checks a healing incision. Mr. Vina has been looking for an assistive device that he can attach to the toilet to help him get up and down. When he asks the visiting nurse if she knows where she can find such a device, the nurse replies, "I'm sorry. I know what you mean, but I don't know where you get them."

Continued

CRITICAL THINKING EXERCISES–cont'd

Note: Exercises followed by asterisks have example responses listed in the Response Key at the back of the book beginning on page 246.

5. Using your own words and giving examples, explain how you use a PPMP approach to health care delivery.*
6. Respond to the following from the prechapter self-test.
   a. Describe what critical thinking and clinical judgment mean to you in relation to the descriptions in this chapter.
   b. Address the implications of the major goals and outcomes of nursing.*
   c. Explain outcome-focused, data-driven, evidence-based care.*
   d. Compare and contrast the *Diagnose and Treat* and the *Predict, Prevent, Manage, Promote* approaches to health care delivery.*

A CHANGING NURSING PROCESS

Use of the nursing process—an organized, systematic approach that consists of five steps (Assessment, Diagnosis, Planning, Implementation, and Evaluation)—is required by national practice standards and is the foundation for clinical judgment. Yet how we teach and use the nursing process is changing, as discussed in the following section.

More Proactive and Dynamic

Today we stress that the nursing process must be proactive, focusing on risk management and health promotion, as well as dealing with problems. We emphasize that the nursing process is a *cycle;* we assess, diagnosis, plan, and intervene, and then we reassess (evaluate) to determine responses. We acknowledge that the nursing process isn't the *only* way to examine patient situations. Other tools can help, as well. For example, also using the 10 key questions for critical thinking on the inside front cover and the tool on the inside back cover (*DEAD ON! A Game to Promote Critical Thinking),* promotes critical thinking.

In the clinical setting, the nursing process is dynamic, unlike how it's described in books or classrooms. If you jump around in books or classrooms trying to explain how things happen dynamically in real life, you confuse people. You have to present content in a logical, step-by-step way. In real life, the nursing process is fluid and changing, with nurses applying principles, but moving back and forth within the steps, and often combining activities from two or more of the steps. Reflect on the following example:

Example: Dynamic Nursing Process
1. You walk into a room and you haven't even said, "Hello." You hardly realize that you have made a quick assessment of the room (the bed

linens are in disarray, there's trash on the floor, and the person is restless with a distressed look on his face). You quickly begin step 2 (*diagnosis*), thinking, *there's a problem here, for sure,* and begin to assess closely to find out exactly what's going on. You may end up deciding that there are signs and symptoms that should be immediately reported to the doctor, or you may simply intervene with a lot of little things, which resolve the overall problem. Either way, you're so busy *doing* that you hardly realize that your brain is assessing and correlating as you go along.

2. Sometimes you deal with standard plans that have already done much of the work of *planning* (step 4) for you. Instead of having to create a plan "from scratch," you must decide whether the standard plan is appropriate for each particular patient. Standard plans don't think for you. You have to think independently, applying principles of the nursing process like assessing and predicting consequences before acting. While the nursing process is certainly dynamic, it's important to remember the following rule:

Rule: ◆ Experts use the nursing process in a very dynamic way because they know what steps can be safely skipped, combined, or delayed—and they can rapidly gather and correlate data in their heads. They also know when situations warrant a rigorous, comprehensive, step-by-step approach.

◆ Beginners often need to follow the steps more rigidly, carefully reflecting on *each* step. Because of their inexperience and lack of knowledge, they take more risks when they skip or delay steps.

Box 3-4 shows use of the nursing process as a tool for clinical judgment. Figure 3-2 shows how a critical thinker uses a more proactive, dynamic approach to the nursing process than a task-oriented thinker does.

Other Perspectives

NURSING PROCESS: LIKE TENNIS?
"It seems to me that learning to use the nursing process is like learning to play tennis. First, you learn basic techniques in a step-by-step way. Then you work at it until you are able to apply the techniques, without having to think about each step. You naturally have a dynamic and fluid approach."

—*Bruce Franklin, One of My Reviewers*

Box 3-4   **THE NURSING PROCESS: A TOOL FOR CLINICAL REASONING (CLINICAL JUDGMENT)**

Assessment. Collecting and recording data to provide the information required to:
♦ Predict, detect, prevent, manage, or eliminate health problems and promote health
♦ Determine expected outcomes
♦ Identify interventions aimed at promoting health and attaining optimum function and independence

Diagnosis. Analyzing data, drawing conclusions, and determining:
♦ Actual and potential health problems and their cause(s)
♦ Presence of risk factors
♦ Resources, strengths, and use of healthy behaviors
♦ Health states that are satisfactory but could be improved

Planning. Determining expected outcomes and interventions by predicting responses. The interventions are designed to:
♦ Detect, prevent, and manage health problems
♦ Promote optimum function and wellness
♦ Achieve the desired outcomes safely and efficiently

Implementation. Putting the plan into action by:
♦ Assessing appropriateness of (and patient readiness for) interventions
♦ Performing interventions, and then reassessing to determine initial responses
♦ Making immediate changes as needed
♦ Charting to monitor progress

Evaluation. Determining whether expected outcomes have been met; modifying or terminating the plan as appropriate; planning for ongoing continuous assessment and improvement

Is the Care Plan Dead?

As critical paths and standard plans replace personally developed care plans, some nurses have begun to say things like, "the nursing process and care planning is dead." However, the care plan is alive and well. It's only changed. Standards in virtually all health care organizations–from hospitals to nursing homes–mandate that clients have a recorded plan of care that demonstrates that their specific needs and problems are being addressed.

Today, you may not find the care plan in one place. Rather, parts of the plan may be addressed in different places of the chart (e.g., the nursing assessment may be in one place, routine interventions may be covered in critical paths or protocols, an individual plan in another, and so on). You must be familiar with principles of the nursing process and care planning to be able to know whether the plan of care is sufficiently

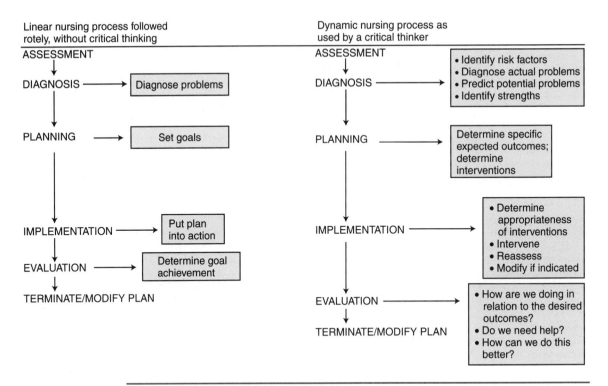

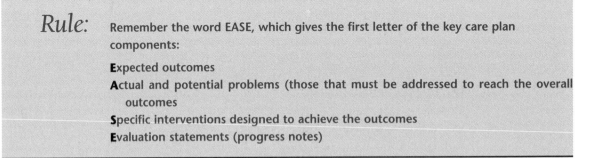

Figure 3-2 ◆ How a noncritical thinker uses the nursing process compared with how a critical thinker uses the nursing process, focusing on the diagnosis, implementation, and evaluation stages.

documented. Whether you're developing a plan yourself or using standard plans, remember the following rule:

Rule: Remember the word EASE, which gives the first letter of the key care plan components:

Expected outcomes

Actual and potential problems (those that must be addressed to reach the overall outcomes

Specific interventions designed to achieve the outcomes

Evaluation statements (progress notes)

What Do Nurses Diagnose?

Another major change in how we use the nursing process is in step 2, *diagnosis*. We have moved from "nurses diagnose and treat only nursing diagnoses" to "nurses diagnose and manage various problems, depending on their knowledge, expertise, and qualifications." For example, advanced practice nurses (APN) and other specially trained nurses may diagnose or manage problems that used to be managed only by physicians (e.g., stable hypertension and common infections).

So then, how do you know when you're accountable for diagnosing and managing a problem? This is a tough question for beginning nurses. It takes varied clinical experiences for the concept of accountability for diagnosis and management to come alive. However, let's begin by considering the following rule:

Rule:　　The terms *diagnose* and *diagnosis* have legal implications. They imply that there's a specific problem that requires management by a qualified expert.

◆ If you make a diagnosis, it means that you accept accountability for accurately naming and managing the problem.

◆ If you treat a problem or allow a problem to persist without ensuring that the correct diagnosis has been made, you may cause harm and be accused of negligence.

◆ You're accountable for detecting, identifying, or recognizing signs and symptoms that may indicate problems beyond your expertise. *Example:* Staff nurses aren't qualified to diagnose and manage pneumonia independently. **However, they *are* accountable for:**

1. **Detecting and reporting signs and symptoms** of pneumonia (for example, fever, productive cough, malaise).
2. **Diagnosing and managing *risk factors*** for pneumonia (for example, weak breathing efforts due to surgical pain, spinal cord injury, or disease (in complicated cases, these risk factors may require medical management).
3. **Diagnosing and managing *human responses*** to pneumonia (for example, fatigue and problems with airway clearance related to pneumonia).
4. **Ensuring that the *medical treatment plan* is implemented** as prescribed.

Nursing Responsibilities Related to Diagnosis

Understanding *conceptually* the types of problems that nurses focus on is an important step toward understanding your responsibilities related to diagnosis and management of health problems. Following are examples of the types of nursing concerns that are clearly nursing responsibilities.

◆ **Monitoring for changes in health status.** Because nurses spend the most time with patients–the ones in the "front line"–they are responsible for detecting signs and symptoms of possible problems requiring medical (or other multidisciplinary) management. For example, in the case of surgery, they're responsible for recognizing and reporting signs of potential complications, such as excessive blood loss.

◆ **Promoting safety and preventing harm; detecting and controlling risks.** At every patient encounter, nurses are responsible for injury or illness. For example, nurses must detect and control risks for falls, skin breakdown, infection, and violence.

◆ **Identifying and meeting learning needs.** Nurses must ensure that patients or their caregivers have the knowledge and ability to manage their own health. For example, diabetic teaching is a nursing responsibility.

◆ **Tailoring treatment and medication regimens for each individual.** Nurses are intimately involved in ensuring that overall regimens are as safe, effective, cost-effective, and convenient as possible, considering the age, culture, religion, roles, occupation, and lifestyles of those involved.

◆ **Promoting comfort and managing pain.** Nurses are accountable for promoting comfort and managing pain through both prescribed medications and holistic therapies.

◆ **Promoting health and a sense of well-being.** Nurses promote health by teaching about health behaviors and detecting and managing risk factors for problems.

◆ **Recognizing and addressing problems that impede ability to be independent and live a healthy lifestyle.** For example, managing problems with performing activities of daily living (ADL), such as bathing and dressing, is a nursing responsibility.

◆ **Determining human responses** (how individuals, families, or groups respond to health problems or life changes). For example, suppose a man has surgery for breast cancer. His human response, how he responds to his medical condition—whether he has problems with self-esteem, sexuality, or whatever—is a nursing concern. The following definition of nursing diagnosis addresses nursing responsibilities in relation to human responses:

   Nursing diagnosis: A clinical judgment about an individual, family, or community response to actual or potential health problems and life processes. Nursing diagnoses provide the basis for selection of nursing interventions to achieve outcomes for which the nurse is accountable.[3]

Now that you have a general idea of common nursing concerns, let's look at how you know what your responsibilities are in relation to specific health problems.

Nursing concerns can be divided into two categories: (1) Those addressed using nursing diagnosis terminology, managed primarily by nurses independently (for example, see Box 3-5 and the nursing diagnoses listed in Appendix D, beginning on page 270) and, (2) Those addressed using medical terminology, often manage by nurses guided by physician-prescribed orders or protocols (see Box 3-6). As you work

Box 3-5 **DIAGNOSES COMMONLY IDENTIFIED IN REHABILITATION NURSING**

Risk for injury	Pressure ulcer
Activity intolerance	Pain
Impaired physical mobility	Deficient knowledge
Colonic constipation	Impaired swallowing
Reflex incontinence	Impaired thought processes
Urinary retention	Body image disturbance
Feeding self-care deficit	Impaired verbal communication
Bathing or hygiene self-care deficit	Ineffective individual coping
Dressing and grooming self-care deficit	Ineffective family coping
	Caregiver role strain
Toileting self-care deficit	Risk for disuse syndrome

Data from Association of Rehabilitation Nurses. (1995). *21 Rehabilitation nursing diagnoses: A guide to interventions and outcomes.* Glenview, IL: Author.

Box 3-6 **COMMON COMPLICATIONS**

Common medical diagnoses (in bold) and their potential complications

Angina/myocardial infarction
Dysrhythmias
Congestive heart failure/pulmonary edema
Shock (cardiogenic, hypovolemic)
Infarction, infarction extension
Thrombi/emboli formation (e.g., pulmonary emboli, cerebrovascular accident)
Hypoxemia
Electrolyte imbalance
Acid-base imbalance
Pericarditis
Cardiac tamponade
Cardiac arrest
Asthma/chronic obstructive lung disease
Hypoxemia
Acid-base/electrolyte imbalance
Respiratory failure
Cardiac failure
Infection

Diabetes
Hyper/hypoglycemia
Delayed wound healing
Hypertension
Eye problems (retinal hemorrhage)
See also Angina/myocardial infarction
Fractures
Bleeding
Fracture displacement
Thrombus/embolus formation
Compromised circulation (pressure points, edema)
Nerve compression
Infection
See also Skeletal traction/casts
Head trauma
Increased intracranial pressure (secondary to bleeding or brain swelling)
Respiratory depression
Shock
Hyper/hypothermia
Coma

Continued

Box 3-6 COMMON COMPLICATIONS–cont'd

Hypertension
Cerebrovascular accident
Transient ischemic attacks (TIAs)
Renal failure
Hypertensive crisis
See also Angina/myocardial infarction
Pneumonia
Respiratory failure
Sepsis/septic shock
Pulmonary embolus
See Angina/myocardial infarction

Renal failure
Fluid overload
Hyperkalemia
Electrolyte/acid-base imbalance
Anemia
See also Hypertension
Trauma
See Anesthesia/surgical or invasive
   procedures
Urinary tract infection
Septic shock

Common treatment and diagnostic modalities (in bold) and their potential complications

**Anesthesia/surgical or invasive
   procedures**
Bleeding/hypovolemia/shock
Respiratory depression/atelectasis
Urinary retention
Fluid/electrolyte imbalances
Thrombus/embolus formation
Paralytic ileus
Incisional complications (infection,
   poor healing, dehiscence/evisceration)
Sepsis/septic shock
Cardiac catheterization
Bleeding
Thrombus/embolus formation
Chest tubes
Hemo/pneumothorax
Bleeding
Atelectasis
Chest tube malfunction/blockage
Infection/sepsis
Foley catheter
Infection/sepsis
Catheter malfunction/blockage

Intravenous therapy
Phlebitis/thrombophlebitis
Infiltration/extravasation
Fluid overload
Infection/sepsis
Bleeding
Air embolism
Medications
Adverse reactions (allergic
   response/exaggerated effects/side
   effects/drug interactions)
Overdose/toxicity
Nasogastric suction
Electrolyte imbalance
Tube malfunction/blockage
Aspiration
Skeletal traction/casts
Poor bone alignment
Bleeding/swelling
Compromised circulation
Nerve compression
See also Fractures

From Alfaro-LeFevre, R. (2002). *Applying nursing process: Promoting collaborative care* (5th ed.). Philadelphia: Lippincott Williams & Wilkins.

in various settings (e.g., pediatrics or maternity nursing), check with experts, up-to-date texts, and policies and procedures to determine the specific problems you're accountable for diagnosing and managing.

Also remember the following rule:

> *Rule:* **To detect *both* possible nursing and medical problems, organize the data you collect in two ways: (1) Use a nursing model (see Box 3-7) to cluster data to help you detect nursing problems and (2) Use a body systems approach (see Figure 3-3) to cluster data to help you detect problems that may require medical management.**

Want to know more about growing knowledge of nursing diagnoses, interventions, and outcomes?

Go online to the following Web sites of organizations working to develop, refine, classify, and standardize nursing terminology (to expand nursing knowledge, and for the purpose of having consistency among terms in computer databases).

♦ North American Nursing Diagnosis Association (NANDA)
   http://www.nanda.org/html/about.html
♦ Nursing Interventions Classification (NIC)
   http://coninfo.nursing.uiowa.edu/nic/overview.htm
♦ Nursing-Sensitive Outcomes Classification (NOC)
   http://coninfo.nursing.uiowa.edu/noc/index.htm
♦ Omaha Nursing Classification System for Community Health
   http://con.ufl.edu/omaha/omahas.htm
♦ Perioperative Nursing Data Set (PNDS)
   http://www.aorn.org/research/pnds.htm
♦ Home Health Care Classification (HHCC)
   http://www.sabacare.com
♦ International Classification for Nursing Practice (ICNP®)
   http://www.icn.ch/icnp.htm

 Other Perspectives

EXPANDING NURSING ROLES: FROM CRITICAL PATHWAYS TO LIFE PATHWAYS
"As people live longer with disabilities, the rehabilitation nurse's role is expanding. We now go beyond traditional, episodic case management to life management, beyond disease management to life care prevention, beyond critical pathways to life pathways."[4]

—Terri Patterson, RN, MSN, CRRN President, LifeTrak Ltd.

Box 3-7 **A FREQUENTLY USED NURSING FRAMEWORK: GORDON'S FUNCTIONAL HEALTH PATTERNS**

Health perception/health management pattern: Perception of health and well-being, knowledge of and adherence to regimens promoting health

Nutritional-metabolic pattern: Usual food and fluid intake; height, weight, age

Elimination pattern: Usual bowel and bladder elimination patterns

Activity-rest pattern: Usual activity and exercise tolerance, usual hours of exercise and rest

Cognitive-perception pattern: Ability to use all senses to perceive environment, usual way of perceiving environment

Self-perception/self-concept pattern: Perception of capabilities and self-worth

Role-relationship pattern: Usual responsibilities and ways of relating to others

Sexuality-reproductive pattern: Knowledge and perception of sex and reproduction

Coping-stress tolerance pattern: Ability to manage and tolerate stress

Value-belief pattern: Values, beliefs, and goals in life; spiritual practices

Summarized from Gordon, M. (2002). *Manual of nursing diagnosis* (10th ed.). St. Louis: Mosby.

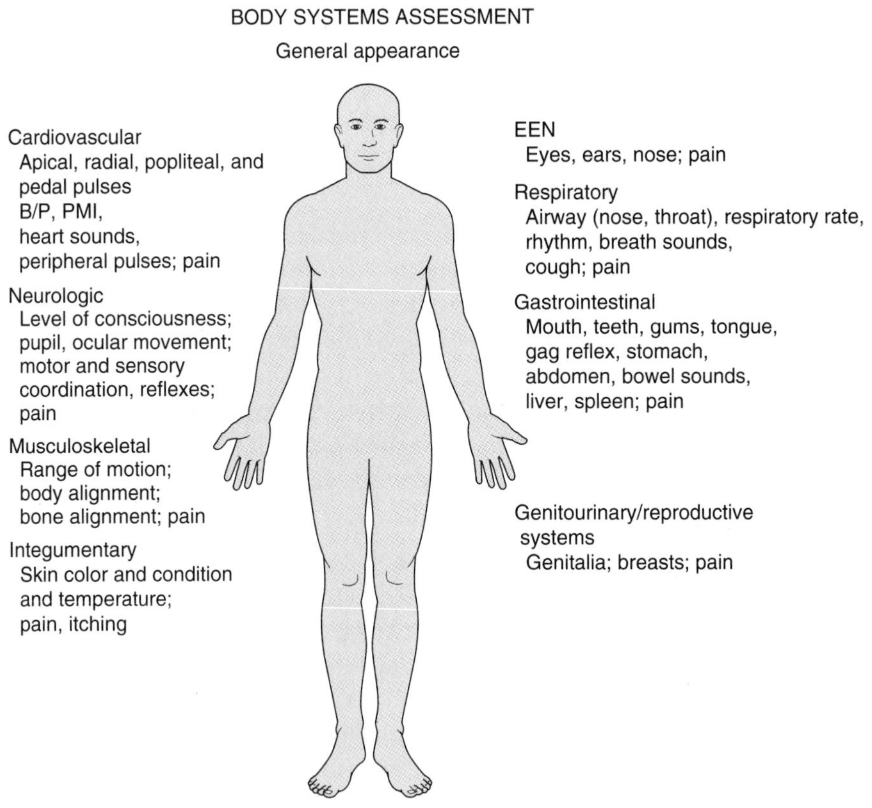

BODY SYSTEMS ASSESSMENT

General appearance

Cardiovascular
Apical, radial, popliteal, and pedal pulses
B/P, PMI,
heart sounds,
peripheral pulses; pain

Neurologic
Level of consciousness;
pupil, ocular movement;
motor and sensory
coordination, reflexes;
pain

Musculoskeletal
Range of motion;
body alignment;
bone alignment; pain

Integumentary
Skin color and condition
and temperature;
pain, itching

EEN
Eyes, ears, nose; pain

Respiratory
Airway (nose, throat), respiratory rate,
rhythm, breath sounds,
cough; pain

Gastrointestinal
Mouth, teeth, gums, tongue,
gag reflex, stomach,
abdomen, bowel sounds,
liver, spleen; pain

Genitourinary/reproductive
systems
Genitalia; breasts; pain

Figure 3-3 ◆ Body systems assessment.

DEVELOPING CLINICAL JUDGMENT (CLINICAL REASONING SKILLS)

Developing clinical judgment—clinical reasoning skills—is one of the most important and challenging aspects of becoming a nurse. It's important because people's lives depend on it. It's challenging because thinking in the clinical setting is often fraught with more anxiety and risks than other situations. For beginners, clinical reasoning is particularly taxing because it requires an ability to recall facts, put them together into a meaningful whole, and apply the information to the real world. For example, you note that someone is pale, sweaty, and has a rapid pulse. To exercise good clinical judgment, you must be able to recall that these are symptoms of shock and that an immediate priority is to take a complete set of vital signs to further evaluate the patient's condition. Keep in mind the following key points:

1. Clinical judgment requires sophisticated critical thinking skills.
2. Clinical judgments (your nursing opinions) are extremely important because they guide nursing care and affect people's lives.
3. Your ability to make clinical judgments depends on theoretical and experiential knowledge (e.g., knowing what to look for, how to recognize when a patient's status is changing, and what to do about it).
4. Using "sound clinical judgment" means drawing valid conclusions and then acting appropriately based on those conclusions. For example, you may conclude that you don't know enough to handle a specific problem and decide the most appropriate immediate action is to consult with a more experienced professional. Remember the following rule:

Rule: Clinical judgment (clinical reasoning) often requires *thinking on your feet*. However, you must also recognize when a situation requires more than *thinking on your feet* (for example, knowing when the situation is so complex that you need to take your time thinking things through, or get additional opinions before drawing a conclusion).

Knowing how to exercise good clinical judgment comes from a "marriage" of theoretical and experiential knowledge—it requires that you apply what you know from class, readings, and simulation exercises to the clinical setting. If you practice without theoretical knowledge, you're unlikely to make sound clinical judgments. If you have only theoretical knowledge, with little clinical experience, you're also unlikely to make sound clinical judgments.

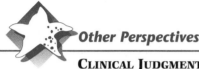

Other Perspectives

CLINICAL JUDGMENT REQUIRES GETTING INVOLVED
"We use the term 'clinical judgment' to refer to the ways in which nurses come to understand the problems, issues, or concerns of clients/patients, to attend to salient information, and to respond in concerned and involved ways.... "[5]

—*Authors Patricia Benner, RN, PhD; Christine Tanner, RN, PhD; and Catherine Chesla, RN, DNSc.*

Where Do Intuition and Logic Fit In?

Increasingly, nurses are addressing the question, What roles do intuition (knowing without evidence) and logic (rational thinking that's based on evidence) play in clinical judgment?[6,7,8,9] Most agree that intuition, an important part of thinking, is often seen in experts, and is the result of years of experience and indepth knowledge of patients. But there is a concern that encouraging the use of intuition sends the message that it's okay to act on gut feelings without evidence, which is risky.

To clarify the use of intuition and logic in clinical judgment, it's important to answer two questions:
1. Is the rapid thinking that goes on in the heads of experts simply the use of intuition?
2. If someone can't explain her thinking, does this mean that she's thinking intuitively?

To the outsider, many experts' actions seem to be based on intuition alone. But this rapid thinking is usually the result of using intuition and logic *together*. Experts move rapidly back and forth between intuition and logic, making leaps in thinking with intuitive hunches, then almost at the same time drawing on logic and past experience to make well-reasoned conclusions.

Experts who juggle several priorities at once often have trouble explaining their thinking at the very moment it's happening. For this reason, it's easy to conclude that this thinking is intuitive. But, if it's really important (for example, if these same experts are challenged in court to explain the actions they took and the reasons behind them) they can readily reconstruct the logic of their thinking (and if they can't, they're in trouble). Remember the following rule:

Rule: **Developing good clinical judgment requires using your whole brain— both the intuitive-right and logical-left sides.** Use intuitive hunches as guides

> *Rule:* **cont'd**
>
> to search for evidence. Use logic to formulate and double-check your thinking, ensuring that your conclusions are based on the best available evidence. In important situations, be careful about acting on intuition alone. Ask questions like, Does this logically make sense? How do I know I'm right? and What could go wrong if I act on gut feelings?

Other Perspectives

USING INTUITION AND LOGIC: DO A LITTLE DANCE

"I agree that nurses must focus on evidence, when available. The ICU nurses say I 'do a dance' when I know something's wrong with my patient but I can't quite figure it out. First, I get quiet (this usually gets attention as I am not really a loud person, just not really silent). Second, I gather all my information—the bedside notes, medication record, etc. Then, I take another set of vital signs, and then sort of slowly pace back and forth, assessing the patient, thinking while standing in the doorway, reassessing the patient, reviewing the trends for the day, reassessing again, checking the lab results, the urine output, etc. Then when I 'get it' I get verbal again. I page the doctor or consult a more experienced nurse or colleague in the unit. Patricia Benner calls this 'thinking in action.' My group calls it my 'intuitive dance.' Once I get the hunch something's up, I keep going until it makes sense."[10]

—*Elizabeth E. Hand, MS, CCRN, Education Specialist*

What about Creativity?

Every so often, I'm asked whether the use of creativity is acceptable in clinical judgment. This question surprised me at first. I wondered, Why *not?* Then clinicians gave me two examples of dangerous or problematic creativity. The first example was of a nurse who was going to administer blood, but found that the blood warmer was broken, so she used a "creative" (and dangerous) approach: She heated the blood in the microwave. The other example is that of nurses who continually reinvent the wheel, creating new approaches that aren't really better, or coming up with ideas that aren't practical or user-friendly. Creativity has an important place in clinical nursing. But, be sure to use *principle-centered* creativity, and evaluate whether your ideas are really useful to the end users. Learn ways to facilitate brainstorming both individually and in a group (e.g., try the *DEAD ON!* game on the inside back cover). Don't be happy with the status quo. Think outside the box and ask questions like, What does the research say on this and how can it be applied to get better results? How can technology help? What human resources might be willing to give their time? and What does the patient or family suggest to make this all better? Think about the following examples of useful creativity.

EXAMPLES OF USEFUL CREATIVITY: SEASHELLS FOR MEDICINE CUPS, AROMA THERAPY, WHAT ELSE? For home care, seashells and party favors make good medicine cups, not to mention conversation pieces. White clamshells—sterilized by boiling for 30 minutes, and then placed in the dishwasher—look great and are functional and fun for the family. For dinner, go formal and put the meds in a tiny gold plastic champagne glass from a party favor store. For bedridden patients, give them a bit of "aroma therapy"—for freshening up, offer them a warm washcloth dabbed with a drop of their favorite perfume (if they don't have a favorite, check for perfume allergies first).

Here are two more examples of useful creativity: I had a colleague who worked in a neonatal ICU. She kept a camera handy, and when she was changing all the tubes on her sick babies, she'd get someone to snap a picture of the baby without all the tubes attached to give to the parents. Another neonatal nurse noticed that the babies under ultraviolet light for high serum bilirubin levels weren't getting much of their trunk exposed to the light because of diapers that were too big for their tiny bodies. She designed a smaller, better-fitting "G-string" diaper that significantly increased exposure, thus reducing the amount of time the babies had to spend under the lights. Eventually, this nurse started her own successful company selling these creative, effective diapers! Box 3-8 shows a reprint of "Critical Thinking Isn't Usually Rapid-Fire," a short article addressing the use of creativity and intuition in nursing.

Scope of Practice Decisions

A key aspect of developing clinical judgment is learning to make decisions about what actions are within your scope of practice: How do you know when you're qualified to give a professional opinion or perform a nursing action? Because laws and standards constantly change, several nursing boards have developed guides to help nurses make these types of decisions (see Fig. 3-4, page 89, an example student guideline).

Box 3-8 **CRITICAL THINKING ISN'T USUALLY RAPID-FIRE***

Too often, nurses want to equate critical thinking with rapid-fire thinking, creativity, and intuition. They seem to say, "Tell us how to diagnose and treat quicker and easier." They're looking for quick fixes and easy outs, which is exactly the opposite of critical thinking. Yes, it's true that when you see experts in action, critical thinking may seem to present itself as "rapid-fire thinking." And it's true that creativity and intuition are an integral part of critical thinking. But critical thinking usually isn't rapid-fire, and it requires much more than creativity and intuition. Let me clarify these three points:

1) **Critical thinking usually isn't rapid-fire.** In fact, experts use rapid-fire thinking only under extreme circumstances. They know that the end result is often "shooting from the hip." We must be clear that critical thinking skills like checking accuracy and reliability, recognizing inconsistencies, and identifying patterns and missing information takes time. We must make time to reflect, evaluating and correcting our thinking, and asking questions like, What am I missing? Do I know what I need to know? What else could be going on here? and How can I do this better?" Too many nurses are at risk for shooting from the hip due to work overloads and pressure from insurance companies to move patients through the system. We must value the need for time to think. Critical thinking requires knowledge, skills, practice, caution, and judgment. It often happens best away from the patient in a quiet place where there are few distractions or in a group, where there is input from various perspectives.

2) **Creativity doesn't necessarily mean critical thinking.** It's true that an essential part of critical thinking is considering many ideas, alternatives, and creative solutions. But if we want to think critically we need to answer questions like, Have I fallen in love with my ideas? Am I re-inventing the wheel? and Whom should I check with to address practical concerns? Too often creativity and brain-storming seminars deal with the creative process, but fail to address the judgment needed to decide how to use creativity in the clinical setting in a safe, sensible way. Applying creativity requires both producing ideas (right-brain function) and evaluating and judging the worth of those ideas (left-brain function).

3) **The problem with equating intuitive thinking with critical thinking.** Much has been written on the power of intuition in the diagnostic process and on the "immediate knowing" of experts. But little is said about how to use intuition or about how experts are able to "immediately know" (other than to say they know it intuitively). As much as possible, critical thinking is based on evidence. When we equate critical thinking with intuitive thinking, we risk sending the message that it's okay to act on gut feelings without much thought. Rather, we need to teach the value of recognizing when we're experiencing gut feelings, and acting appropriately (e.g., using intuition as a guide for looking for evidence or as a trigger to monitor more closely).

Critical thinking requires you to be able to explain how you know what you know. Push any nurse who tells you about a time that he "immediately knew something" to closely examine how he knew it. More likely than not, he will be able to give you a simple answer (e.g., I saw it happen before in a similar case, or things were just a little different). The point is that nurses who "know immediately" usually know because they are able to match the present situation with previous knowledge and experience (or perhaps they have taken the time to know the patient better than others have). We don't serve our profession by teaching nurses that some clinicians "just know" because of the mystery of their intuition. These mysterious instances are the exception. By emphasizing that in most cases, "immediate knowing" is a result of previous experience and getting to know patients and their problems well, we teach the importance of gaining knowledge and experience, of making time to monitor closely and assess comprehensively, and of aiming for continuity of care. Without respect for the knowledge, experience, caution, judgment, and time required to think critically, creativity and intuition are wasted. And we're likely to see more "casualties at the OK Corral" due to shooting from the hip.

*Adapted with permission from: R. Alfaro-LeFevre, (2000). Critical thinking isn't usually rapid-fire. AACN News, 2, 12.

Critical Moments

BEING CREATIVE AND APPLYING PRINCIPLES WORKS
Sometimes simple, principle-centered ideas get you the best results. Be creative and apply principles when searching for solutions.

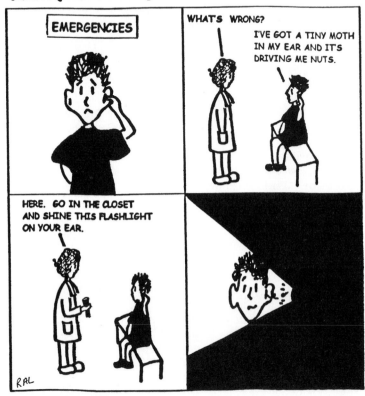

© Alfaro-LeFevre 1998.

Decision Making and Nursing Standards and Guidelines

As noted in my description of critical thinking and clinical judgment at the beginning of this chapter, critical thinking in nursing is guided by professional standards. Let's look at how clinical judgment in nursing is influenced by broad and specific standards. National practice standards provide broad standards that address how nurses are expected to plan and give care (see Standards for Practice, Appendix C, page 263). Each specialty organization (for example, American Association of Critical-Care Nurses, Association of Rehabilitation Nurses, Association of Operating Room Nurses) develops its own standards for specialty

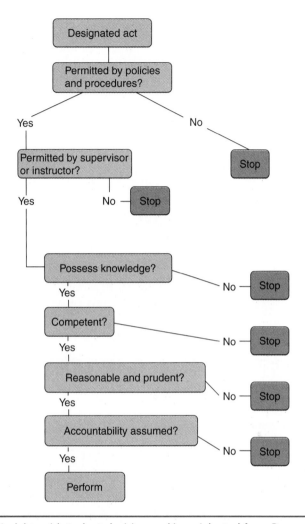

Figure 3-4 ◆ Model to aid student decision making. Adapted from Pennsylvania State Board of Nursing Decision-Making Model.

practice. Each health care organization develops numerous specific standards and guidelines (in the form of standards of care, policies, protocols, procedures, care plans, and critical paths) that guide decision making in specific situations.

Three main questions to raise when deciding how to manage care are:

1. Has this facility developed specific standards, guidelines, or policies for the care of this specific situation? For example, if you're caring for someone with a mastectomy, you need to ask, Has this facility developed any type of guidelines for someone undergoing a mastectomy?
2. Are there national or local evidenced-based practice guidelines relating to this particular problem?

3. To what degree do these standards and guidelines apply to my patient's situation?

Organizational, national, and local practice standards are valuable tools to help you make care decisions. However, don't follow guidelines blindly. An essential part of decision making is using critical thinking to recognize when the situation at hand *differs* from the standards or guidelines. Carefully compare your patient's situation with the information presented in the guideline and decide whether they indeed apply to your specific patient. For example, suppose that you're looking after a man following prostate surgery and the critical path for this problem states that on the first postoperative day, the patient gets out of bed twice. On the first postoperative day, you assess the man and find he has chest pain. This finding is significant enough for you to question whether he should indeed get out of bed. Could this man be suffering a complication such as myocardial infarction or pulmonary embolus? In this case, you need to report the symptoms and keep the man in bed until a physician or more qualified nurse evaluates him.

Critical Moments

CRITICAL PATHWAYS: NOT LIKE IN THE LAND OF OZ

Critical pathways, protocols, and standard plans aren't meant to be like the yellow brick road in the land of Oz, which allowed Dorothy to find the wizard without much thought. Use critical pathways as maps, carefully considering how they apply to your particular patient situation. Think about this analogy: Imagine you're driving down the road, and you come to a temporary roadblock. Even though the map says you have to go straight, you clearly have to figure out another way. Whether talking about care maps or road maps, you are the one who has to assess the actual "road conditions," taking detours and changing speed as needed. When using standard plans, don't be a task-oriented thinker. Approach situations with a critical mind. Consider the two examples that follow:

Task-Oriented Thinking	**Critical Thinking**
"I have a path for this patient so this will be easy and straightforward because I already know what the problems are going to be."	"I'm familiar with this path…I wonder how this particular patient is doing in relation to the predicted care for this problem."

How to Develop Effective Clinical Judgment

Developing clinical judgment skills takes time. It requires a commitment to study common health problems, seek out clinical experiences, and come prepared to the clinical setting. In Chapter 5, you'll have opportunities to practice skills that are essential to developing clinical judgment (e.g., drawing valid conclusions and setting priorities). For now, study the following 10 strategies for developing clinical judgment.

10 Strategies for Developing Clinical Judgment

1. Until you have enough repeated experiences with diagnosis and management of commonly encountered health problems, keep references such as notes, texts, and pocket guides readily available. Unless you have repeated experiences, you're unlikely to be able to recall the information you need to think and act appropriately.

   ◆ **Learn terminology and concepts.** If you encounter words like embolus, thrombus, or phlebitis and you don't know what they mean, look them up as you encounter them, and they'll soon become part of your long-term memory. Learning the terms in *context* helps you store information in related groups, rather than as isolated facts.

   ◆ **Become familiar with normal findings** (e.g., normal lab values, assessment findings, disease progression, growth and development) before being concerned with abnormal findings. Once you know what's normal, you'll readily recognize when you encounter information that's outside the norm (abnormal).

   ◆ **Ask, Why?** Find out what theories or principles explain why normal and abnormal findings occur.

   ◆ **Learn problem-specific facts.** You need to know how problems usually present themselves (their signs and symptoms), what usually causes them, and how they're managed. For instance, if you're going to take care of someone who has a medical diagnosis of diabetes and a nursing diagnosis of ineffective individual coping, become familiar with the common signs, symptoms, causes, complications, and management of these two problems before caring for the person. Box 3-9 provides questions you should ask to gain the facts you'll need to know to reason well in the clinical setting.

2. Apply principles of nursing process. For example, assess before acting, stay focused on outcomes, anticipate and change approaches as needed. Make judgments based on evidence rather than emotions or hearsay, and remember the following rule:

Rule: Comprehensive assessment means getting information from patient records, caregivers, significant others, and applicable literature (e.g., information from a drug manual about medications being taken). But *always consider your direct assessment of the patient to be your primary source of information.*

Box 3-9   QUESTIONS YOU NEED TO ANSWER TO GAIN PROBLEM-SPECIFIC
KNOWLEDGE BEFORE GOING TO THE CLINICAL SETTING

1. Based on this particular clinical setting, what common problems are seen, and what problems do I know or suspect my patients have?
2. What are the signs and symptoms of these problems?
3. What risk factors do I know or suspect my patients have?
4. What must I assess to determine the status of these signs, symptoms, and risk factors?
5. What are the usual causes of these problems?
6. What must I assess to determine the status of the causes of the problems?
7. How do these problems usually progress, and how are they managed?
8. How can these problems be prevented?
9. What are the signs and symptoms of potential complications of these problems and how will I monitor for these signs and symptoms?
10. How can I be prepared to manage potential complications if they should occur?
11. What medications and treatments are likely to be used, and why?
12. What medication-related or treatment-related problems might I encounter, how will I monitor to detect them, and how are they usually managed?
13. What cultural factors, values, or beliefs might have bearing on health practices in relation to these health problems?
14. What are the key things people need to know to manage these problems independently, and what will I do to ensure that this knowledge is gained?

3. Follow policies, procedures, and standards of care carefully with a good understanding of the reasons behind them. Policies, procedures, and standards of care are designed to help you use good judgment, but you must know the reasons behind them to know when and how to adapt them.
4. Develop a systematic and comprehensive approach to assessment, so that you're more efficient and less likely to overlook anything (see Assessing Systematically and Comprehensively in Chapter 5, pages 142-146).
5. Determine a system that helps you make decisions about what must be done now and what can wait until later (see Setting Priorities in Chapter 5, pages 167-171).
6. Never perform actions (interventions) if you don't know why they're indicated, why they work (the rationale), and whether there are risks of harm *in the context of the current patient situation.* Only when you know the reasons behind interventions can you decide if they are still appropriate. Only when you know risks of interventions can you identify ways of preventing harm. For example, if you're aware of the risks of introducing an air embolism into an IV line, you find ways to reduce that risk (e.g., taping connections together).

7. Learn from human resources (e.g., educators, preceptors, class-mates, other nurses) and when in doubt, get help from a qualified professional. Your patients' rights to timely care take precedence over your need to learn independently. Other professionals can help you decide whether you have time to look up your concerns in a reference. Also learn from your peers' experiences. Collaborating with classmates is a win-win situation: Asking questions like, What did you look for in that patient? How did you know? and What was the biggest thing you learned? will help your classmates clarify their knowledge and help you learn from being involved in real situations. Keep in mind the ethics of discussing patient care: Don't use names or talk about patients in public places where others might overhear (e.g., cafeteria, elevators).

8. To avoid the "brain drain" of learning new technology, become familiar with the technology you'll use (for example, IV pumps, computers, heart monitors) *before* you go to the clinical setting.

9. Remember the importance of caring. Patients describe caring as vigilance (attentiveness, highly skilled practice, basic care, nurturing, and going the extra mile); mutuality (building relationships among nurses, patients, and families); and healing (lifesaving behaviors and freeing the patient from anxiety and concerns).[11]

10. When estimating time needed for nursing care, consider the time required for *direct care interventions* (things you do directly for or with the patient, such as helping someone ambulate) and *indirect care interventions* (things you need to do away from the patient, such as consulting with the pharmacist or analyzing lab study results).

Box 3-10 shows 10 key questions to consider to promote clinical judgment (clinical reasoning). While the nursing process provides the

---

Box 3-10 **CLINICAL JUDGMENT (CLINICAL REASONING): 10 KEY QUESTIONS***

1. **What major outcomes (observable beneficial results) do we expect to see *in this particular person, family, or group* when the plan of care is terminated?**
   Example: The person will be discharged infection-free, able to care for himself, three days after surgery.
   Outcomes may be addressed on a standard plan or you may have to develop these outcomes your-self. Be sure that you check that any predetermined outcomes in standard plans are *appropriate* to your patient's specific situation. (Chapter 5 gives guidelines and practice exercises for developing outcomes.)

2. **What problems, risks, or issues must be addressed to achieve the major outcomes?**
   Answering this question will help you set priorities. You might be faced with a long list of actual or potential health problems. You need to narrow down your list to those that *must* be addressed.

Continued

Box 3-10 CLINICAL JUDGMENT (CLINICAL REASONING): 10 KEY QUESTIONS*–cont'd

3. **What are the circumstances (what is the context)?** Who's involved (e.g., child, adult, group)? How urgent are the problems (e.g., life-threatening, chronic)? What are the factors influencing their presentation (e.g., when, where, and how did the problems develop)? What are the patient's values, beliefs, and cultural influences?

4. **What knowledge is required?** Required knowledge includes problem-specific facts (e.g., how health problems usually present, how they're diagnosed, what their common causes and risk factors are, what common complications occur, and how these complications are prevented and managed); the nursing process and related knowledge and skills (ethics, research, health assessment, communication, priority setting); related sciences (anatomy, physiology, pathophysiology, pharmacology, chemistry, physics, psychology, sociology). You must also be clearly aware of the circumstances, as addressed in Question 3 above.

5. **How much room is there for error?** In the clinical setting, there is usually minimal room for error. However, it depends on the health of the individual and risks of interventions. *Example:* In which of the following cases do you think you have more room for error?
    ◆ You're trying to decide whether to give a healthy child a one-time dose of acetaminophen for heat rash without checking with the doctor.
    ◆ You have a child who's been sick for three days with a fever and the mother wants to know if she should continue giving acetaminophen without checking with the doctor.
        If you thought *the first one* above, you're right. In the second case, the symptoms have continued for three days without a diagnosis. If you continue to give acetaminophen without checking with a physician, you might be masking symptoms of a problem requiring medical management.

6. **How much time do I/we have?** Your time frame for decision making depends on a) the urgency of the problems (e.g., there's less time in life-threatening situations, such as cardiac arrest), and b) the planned length of contact (e.g., if your patient will be hospitalized only for two days, you have to be realistic about what can be accomplished, and key decisions need to be made early).

7. **What resources can help me?** Human resources include clinical nurse educators, nursing faculty, preceptors, more experienced nurses, advance practice nurses, peers, librarians, and other health care professionals (e.g., pharmacists, nutritionists, physical therapists, physicians). The patient and family are also valuable resources (usually they know their own problems best). Other resources include: texts, articles, references, and computer databases and decision-making support; national practice guidelines; and facility documents (e.g., guidelines, policies, procedures, assessment forms).

8. **What perspectives must be considered?** The most significant perspective to consider is that of the patient. Other important perspectives include key stakeholders (e.g., significant others, caregivers), relevant third parties (e.g., insurers), and standards that apply to the patient's problems.

9. **What's influencing my thinking?** Be sure you identify personal biases. Thinking may also be influenced by any of the factors listed in Table 2-2, Factors Influencing Critical Thinking Ability (page 30).

10. **What must we do to prevent, manage, or eliminate the problems, issues, and risks identified above in Question 2?** Identify specific interventions aimed at achieving the outcomes and managing or eliminating the problems, issues, and risks. Focus on eliminating or managing the underlying cause(s) of the problems. Also identify interventions that promote function (e.g., adequate nutrition, rest, and exercise, if possible). Including key caregivers, develop approaches by considering patient needs and desires. Be sure to weigh risks and benefits of approaches, and to include patient, significant others, and caregivers in determining interventions.

*The nursing process (Box 3-3) provides the foundation for clinical reasoning. These questions offer an additional perspective for examining thinking in clinical reasoning.

foundation for clinical reasoning, these questions offer an additional approach to examining thinking in clinical reasoning.

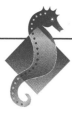

Critical Moments

IT'S HARD TO THINK CRITICALLY WHEN YOU'RE STRESSED OUT

One of the biggest challenges nurses face is stress management. When you're constantly stressed out, you're not only unlikely to be thinking critically, you're setting yourself up for other health problems like high blood pressure and depression. Studies show that 60% to 90% of visits to primary care providers are for stress-related conditions.[12] Learn about stress management. Pay attention to things that add stress to your life, and find out what you can do about them. If you can't do much about the stressful situations around you, do things to help yourself (for example, get enough rest, eat well, exercise, and learn biofeedback and relaxation strategies). For more on stress management, read Stress Management, *at http://nsweb.nursingspectrum.com/ce/ce88.htm or go to http://www.teachhealth.com where you can take a test to determine your stress level and also get some stress management tips (available in English and Spanish). Also recommended:* The Wellness Book *by Herbert Benson, MD and Eileen Stuart, RN, MS.*

MAKING SURE YOUR CHARTING REFLECTS CRITICAL THINKING

Finally, it seems appropriate to end a chapter on critical thinking and clinical judgment with a few words of caution: Be sure your charting reflects critical thinking. Realize that your nursing records are a major factor in helping others judge whether or not you're a critical thinker. If your supervisor or instructor picks up several of your charts and sees nothing but rote repetition of what the person ahead of you charted, a flag goes up that says, This person never seems to have a thought of her own. Follow policies and procedures for charting—these may include a system of flow charts and check marks—but always ask yourself whether there is something *different* today that you should record. When entering individualized notes, use your best words and handwriting to clearly record:

1. what you assessed in the patient (consider both what you observed and what the patient reports);
2. what you concluded, stating facts to support your conclusions;
3. what you did, and how the patient responded; and
4. anything you did to correct any adverse responses.

Example: *Appears anxious. States he's concerned because his wife just called and said a check had bounced. Briefly discussed financial situation with him. Apparently, this was a simple oversight—pointed this out to him. He seems calmer (says his wife can handle this).*

If you chart early and *think* when you chart, it's your opportunity to pick up trends, problems, and things you may have forgotten to do or assess. It's your opportunity to not only show reasonable thinking, but also improve patient care through communication of problems to others.

KEY POINTS

Because the conclusions and decisions we as nurses make affect people's lives, our thinking must be guided by sound reasoning—precise, disciplined thinking that promotes accuracy and depth of data collection and that seeks to clearly identify the issues at hand. To bring your understanding of this chapter together as a whole, see Table 3-3, page 97.

Understanding how novice thinking differs from expert thinking helps us set realistic goals for developing critical thinking and clinical judgment skills. Care delivery has moved from a *diagnose and treat (DT)* to a *predict, prevent, manage, and promote (PPMP)* approach that focuses on disease management and holistic health promotion through identification of risk factors and early intervention. To think critically you must be very clear about the outcomes you expect *and* the problems, issues, and risk factors you need to manage to achieve the outcomes. Experts use the nursing process in a very dynamic way because they know what steps can be safely skipped or delayed, and when situations warrant a rigorous, comprehensive, approach. Developing clinical judgment requires you to nurture your ability to use both the *intuitive right* and *logical left* side of the brain.

Because care plan components (expected outcomes, actual and potential problems, specific interventions, and evaluation or progress notes) may be in various parts of the chart, you must be familiar with principles of the nursing process to be able to know whether the plan of care is sufficiently documented. The terms *diagnose* and *diagnosis* imply there's a specific problem that requires management by a qualified expert. To be sure to detect both possible nursing and medical problems, use both a nursing model and a body systems approach to organize data (see Box 3-7 and Fig. 3-3). Ability to make clinical judgments depends on theoretical and experiential knowledge (e.g., knowing what to look for, how to recognize when a patient's status is

Table 3-3   APPLIED DEFINITION OF CRITICAL THINKING WITH CORRESPONDING STRATEGIES

Key Points on Critical Thinking in Nursing	Strategies
◆ Entails purposeful, informed, outcome-focused (results-oriented) thinking that requires careful identification of key problems, issues, and risks involved	◆ Determine overall client-centered outcomes: describe exactly what will be observed in the patient, family, or group to show the benefit of nursing care. Be sure your data are accurate and complete.
◆ Is driven by patient, family, and community needs	◆ Decide what specific patient, family, or group needs, problems, issues, or risks *must* be managed to achieve the overall outcomes.
◆ Is based on principles of nursing process and scientific method	◆ Follow principles of assessing, diagnosing, planning, implementing, and evaluating care; focus on evidence-based care.
◆ Uses both intuition and logic, based on knowledge, skills, and experience	◆ Apply related theoretical and experiential knowledge; consult experts and other disciplines as needed.
◆ Is guided by professional standards and ethics codes	◆ Plan and give care in accordance with professional standards and ethics codes (e.g., national, local, and facility standards, practice guidelines, ethics codes).
◆ Requires strategies that maximize human potential and compensate for problems created by human nature	◆ Use client, family, and community strengths; identify ways to maximize human potential (e.g., promote independence by facilitating learning); be cognizant of how your own perspective may be influencing care (e.g., personal biases or dislikes).
◆ Is constantly reevaluating, self-correcting, and striving to improve	◆ Monitor outcomes closely, reflecting on how things could be done more efficiently; think out of the box—what new or innovative approaches can improve care.

changing, and what to do about it). Clinical judgment includes knowing when the situation requires more than "thinking on your feet" (for example, knowing when you need to take more time or get additional opinions). Finally, be sure your charting shows independent critical thinking, rather than repeating previous entries from others.

CRITICAL THINKING EXERCISES

Note: Exercises followed by asterisks have example responses listed in the Response Key at the back of the book beginning on page 246.

1. Clarify how the terms *clinical judgment, clinical reasoning,* and *critical thinking* are related (five or fewer sentences).*
2. Write a paragraph describing what clinical judgment entails.*
3. Give at least one reason health care delivery today is focused on customer satisfaction.*
4. Figure 3-4 (page 89) provides a model to help students decide whether an act is within their scope of practice. Using this model, decide whether you're allowed to irrigate a nasogastric tube in the clinical setting.*
5. An important aspect of developing clinical judgment is being willing to place great importance on the wants and needs of patients and their significant others. Keeping this in mind, how would you interpret the statements made by the off-going nurse below?*
   Oncoming nurse: "How is the family doing?"
   Off-going nurse: "They seem to be fine. They're sticking to visiting hours and have been in to visit 15 minutes this morning and 15 minutes this afternoon."
6. Critical thinking is a complex process that sometimes requires more than one way of looking at things. The inside back cover of this book offers a game that can facilitate a systematic, comprehensive, approach to critical thinking. With at least one other person, pick a situation you need to think critically about—a patient, a presentation, a dilemma, or problem you have. Play the game and evaluate your results.
7. Go to http://www.teachhealth.com and take the stress test. What are the stressful things in your life, and how are you handling them? What healthy behaviors might help?
8. Respond to the following from the prechapter self-test.
   a. Clarify your responsibilities related to diagnosis and management of medical and nursing problems.*
   b. Explain the role of ethics codes and national and organizational standards and guidelines in making decisions.*
   c. Identify three things you will begin doing immediately to develop your clinical reasoning skills.*

References

1. Beckman, D. (1993). Andrew's not-so-excellent adventure. *Healthcare Forum J., May/June,* 90–96.
2. Norman, G. (1988). Problem-solving skills, solving problems and problem-based learning. *Medical Education, 22,* 280.
3. North American Nursing Diagnosis Association. *Nursing diagnosis: Definitions and classifications 2001-2002.* Philadelphia: Author.
4. E-mail communication. (April 2002).
5. Benner, P., Tanner, C., & Chesla, C. (1996). *Experience in nursing practice: Caring, clinical judgment and ethics.* New York: Springer.

6. Lamond, D. & Thompson, C. (2000). Intuition and analysis in decision making and choice. *Journal of Nursing Scholarship, 32*(3),411–414.
7. Benner, P., Tanner, C., & Chesla, C. (1996). *Experience in nursing practice: Caring, clinical judgment and ethics.* New York: Springer.
8. Hansten, R., & Washburn, M. (2001). Intuition in professional practice: Executive and staff perceptions. *Journal of Nursing Administration, 30*(4),185–188.
9. Scheffer, B., & Rubenfeld, M. (2000). A consensus statement on critical thinking in nursing. *Journal of Nursing Education, 39*(8),353.
10. E-mail communication. (April 2002).
11. Burfitt, S., Greiner, D., & Miers, L. (1993). Professional nurse caring as perceived by critically ill patients: A phenomenologic study. *American Journal of Critical Care, 2*(6),489–499.
12. Nursing Spectrum E-zine, June 24, 2002.

See comprehensive bibliography beginning on page 286.

Critical Thinking in Nursing: Beyond Clinical Judgment

THIS CHAPTER at a Glance ...

◆ Moral and Ethical Reasoning
   Moral versus Ethical Reasoning
   How Do You Decide?
   Seven Ethical Principles
   Standards, Ethics Codes, Patients' Rights, Advance
      Directives
   Steps for Moral and Ethical Reasoning
◆ Nursing Research
   Frequently Asked Questions on Beginning Nurses'
      Research Role
   Scanning Before Reading Research Articles
   Getting Research into Practice
   Quality Improvement
◆ Teaching Others
◆ Teaching Ourselves
   Memorizing Effectively
◆ Test-Taking
◆ Key Points

Read the following Learning Outcomes and decide whether you can readily achieve each one. If you can, you don't need to read this chapter and can go on to Chapter 5. Don't be concerned if you can't achieve any of the objectives at this time. We'll come back to these outcomes later in the chapter, in Critical Thinking Exercises.

Learning Outcomes

After completing this chapter, you should be able to:

- Give a description and an example of the terms *moral uncertainty, moral dilemma,* and *moral distress.*

- Make prudent decisions based on ethical principles, codes, and practice standards.

- Develop a personal code of conduct based on your personal values and content in this chapter.

- Describe your responsibilities in relation to nursing research and quality improvement.

- Explain why it's important to choose refereed or peer-reviewed journals when looking for research articles.

- Explain how to decide whether you know enough to apply research findings to practice.

- Use critical thinking to create individualized teaching plans.

- Address the roles of memorizing and reasoning in teaching ourselves.

- Describe five strategies that can help you improve your test scores.

Having examined how to promote critical thinking in clinical judgment in Chapter 3, let's go on to examine reasoning in the five other common nursing situations:

◆ Moral and ethical reasoning
◆ Nursing research
◆ Teaching others
◆ Teaching ourselves
◆ Test-Taking

You may think that the above skills seem like *extra* skills when compared to clinical judgment. But they're actually *central* to demonstrating good clinical judgment. In the clinical setting, you must be able to reason about ethical issues, apply research, and teach others and yourself. Often your ability to pass tests will be the only way you can validate that you have the clinical judgment skills needed to function safely and effectively in the clinical setting.

MORAL AND ETHICAL REASONING

Treatment advances, longer life spans, and a greater emphasis on patient rights and autonomy create new challenges. For example, questions related to end-of-life care, genetic advances, quality of life, and resource allocation are commonplace. We nurses are often "front and center" when patients, families, and other health care professionals struggle with ethical dilemmas. Knowing how to deal with these issues is a cornerstone of competent nursing practice. Learning to apply basic principles of moral and ethical reasoning will help you feel more confident and *be* more competent when faced with ethical quandaries. Ultimately, it will help your patients receive care that's consistent with nursing's mission—to help people help themselves. Think about the following Other Perspectives, and then go on to think more about how to respond to difficult ethical situations.

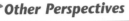

Other Perspectives

WHAT ETHICS GUIDE YOUR CONDUCT?

"Everyone has an ethical framework—the question is how aware of it are they? We all need to clarify our ethical frameworks before we're faced with dilemmas. Just as we're too late if we're flipping through our advanced life support book during a code, we can make some regrettable decisions if we haven't given thought to how we'll respond to difficult situations."[1]

—*Michael Riley LMSW, LPC, EMT-Paramedic*

WHAT ETHICS GUIDE YOUR CONDUCT?

"An ethic of care respects individual uniqueness, personal relationships, and the dynamic nature of life. Essential to an ethic of care are compassion, collaboration, accountability, and trust."[2]

—*The American Association of Critical Care Nurses*

Moral versus Ethical Reasoning

Moral reasoning and *ethical reasoning* are often used interchangeably. However, there is a slight difference between these two terms. Consider the difference in the following descriptions.

◆ **Moral reasoning:** Refers to judgments made based on *personal* standards of right and wrong (e.g., I personally believe it's okay to tell little white lies now and then).

◆ **Ethical reasoning:** Refers to judgments made by applying standards *derived from the formal study of what criteria ought to be used to determine whether actions are justified,* and therefore morally right or wrong (for example, I personally don't think that there's anything wrong with little white lies now and then, but most ethicists will tell you it's wrong to lie to patients).

Here's another example:

Case scenario | Suppose you're admitting a young woman who is freely and knowledgeably seeking a tubal ligation. Morally (according to your personal standards), you believe sterilization is wrong. However, as a nurse, you realize that ethically this woman has a right to make this choice and that it would be inappropriate for you to tell her sterilization is wrong or for you to try to get her to change her mind.◆

How Do You Decide?

So how *do* you make decisions about moral and ethical issues? The answer is *with great difficulty.* Okay, so I'm only kidding, but sometimes thinking about these types of issues is so stressful that you need a little humor. Let's get serious and look at what to do when you face situations that have no easily agreed upon *right* answers—when each answer has its own merits and drawbacks, and it's difficult to say that one is better than another.

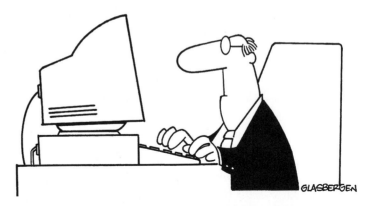

Copyright 2002 by Randy Glasbergen.
www.glasbergen.com

"MEMO: It has come to my attention that every time we solve one problem, we create two more. From now on, all problem solving is forbidden."

Cartoon by Randy Glasbergen, Copyright 2002. Reprinted with special permission from www.glasbergen.com

Moral and ethical problems may be divided into three categories:

◆ **Moral uncertainty:** You aren't sure which moral principles or values apply. *Example*: A patient asks you whether you think his doctor is a good doctor. You don't think the doctor is very competent. Do you tell him?

◆ **Moral dilemma:** You're faced with a situation in which you have two (or more) choices available, but neither (or none) of them seems satisfactory. *Example:* A doctor takes you aside and tells *you* she's sure your friend has cancer but tells *your friend*, "I won't know anything until the diagnosis is made by the lab, next week." When your friend begs you to tell him what the doctor knows, what do you do? If you tell him you don't know, you're lying. If you tell him what the doctor told you, you risk breaking his trust in his physician.

◆ **Moral distress:** You know the right thing to do, but institutional constraints make it nearly impossible to do what is right. *Example:* You think a patient isn't ready for discharge because his wife is unprepared to care for him. When you report this problem to the physician, you're told the hospital has "no choice" but to discharge him. What do you do?

Did you know what to do in the above examples? If so, on what did you base your decisions? Gut feelings? Personal values and standards? Professional standards?

Making moral and ethical decisions requires knowledge of ethical principles and codes. You can't be impulsive or act on the basis of feelings.

As a nurse, you must clearly understand standards and principles that guide moral and ethical decision making. You must be able to justify your actions to others by ethical argumentation.

Seven Ethical Principles

Seven principles guide ethical decision making:
1. **Autonomy.** Believing that people have the right to be self-determining and to make legally acceptable decisions based on:
   ◆ their *own* values and beliefs
   ◆ adequate information that is given free from coercion
   ◆ sound reasoning that considers all the alternatives
2. **Beneficence.** Aiming to benefit others and avoid harm.
3. **Justice.** Treating all people fairly and giving what is due or owed.
4. **Fidelity.** Keeping promises and not making promises you can't keep.
5. **Veracity (Truth Telling).** Being honest and telling the truth.
6. **Confidentiality.** Keeping information private.
7. **Accountability.** Being willing to accept responsibility for the consequences of your actions.

Standards, Ethics Codes, Patients' Rights, Advance Directives

Standards, ethics codes, codes of conduct (see Box 4-1) and official statements of patients' rights (see page 107) also guide ethical conduct. For example, the American Nurses Association publication, *Standards of Nursing Practice,* states that the nurse makes decisions and actions on behalf of clients. The *Code of Ethics for Nurses* states that the nurse:
◆ maintains client confidentiality
◆ acts as client advocate
◆ delivers care in a nonjudgmental and nondiscriminatory manner that's sensitive to client diversity
◆ preserves/protects client autonomy, dignity, and rights
◆ seeks resources to help formulate ethical decisions.[3]

Ethically, you're required to maintain acceptable standards of practice. By taking the nursing role, you must see that your patients and clients receive competent care. Therefore, standards addressing how care should be given in specific situations (e.g., policies, procedures, and specialty practice standards) play an important part in delivering ethical care.

Other bills of rights (e.g., Pregnant Patient's Bill of Rights, Indian Patient's Bill of Rights, a Nursing Home Bill of Rights, and Veteran's Administration Code of Patient Concern) also act as guides for how you respond to ethical issues.[4]

Box 4-1 **EXAMPLE CODE OF CONDUCT**

As a member of the NPCU (Neuroscience Progressive Care Units) Meyer 7 Team, I agree to commit to learning to make the following a part of my daily routine.

I. To value who you are and the relationship we have by:
   ◆ Always treating you with respect and courtesy
   ◆ Using the concept of the Golden Rule in my interactions with you
   ◆ Maintaining confidentiality when I am utilized as a sounding board
   ◆ Dealing with issues and behaviors, not the person
   ◆ Listening openly
   ◆ Attempting to walk a mile in your shoes to gain understanding
   ◆ Accepting personal diversity in our styles

II. Optimizing a positive work environment and facilitating appropriate communication by:
   ◆ Searching for a solution that is acceptable for both of us
   ◆ Committing to resolving each conflict without resorting to the use of power to try to win at the expense of the other person losing
   ◆ Doing my "homework" before I draw conclusions
   ◆ Using only ONE person as my sounding board before I decide to either give feedback or drop the issue
   ◆ Validating any rumors I hear
   ◆ Redirecting coworkers who are talking about someone to speak directly to the person
   ◆ Giving feedback as we agreed to do:
     –Within 72 hours
     –Using "I" statements
     –Describing behaviors and painting a picture with my words instead of labeling
     –Limiting my discussion to the event at hand and not discussing past history
     –Telling you honestly and openly the effect the behavior had on me

III. Be approachable and open to feedback from others by:
   ◆ Taking personal responsibility for my words and behaviors as well as my responses to people and events
   ◆ Taking time to reflect on what was said rather than blaming, defending, or rejecting
   ◆ Seeking clarification and validation of the perceived behaviors

Developed: May 1996 (courtesy Ski Lower and Neuroscience Critical Care and Progressive Care Units, Johns Hopkins Hospital).

Advance Directives (see Box 4-2) help us make decisions about cardiac resuscitation and other end-of-life treatments as noted in the Critical Moments that follow.

Critical Moments

Don't Wait Too Late
Too many people wait until it's too late to address advance directives. Encourage people to talk with loved ones about what they would want if they were unable to speak for themselves. This eases the burden of making tough decisions about whether to refuse aggressive treatment that merely prolongs dying.

PATIENTS' RIGHTS*

Dear Consumer:

State law requires that your health care provider or facility recognize *your rights* while receiving medical care and that you respect *their right* to expect certain behavior on the part of patients. You may request a copy of the full text of this law from your health care provider or facility.

YOU HAVE THE RIGHT TO:

❑ Be treated with courtesy and respect with appreciation of dignity and protection of your need for privacy.
❑ Prompt and reasonable response to questions and requests.
❑ Be informed of:

❑ who is providing medical services and who is responsible for your care.
❑ what patient support services are available, including whether an interpreter is available if you have communication problems.
❑ your diagnosis, planned course of treatment, alternatives, risks, and prognosis.
❑ whether treatment is for purposes of experimental research (and to give or refuse your consent to participate in such research).

❑ Refuse treatment, except as otherwise provided by law.
❑ Have impartial access to medical treatment or accommodations, regardless of race, national origin, religious, physical handicap, or source of payment.
❑ Be given treatment for any emergency condition that will deteriorate from failure to receive treatment.
❑ Express any grievances about any violation of your rights as stated by state law, through the grievance procedure of your health care provider or facility and appropriate state licensing agency.
❑ File complaints against a health care professional, hospital, or ambulatory surgical center with the Agency for Health Care

Administration. (Appropriate information for how to reach each state's agency must be listed here).
❑ Receive (upon request):

❑ full information and necessary counseling on the availability of financial resources for your care.
❑ a reasonable estimate of charges for medical care before treatment.
❑ information about whether your health care provider or facility accepts the Medicare assignment rate before treatment.

❑ Be given a copy of a reasonably clear and understandable, itemized bill, and upon request, to have charges explained.

YOU HAVE THE RESPONSIBILITY TO:

❑ Provide your health care provider, to the best of your knowledge, accurate and complete information about your complaints, past illnesses, hospitalizations, medications, and other matters relating to your health.
❑ Follow the treatment plan recommended by your provider.
❑ Report unexpected changes in your condition to the health care provider.
❑ Keep appointments. And, if you're unable to do so for any reason, notify your provider or facility.
❑ Ensure that the financial obligations of your health care is fulfilled as soon as possible.
❑ Comply with health care provider and facility rules and regulations affecting patient conduct.

---

* This is an example form and summary of rights. Rights may vary from state to state. Forms may vary from facility to facility.

Box 4-2 WHAT ARE ADVANCE DIRECTIVES?*

Advance directives include two documents:*

Living Will: Designates the types of medical treatments you would or wouldn't want in specific instances (e.g., whether you want to continue ventilator support if you become permanently unconscious).

Durable Power of Attorney for Health Care (DPAHC): Identifies who you want to make treatment decisions if there comes a time when you aren't able to do so.

*These two documents may be combined into one document called a *combination directive.*

You now have an idea of the principles and standards that guide moral and ethical decision making. Let's go on to some steps that can help you develop a comprehensive, thoughtful approach to moral and ethical reasoning.

Steps for Moral and Ethical Reasoning

1. **Clearly identify the problem or issue based on the perspectives of the key stakeholders (those who will be most affected by the results of the decision).** For example, Mrs. Morris, an elderly woman who lives alone, tells you she doesn't want her leg amputated and that she'd rather die than live as an amputee. Her daughter tells you her mother is incompetent to make this decision. *Problem:* Who has the right to make this decision? Is Mrs. Morris competent? Does she have the right to refuse surgery? Does the daughter have the right to overrule her mother?

2. **Decide what your role will be.** For example, is an ethical board involved? Does this family rely heavily on your judgment? Do you just need to listen?

3. **Recognize your personal values and how they influence your ability to participate in health care decision making.** For example, in Mrs. Morris's case, do you believe no one has the right to refuse lifesaving surgery? If so, how would this affect your ability to help Mrs. Morris with this decision? If you can't be objective, let your supervisor know so that another caregiver can assist with decision making.

4. **Identify the alternatives.** For example, is it possible to delay this decision? Would Mrs. Morris be willing to have the surgery if the daughter commits to caring for her? Could social services help? Should you request an ethics consult?

5. **Determine the outcomes (consequences) of the alternatives.** For example, if the decision is delayed, will it be detrimental to health? Would the daughter indeed be able to care for her mother?

6. **List the alternatives and rate them according to which would produce the least harm or greatest good, based on client and**

family values. To do so, don't consider good versus bad. Instead, ask where each fits on the following scale:

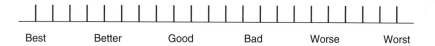

Best   Better   Good   Bad   Worse   Worst

The above scale will help you distinguish between choices that at first glance might seem equally moral.

7. **Keeping the key stakeholders in mind, develop a plan of action that will facilitate the best choices.** In situations where the choices are all good, choose the one that is the *greater good*. In situations where none of the choices are really good, choose the one that is the *lesser evil*.

8. Put the plan into action and monitor the response closely.

To complete this section on moral and ethical reasoning, study Box 4-3, which answers key critical thinking questions in relation to moral and ethical decision making.

Critical Moments

PRIVACY BREECH MAY CAUSE LEGAL PROBLEMS
We know that ethically, nurses are bound to keep patient information private. Patient privacy is also a legal concern. If you divulge private information, you could find yourself involved in a lawsuit. Carefully guard patients' rights to privacy.

Want to Know More?

Here are some resources you can contact to learn more about how to get help, publications, and educational programs on moral and ethical reasoning:

◆ American Nurses Association, Center for Ethics and Human Rights (http://www.nursingworld.org/ethics/)
◆ National Reference Center for Bioethics Literature (http://georgetown.edu/research/nrcbl/)
◆ American Society of Law and Ethics (http://www.aslme.org)
◆ American Society of Bioethics & Humanities (http://www.asbh.org)
◆ Nursing Ethics of Canada http://www.nursingethics.ca
◆ Markkula Center for Applied Ethics, Santa Clara University (http://www.scu.edu/SCU/Centers/Ethics/)

* This is the common utilitarian approach. Other approaches that may apply are listed in Table 4-1.

Table 4-1   APPROACHING ETHICS*

Approach	Focus	Principle
Virtue Approach	Attitudes, dispositions, or character traits that enable us to act in ways that develop our human potential (e.g., honesty, courage, integrity).	What is ethical is what develops moral virtues in ourselves and our communities.
Utilitarian Approach	Consequences that actions or policies have on the well-being ("utility") of all persons directly or indirectly affected by the action or policy.	Of any two actions, the most ethical one will produce the greatest balance of benefits over harms.
Rights Approach	Identifies interests or activities that our behavior must respect, especially those areas of our lives that are of such value to us that they merit protection from others. Each person has a fundamental right to be respected and treated as a free and equal rational being capable of making his or her own decisions. This implies other rights (e.g., privacy, free consent, freedom of conscience) that must be protected if a person is to have the freedom to direct his or her own life.	An action or policy is morally right only if those persons affected by the decision are not used merely as instruments for advancing some goal, but are fully informed and treated only as they have freely and knowingly consented to be treated.
Fairness (Justice)	How fairly or unfairly our actions distribute benefits and burdens among the members of a group. Fairness requires consistency in the way people are treated.	Treat people the same unless there are morally relevant differences between them.
Common Good Approach	Presents a vision of society as a community whose members are joined in a shared pursuit of values and goals they hold in common. The community is composed of individuals whose own good is inextricably bound to the good of the whole.	What is ethical is what advances the common good.
Care-Based Approach	Source of the moral life is in the human capacity to extend care to others, to nurture relationships and to develop the communication, psychological skills and responsibility needed to sustain these networks of care. Moral problems arise out of disruptions in or conflicts between responsibilities to self and others and they require a type of thinking that is contextual and narrative.	What is ethical is what best responds to the individualized needs of those with whom I live in relationship, people with unique life narratives and plans.

* Adapted with permission from "Approaching Ethics," by the Markkula Center for Applied Ethics at Santa Clara University, www.scu.edu/ethics. Care-based approach added by Carol Taylor, PhD, MSN, Director, Center for Clinical Bioethics and Assistant Professor of Nursing, Georgetown University, Washington, DC.

Box 4-3   **MORAL AND ETHICAL REASONING: 10 KEY QUESTIONS***

1. **What major outcomes (observable results) do I/we expect to see in this particular person, family, or group?** The patient (or person designated to make treatment decisions) will be able to express that he has made an informed, uncoerced, well-reasoned, legally acceptable decision based on his values and believed to promote his interests.

2. **What problems, risks or issues *must* be addressed to achieve the major outcomes?** *What's* the main issue (be sure you understand *when, where,* and *how* the issue developed)? How can we be sure the key players are well informed, have considered all the alternatives, and understand the short- and long-range consequences of each alternative?

3. **What are the circumstances (what is the context)?** *Who* are the key players (e.g., patient, family, caregivers, payors)? *What* is your role (policies and procedures are likely to affect your role)? What are the morally significant variables present (e.g., beliefs, values, and preferences of the participants; cultural, religious, and economic considerations; interests of all involved parties)?

4. **What knowledge is required?** Required knowledge includes:
   ◆ Ethical theory and related principles, standards of care, professional codes of ethics (e.g., ANA and CNA codes of ethics, Bills of Rights).
   ◆ Ethical decision-making framework and approaches (see steps on page 108 and Table 4-1).
   ◆ Communication and interpersonal skills.

5. **How much room is there for error?** Room for error *varies* according to the consequences of the decision. For example, in which of the following situations do you have more room for error?
   a. Deliberating about a patient's capacity to make an informed, voluntary decision about stopping life-sustaining therapies.
   b. Deliberating about a patient's capacity to make an informed, voluntary decision about choosing among chemotherapies with different probabilities of success and side effects.
   If you thought *b,* you're correct. In situation *a,* you're deciding whether the person has the capacity to decide whether to live or die, leaving little room for error. In situation *b,* you're deciding whether the person has the capacity to choose among therapy options, some of which may be better matched to his values and interests.

6. **How much time do I/we have?** The time frame for decision making is also a factor of the consequences of the decision at hand. For example, if the parents of a sick child withhold consent for treatment, there's more time to deliberate if the child's life isn't in immediate jeopardy.

7. **Who and what resources can help?** Human resources include clinical ethicists, ethics committees, clinical nurse educators, nursing faculty, facility policies on ethics, and librarians. Other resources include articles, ethics texts, computer databases, and organizations that promote the study of ethics (see *Want to Know More?,* page 109).

8. **Whose perspectives must be considered?** The most significant perspective to consider is that of the patient. Other important perspectives include key stakeholders (e.g., significant others, caregivers), relevant third parties (for example, insurers), and professional groups who have addressed the issues (for example, those who have developed professional ethics codes and patient rights statements).

9. **What's influencing thinking?** Thinking may be influenced by conscious or subconscious bias, discrimination, personal motives, or fear of legal liability (e.g., I've got to restrain this person or he may fall, and I'll be sued). Thinking may also be influenced by any of the factors listed in Table 2-1, Factors Influencing Critical Thinking Ability (page 30).

10. **What must we do to prevent, manage, or eliminate the problems, issues, and risks identified above in Question 2?** Interventions such as teaching and counseling (including all key stakeholders) about options (benefits, risks, and short- and long-term consequences) are common. Complex issues may require consulting with a multidisciplinary group or ethics board.

*Answers to questions provided by Carol Taylor, PhD, MSN, Director, Center for Clinical Bioethics and Assistant Professor of Nursing, Georgetown University, Washington, DC.

◣ NURSING RESEARCH

Based as much as possible on strict rules of the scientific method, research is one of the most rigorous and disciplined uses of critical thinking in nursing. Researchers must have a variety of highly developed critical thinking skills, from knowing how to clearly identify the problem or issue to be studied to determining the best way to collect meaningful data, to analyzing and interpreting statistical data. Think about the following definition:

Research is diligent, systematic inquiry or investigation to validate and refine existing knowledge and generate new knowledge. The concepts *systematic* and *diligent* are critical to the meaning of research because they imply planning, organization, and persistence.[5]

As in many professions, nursing research is done by a comparatively small group of dedicated, highly qualified nurses who are willing to commit themselves to a lengthy, sometimes costly process.

So, you might wonder, if research is conducted by a relatively small group of expert nurses, how important is it for staff nurses and students? The answer is, *very important*. Research is essential to advancing nursing practice. It helps us generate a body of knowledge that provides a basis for planning, predicting, and controlling the outcomes of nursing practice. Its importance is emphasized by the inclusion of using research as a standard of performance set forth by the American Nurses Association (ANA). By listing research as a *standard of performance*, the ANA sends the message that all nurses are expected to use research findings whenever appropriate.

Although it's beyond the scope of this chapter to address how to actually *conduct* research studies, this section focuses on how to *use* research findings. Let's begin by addressing two frequently asked questions.'

Frequently Asked Questions on Beginning Nurses' Research Role

Q. What's the role of beginning nurses in relation to nursing research?
A. Beginning nurses have four main responsibilities:

   1. To think analytically about the situations they encounter and seek out research results that might improve nursing care. For example, if you frequently care for people with postoperative leg edema after heart bypass surgery, you should be thinking, I wonder if there are any new studies explaining why this happens and what can be done about it?

2. To raise questions about their practice that might prompt a researcher to formulate a question to guide a study. For example, you could ask your manager, "Since we seem to be having an increase in infections, would it be worthwhile to study whether our procedure for hand washing is really effective?"

3. To help researchers collect data. If you're asked to complete a questionnaire or to chart specific data for research purposes, it's your professional responsibility to do so, diligently and accurately, as long as it doesn't interfere with nursing care.

4. To continue to acquire and share knowledge related to research. We must constantly ask ourselves questions like, Am I making time to become familiar with research related to the clinical situations in which I'm involved? and Do I interact with others (peers, educators) to learn more about research? For those of you who find reading research articles tedious, get started by talking with peers and educators or perhaps joining a journal club. This helps you to learn in a dynamic, stimulating environment. Once you learn the basics, meeting your responsibilities in relation to research becomes easier, more interesting, and even an enjoyable challenge!

Q. If I have limited knowledge of research, how do I know whether there are research studies I should be using in my practice?

A. Recognize that you can't use research findings indiscriminately:

1. Before using research results, decide whether the study is valid and reliable (i.e., whether it was conducted in such a way that you can trust that the results are accurate). For example, how often have you heard a commercial that proclaims, "In a recent research study, our product was proven to be more effective than the other leading products."? Do you believe every one of these commercials? Probably not. Think independently. Ask questions to determine whether you can apply the results of any research study.

2. Search the literature for research articles related to your area of practice. The first time you do this, take a partner with you to the library and tackle the search collaboratively.

3. Choose refereed or peer-reviewed journals (journals that publish articles only after they've been reviewed by peer experts). Whether or not a journal is peer-reviewed usually is found in the front of the journal where you find information like who's on the editorial board, who's the publisher, and so on. These journals are more likely to have reliable information.

4. Scan first to eliminate irrelevant articles; then read the ones that seem as though they'd be most useful. Learning how to scan, and then read research articles efficiently helps you avoid becoming overwhelmed trying to do too much at one time.

Scanning Before Reading Research Articles

Scanning research articles before reading them saves time by helping you eliminate irrelevant articles without having to read them in their entirety. Here are some steps to systematically scan articles to choose the ones most relevant to your needs.

1. **Read the abstract first: This summarizes the issues, methods, and results.** If the abstract isn't applicable to your clinical problem, you might choose to read no further.
2. **If the abstract seems applicable, skip to the end of the article,** then scan the article by reading the information under the following headings in the order listed below:
   a. Summary (may also be listed as *Conclusions*)
   b. Discussion
   c. Nursing Implications
   d. Suggestions for Further Research

   You may be able to eliminate articles just by reading any of the above headings.
3. **If the information you scanned is relevant, go on to read the entire study.** Give yourself plenty of time and don't be discouraged if you find sections you don't understand. Instead, take notes on what you *do* understand. Come back to the more difficult sections at another time, after getting help from an expert or textbook (or both).
4. **If you decide the article is relevant to your needs, ask the questions in Box 4-4 to decide if you have enough knowledge to apply what you learned from your readings.**

Box 4-4   QUESTIONS TO ASK YOURSELF TO DECIDE WHETHER YOU KNOW ENOUGH ABOUT A RESEARCH ARTICLE TO USE THE RESULTS

1. **Have I checked whether the article comes from a journal that's peer or expert reviewed?**
2. **Do I understand:**
   ◆ What's already known about the topic?
   ◆ What the researchers studied and why and how they studied it?
   ◆ What they found out and whether the results are valid?
   ◆ What the results imply and how they apply to my particular clinical situation?
   ◆ Whether the study may be biased (for example, when drug companies fund a study, there may be a vested interest)?
3. **Do I know how the results of this study compare with the results of other, similar studies?** If other studies produced similar findings, the probability that the results are *reliable* increases.

Getting Research into Practice

In these times of high demand on nursing time, we must be careful not to fall into the trap of doing things because of tradition, rather than research. Too many nurses continue to do things because "That's how we've always done it" without "going out of the box" and questioning care practices. Keep the importance of questioning what we do and how we do it in the forefront by using some of the following strategies:

1. **On a bulletin board in a convenient place, post a blank paper with "What Do You Want to Know?" at the top.** For example, someone might write, "Does anyone know the most recent information on managing infected wounds after surgery?"

2. **Make reading research articles convenient.** If you find a good article, post it on the bulletin board and ask people to initial that they've read it. Reward nurses who bring in useful literature.

3. **Develop protocols for placing research into practice, including making sure you have defined expected outcomes.**

4. **Encourage nurses to critique practice protocols and make suggestions for improvement.**

5. **Reward the use of research on performance evaluations.**

Other Perspectives

NURSES QUESTIONING CARE PRACTICES IMPROVE OUTCOMES

"Three nurses in one hospital questioned the use of large bore central venous lines on one acute care surgery unit. They did an extensive literature review and analysis of the use of these types of lines. They also queried 81 university hospitals about their use of these lines in acute care surgery units. Their study showed that the use of these large bore central lines in the general acute care setting increased risks of untoward patient outcomes. They pointed out that staffing ratios in acute care settings made it difficult to monitor patients closely enough to prevent and detect complications such as hemorrhage or air emboli. Based on evidence from this study, a policy restricting use of these lines in non-ill settings was written, thereby promoting patient safety and positive outcomes."[6]

—Nurse Investigators Beth Dierdorf, Kim Elgin, and Kathleen Rea

Quality Improvement

In the clinical setting, quality improvement (QI), a responsibility of all nurses, is perhaps the most frequently encountered type of research. Most facilities have a department that is responsible for ongoing studies designed to improve outcomes. For example, through quality improvement studies, some nurses have shown that delays in medications coming from pharmacy may significantly increase lengths of hospital stays. As a result policies and procedures have changed to ensure that medications come to the units in a timely way, and lengths of stays have decreased.

QI studies usually study information from three different perspectives:

1. **Outcome evaluation (focuses on results).** For example, asking, How many of our patients undergoing bowel surgery experienced an infection that was serious enough to delay discharge?

2. **Process evaluation (focuses on how care was given).** For example, asking, At what point were our patients undergoing bowel surgery first given antibiotics?

3. **Structure evaluation (focuses on setting).** For example, asking, In what setting were antibiotics first given (emergency department? operating room? surgical unit?)?

Your responsibilities in relation to QI are the same as the previously listed responsibilities for research.

To complete this section, review Box 4-5, which answers key critical thinking questions in relation to using nursing research.

Box 4-5 USING NURSING RESEARCH: 10 KEY QUESTIONS

1. **What major outcomes (observable results) do I/we plan to achieve?** After studying available nursing research, I/we will be able to improve nursing practices or understand more about a nursing concern.

2. **What problems, risks, or issues *must* be addressed to achieve the major outcomes?** Example problems or issues include, How can we find the most current research articles for this particular information? How can we make time to do the work involved? Are there policies and procedures on putting research into practice we must follow? What are the risks of applying this research to our practice? How can we ensure that we proceed safely, keeping an eye on ethical concerns?

3. **What are the circumstances (what is the context)?** For example, how urgent is the problem? In what setting are you planning to use the research findings? What are the characteristics of your patient population (age, sex, etc.)?

4. **What knowledge is required?** Required knowledge includes knowing whether the research article comes from a refereed or peer-reviewed journal, familiarity with previous research on the topic, research methods, and (for some studies) statistical analysis. You also need to know how to use the following library resources: indexes, catalogs, computer search services, interlibrary loan services, circulation department, reference department, and audiovisual services.

Continued

Box 4-5 USING NURSING RESEARCH: 10 KEY QUESTIONS–cont'd

5. **How much room is there for error?** Room for error depends on how you plan to use the research results. For example, in which of the following situations do you think you have more room for error?
   a. You're reviewing available research to determine what colors have a calming effect so that hospitals can choose calming colors for their walls.
   b. You're reviewing research to determine the best ways to prevent postoperative breathing complications so that you can include these methods in guidelines for postoperative care.

   If you thought *a*, you're correct. Little harm can occur if you're incorrect about the best colors, but if you're incorrect about how to best manage postoperative breathing complications, lives may be in jeopardy.

6. **How much time do I/we have?** The time frame depends on deadlines. Be careful to be realistic. Reviewing and analyzing research studies for application to practice is time-consuming.

7. **Who and what resources can help?** Human resources include nurse researchers, clinical nurse educators, clinical nurse specialists, faculty, preceptors, peers, journal clubs, and librarians. Other resources are research texts, journal articles, and computer databases.

8. **Whose perspectives must be considered?** Carefully consider patient, nursing, and financial perspectives of using the research.

9. **What's influencing my thinking?** Thinking may be influenced by a vested interest in the results or by a feeling of being too overwhelmed with other nursing duties to devote time to applying research. It may also be influenced by any of the factors listed in Table 2-1, Factors Influencing Critical Thinking Ability (page 30).

10. **What must we do to prevent, manage, or eliminate the problems, risks, or issues identified above in Question 2?** Check for policies and procedures for using research findings in practice. Identify ways to deal with safety and ethical concerns. Double-check with experts (e.g., quality improvement nurses, researchers, ethicists, librarians) if unsure about where to find the best information or how to use it.

Other Perspectives

IMPROVING END-OF-LIFE CARE: SOMETIMES LESS IS MORE

"We decided our role is to be a patient advocate and to be able to help patients have what they think is most important in the dying process.... (When patients are terminal) vital signs are measured only once a day. Daily weights aren't done and blood for tests isn't routinely drawn. IVs aren't restarted unless needed for pain relief medication. Patients aren't routinely turned except when it will ease pain."[7]

—K. Janssen, RN, Case Manager and Quality Improvement Nurse

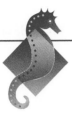

Critical Moments

STUDY CHANGES THINKING ON USING RESTRAINTS
We often assume that restraining patients protects them from injury and prevents complications. But evidence shows that restrained patients are more likely to sustain serious injury when they fall, that they are hospitalized twice as long as those who aren't restrained, and that they are eight times more likely to die during hospitalization than non-restrained patients. It also shows that restraints contribute to depression, anger, nosocomial (hospital-acquired) infection, pressure ulcers and deconditioning—all of which leave patients in a worse condition than before they were admitted.[8] Think twice before you restrain someone.

CRITICAL THINKING EXERCISES

Note: Exercises followed by asterisks have example responses listed in the Response Key at the back of the book beginning on page 246.

Moral and Ethical Reasoning Exercises

1. Decide what you'd do if you had been "Me" in the following scenario*:

    CASE SCENARIO: What Would You Do? My father was admitted to an intensive care unit and wasn't expected to live. I was approached by a physician, who asked, "Do you want us to resuscitate him if he arrests again?" Since my father never wanted to talk about these things, I didn't know what he'd want. I also didn't feel it was my place to answer. I called my mother and asked her the question. Here's how the conversation went.

    Me: "Mom, they want to know if they should resuscitate Dad if he arrests again."

    Mom: "You don't know what you're asking me."

    Me: "Yes, I do. I know it's hard, but you're supposed to speak in his voice. Not what *you* want—what you think *he* wants."

    Mom: "That's the problem. You see, all my life when I've tried to guess his decisions, he's always done just the opposite. Even when I've said to myself, 'I think he'll do (whatever) only because it's the opposite of what I think he'd do,' I've still been wrong."

2. Which of the seven moral and ethical principles (autonomy, beneficence, justice, fidelity, veracity, confidentiality, accountability) apply to the following statement? (More than one may apply.)*

    By choosing the role of a nurse, you must see that your patients and clients receive competent care.

CRITICAL THINKING EXERCISES–cont'd

Note: Exercises followed by asterisks have example responses listed in the Response Key at the back of the book beginning on page 246.

3. Respond to the following outcomes from the prechapter self-test.
   a. Give a description and an example of the terms *moral uncertainty, moral dilemma,* and *moral distress.*
   b. Will you be able to make prudent decisions based on ethical principles, codes, and practice? To show that you can achieve this outcome, together with a partner or in a group, consider the following situation:

   > **CASE SCENARIO:** What Would You Do? The LaRusas have cared for their 40-year-old daughter, Marilou, at home for 20 years, since she became totally comatose after a car accident. All diagnostic studies indicate that Marilou will never regain consciousness. The LaRusas are almost 80 years old. Because they are concerned that they won't be able to care for her, they are considering stopping tube feedings and allowing her to die. Because the family has relied heavily on your decisions for the past 5 years, they ask you what to do. Decide how you can best help the LaRusas make this decision.

   c. Develop a personal code of conduct based on your personal values and content in this chapter.

Nursing Research Exercises
1. Acquaint yourself with "big picture" research reviews. Scan the section called Research for Practice in recent issues of the *American Journal of Nursing.* Choose one that you find interesting. Then:
   a. Summarize in your own words what the researchers studied, what they found, how it *might* be used in practice, and what questions are raised by the summary.
   b. Determine where you can find out more about the research topic, so that you can apply the study to practice.*
2. Analyze a research article to apply the findings to practice. Find an article that sounds interesting. Decide:
   a. Whether you can safely apply the findings to practice.
   b. Where you can find more information on the topic.
   c. What questions reading the article raises.
3. Respond to the following from the prechapter self-test.
   a. Describe your responsibilities in relation to nursing research and quality improvement.
   b. Explain why it's important to choose refereed or peer-reviewed journals when looking for research articles.*
   c. Explain how to decide whether you know enough to apply research findings to practice.

◆ TEACHING OTHERS

Creative critical thinking is key to helping people master the information they need to be independent. People today are discharged quicker and sicker than they were in the past, and many must manage complex problems independently at home. Our teaching must be timely and effective. We must be able to clearly identify what *must* be learned and then initiate a plan that draws on client strengths.

The following steps can help you think critically about how to teach others:

1. **Be clear about the desired outcome: What exactly will the person be able to do when you complete your teaching?** Example: The person will be able to regulate insulin dosage based on blood glucose readings.

2. **Decide (1) *what* exactly the person must learn to achieve the desired outcome and (2) what the best way is for him to learn it.**

◆ Clarify *with the person* what is already known.
◆ Determine readiness to learn: Ask what the biggest concerns are and *listen carefully.*
◆ Determine preferred learning styles (for example, doing, observing, listening, or reading) and use this information to plan teaching. For example, if you're teaching injection technique to doers, have them start by *doing* something, like handling a syringe. If they'd rather read, start by giving them a pamphlet.
◆ Identify barriers to learning (for example, consider language, reading skills, developmental problems, or problems with motivation).
◆ Encourage others to ask questions, get involved, and let you know how they'd like to learn. For example, you could say, Let me know if you have a better way of learning this. Not everyone learns the same way.

3. **Reduce anxiety by offering support.** An example is saying something like, "Everyone is nervous when first learning to change dressings, but once you've done it a couple of times, it will be much easier."

4. **Minimize distractions and teach at appropriate times.** For example, pick a quiet room and choose times when the learners are likely to be comfortable and rested.

5. **Use pictures, diagrams, and illustrations.** These visual aids enhance comprehension and are better remembered.

6. **Create mental images by using analogies and metaphors.** For example, insulin is like a key that opens the cell's door to allow sugar to enter. If you don't have the key (insulin), the sugar can't get into the cell. The cell starves, and sugar accumulates in the blood.

7. **Encourage people to remember by using whatever words best trigger their mind.** For example, someone might say, I need to have three things: the *soaking-dressing stuff*, the *scrubbing stuff*, and the *after-dressing* stuff.

8. **Keep it simple.** The explain-it-to-me-as-if-I-were-a-4-year-old approach works especially well for complex situations. If you can't make it simple, you're not ready to teach it.

9. **Tune into your learners' responses and change the pace, techniques, or content if needed.** For example, if they don't remember important content, take time to review it; if they don't seem to understand what you're saying, write it down or draw a picture.

10. **Summarize key points and don't leave learners empty-handed.** Even the best learners may have trouble remembering what they just learned. Give them the important points in writing so they can refresh their memory later.

To complete this section, review Box 4-6, which answers key critical thinking questions in relation to teaching others.

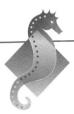

Critical Moments

TEACHING "WHY" PROMOTES INDEPENDENCE
Knowing why something must be done empowers people to problem-solve for themselves. Always explain the principles and rationales for treatments. If they know the reasons behind the treatments, they'll be able to make decisions about what to do when things go wrong.

Box 4-6   TEACHING OTHERS: 10 KEY QUESTIONS

1. **What major outcomes (observable results) do I/we plan to achieve?** After I/we finish teaching, and with the help of notes if needed, the person (or caregiver) will be able to demonstrate mastery of the required information or skill.

2. **What problems, issues, or risks *must* be addressed to achieve the major outcomes?** What exactly must be learned? Is the person ready to learn or are there other issues to be dealt with, such as anger, denial, or anxiety? What's this person's motivation (does he or she understand why it is necessary to learn the information or skill)? What's this person's preferred learning style? Are there other barriers to learning (e.g., language or literacy)?

Continued

Box 4-6   TEACHING OTHERS: 10 KEY QUESTIONS–cont'd

3. **What are the circumstances (what's the context)?** Who must you teach (adult, child, elderly person)? How complex is the information to be learned? Are you dealing with real or simulated situations? Does the person have previous experiences related to what must be learned?

4. **What knowledge is required?** Required knowledge includes familiarity with content to be taught, communication skills, and teaching and learning principles.

5. **How much room is there for error?** Room for error varies according to the consequences of what happens if the learner doesn't master the information. For example, in which situation below do you think you have more room for error?

   a. You're teaching insulin injection technique to someone who's basically healthy and whose daughter is an ICU nurse who's willing to monitor injection technique at home.

   b. You're teaching insulin injection technique to someone who has a compromised immune system and lives alone with no relatives.

   If you thought *a*, you're correct. If the person in situation *b* goes home without mastering insulin technique, he may not manage his diabetes, and he may also develop an infection. Therefore, you must be sure his injection technique is meticulous.

6. **How much time do I/we have?** The time frame for teaching depends on when the patient will be discharged from care. For example, if by day three the person is expected to be discharged, you have 3 days to teach the required information, or home care visits will be required.

7. **What resources can help me?** Human resources include clinical nurse educators, clinical nurse specialists, preceptors, more experienced nurses, peers, librarians, and other health care professionals (e.g., pharmacists, nutritionists, physical therapists, physicians). The learners are also valuable resources (it's not unusual for them to be the ones who can best identify what must be learned and how they can best learn it). Other resources include texts, Internet Web sites, articles, computerized learning packages, pamphlets, audiovisuals, and facility documents (e.g., teaching guidelines, standards of care).

8. **Whose perspectives must be considered?** The most significant perspective to consider is that of the learners: What is it they think they need to learn? How do they learn best? What are motivating factors for them to learn (e.g., some people need a deadline or a test)? Another perspective to consider is your own (e.g., how you feel you can best teach the material).

9. **What's influencing my thinking?** A major influencing factor is whether the learners believe they can learn and whether you believe you can be successful in helping them (both can be self-fulfilling prophecies). Thinking may also be influenced by any of the factors listed in Table 2-1, Factors Influencing Critical Thinking Ability (page 30).

10. **What must we do to prevent, manage or eliminate the problems, risks, or issues identified above in Question 2?** Assess what the person already knows, what he needs to know more about, whether he's ready to learn, and how he'd like to learn it. Identify available teaching aids (videos, pamphlets, etc.). Include key caregivers in developing approaches.

TEACHING OURSELVES

Today's challenging workplace requires that we know how to teach ourselves. We must be able to identify what it is we must learn and then find ways to learn it efficiently.

Using critical thinking when we learn, or figuring things out for ourselves in our own way, helps us connect with our own unique way of making information *ours*. Think about the following description.

Other Perspectives

FIGURING THINGS OUT FOR YOURSELF: THE BEST WAY TO LEARN
(Figuring things out for yourself goes something like this) "Let's see, how can I understand this? Is it to be understood on the model of this experience or that? Shall I think of it in this way or that? Let me see. Ah, I think I see. It's just so ... but, no, not exactly. Let me try again. Perhaps I can understand it from this point of view. ... OK, now I think I'm getting it."[9]

—*Author Richard Paul*

When you encounter something new, take charge and reason your way through the learning experience. Be confident in your ability to learn. Don't be afraid to ask questions. Remember, you are your own best teacher.

Memorizing Effectively

As much as experts emphasize that critical thinking is *more* than memorizing (remembering facts), learning how to memorize effectively enhances your ability to think critically: You must be able to recall facts to progress to higher levels of thinking, such as knowing how to apply and analyze information. For example, if you aren't able to *recall* what *normal* health assessment findings are, you won't be able to analyze your patient's data to decide whether there are any *abnormal* findings.

Some disciplines require more memorization than others. Nursing is a discipline that requires a considerable amount of memorization, especially in the beginning. The following strategies are suggested to help you memorize effectively:

1. **Try to understand before you try to memorize.** Once you make sense of the information, you begin to realize what's most important and how you can organize it to make remembering easier.

2. **Don't try to memorize everything.** Take the time to identify what's most important; then separate this information from all the

other information. This keeps you from trying to memorize too much. Your brain can only take so much new information at a time.

3. **Work to find relationships between the facts, rather than trying to just remember a list of facts.** You can remember *groups of information* easier than isolated facts. The process of trying to understand how the facts relate to each other will also help you *remember* the facts. Mind mapping, or concept mapping, is especially helpful for determining relationships (see page 260.)

4. **Create a memory hook.** Put the information into context. For example, if you looked after someone with the diagnosis you're studying in class, visualize the patient and how the situation compares with the information given in class (the patient becomes your memory hook). If you don't have a real situation to connect with, play around with the information until something comes to mind that helps you remember (e.g., a rhyme, a picture, a story, a mnemonic). For example, consider the following techniques:

◆ Use a mnemonic (organize what you're trying to remember in such a way that each word's first letter makes a real or nonsensical word). *Examples:*
TACT helps you remember what you should be monitoring when you're giving medications:
T = Therapeutic effect
A = Adverse reactions
C = Contraindications
T = Toxicity/overdose
PERRL (Pupils Equally Round and Reactive to Light) helps you remember to check the pupils to make sure they react equally to light when doing a neurologic assessment.

◆ **Use an acrostic** (create a catchy phrase that helps you remember the first letters of the information you're trying to remember).
Example: **M**aggie **c**hewed **n**uts **e**very **p**lace **s**he **w**ent provides the first letters of things you need to assess when performing a neurovascular assessment: **m**ovement, **c**olor, **n**umbness, **e**dema, **p**ulses, **s**ensation, **w**armth.

5. **In addition to using your preferred learning style, use as many senses as possible.** If you use other senses together with your preferred style, you remember even more. For example, use all three senses by saying the words as you write and read them. Sing what you're trying to remember to the tune of a favorite song.

6. **Organize the information, then see if you can organize it a different way.** By mentally using the information in different ways, you'll remember it better.

7. **Review the information briefly before going to sleep.** Studies show that even if you're a "morning person," information moves into long-term memory better if reviewed late in the day, immediately before going to bed.

8. **Put the information on tape.** Tapes can be played almost anywhere, anytime. Those minutes driving, walking, or riding a bicycle can be valuable time to load information into long-term memory.

9. **Use the information and quiz yourself periodically ("use it or lose it").** Remember, just because you can recognize information in your notes, it doesn't mean you'll be able to recall the information without your notes.

10. **Know yourself and use self-discipline.** Identify the circumstances that help you retain information and plan your schedule to include those circumstances. For example, if you study better in the morning, go to bed early enough that you can get up early and feel rested. If you're easily distracted or sidetracked, go to the library or put a Don't Disturb sign on your door.

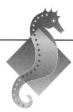

Critical Moments

THE BENEFITS OF MENTORS AND ROLE MODELS
Seek out mentors and role models—teachers, other nurses, friends, and peers. They help you clarify your thoughts and set goals better than any textbook.

TEACHING OTHERS HELPS YOU LEARN
When you want to know something well, offer to teach it to someone else. You learn and recall best what you teach someone else.

TEST-TAKING

Test-taking can be frustrating and anxiety producing. Almost everyone can identify with being in the position of knowing information well yet not being able to perform on the test. Lots of us can reason well in real situations but are stumped when it comes to reasoning our way to a correct test answer. For example, someone once said to me, "I need to be in real situations to think well." If you're one of those people (as I am), this section should be helpful to you.

Using critical thinking to identify the best way to prepare for and take tests reduces your anxiety and improves your test scores. Being successful at test-taking requires more than knowledge about the content. It also requires knowing yourself, the test format, and test-taking skills. The following strategies are suggested to help you improve your test scores:

1. **Know yourself.** Identify your usual test-taking behaviors (e.g., Do you get overly anxious? Do you frequently run out of time? Are you more successful at one type of test than another?) Seek help for areas you'd like to change.

2. **Know the test plan.** Find out what types of questions (multiple-choice, short-answer, essay) are going to be asked and what information is most important to study. If the teacher doesn't share this information, review course objectives, text objectives, and summaries—often these will help you decide.

3. **Start preparing with an attitude of, I can do this–I just have to figure out how.** You are capable. Sometimes you need to remind yourself of this to acquire the positive attitude we all know is so important.

4. **Get organized and plan ahead.** Decide what you need to study, what your resources are (for example, notes, books, tutors), and when and how you'll prepare for the test.

5. **Learn how to read questions and make educated guesses.** See Boxes 4-7 and 4-8.

6. **Practice answering the types of questions you expect to take on the test.** For example, practice multiple-choice questions for state board exams. One reason some of us don't do well on tests is because we don't take them every day. Often, answering discussion questions and end-of-chapter exercises are also good ways to practice. If you're going to take the test on a computer, practice on the computer. For state board exams, take a review course.

7. **Arrive early for warm-up.** Give yourself time to calm down, get focused, and mentally go through information you've decided is important. Reviewing practice questions is also a good way to get your brain in test-taking gear.

8. **If possible, skim the whole test and plan your approach.** For example, you might begin by answering the types of questions you like before tackling types you don't like (for example, you may like matching better than essay). Completing what you like and know first reduces anxiety and gets your brain in the test-taking mode before you tackle more difficult questions.

Box 4-7 **TEST QUESTION COMPONENTS**

1. **The background statement(s).** The statements or phrases that tell you the context in which you're expected to answer the question (e.g., the words in italics below):

     Example Test Question: *You're caring for someone who has severe asthma, is wheezing loudly, is confused, and can't sleep. You check the orders and note that a sedative can be given for sleeplessness.* Knowing the possible effects of giving a sedative to an asthmatic, <u>what would you do</u>?
     a. Give the sedative to help the patient relax.
     b. Withhold the sedative because it aggravates asthma.
     c. Withhold the sedative and monitor the patient closely.
     d. Give the sedative but monitor the patient carefully.
2. **The stem.** A phrase that asks or states the intent of the question (e.g., the underlined words above).
3. **Key concepts.** The most important *concepts* addressed in the background statement(s). In the above example the key concepts are severe asthma, wheezing loudly, and effects of giving a sedative to an asthmatic.
4. **Key word(s).** The words that *specify* what's being asked and what's happening. In the example above the key words are "severe," "loudly," and "confused." These words specify that the asthma problem is severe. "Would you do" specifies that you're being asked for an appropriate action to take.
5. **The options (choices).** These include one correct answer (called the *keyed response*) and three to five *distractors* (incorrect answers). In the example above, *c* is the keyed response, and the rest are distractors.

9. **Focus on what you know.**
◆ **Skip more difficult questions and come back to them later.** For example, put a question mark next to questions you might be able to answer and an "X" next to the toughest questions. Go back to the question mark questions before the "X" questions.
◆ **For essay tests,** jot down key points you know you want to address before writing your essay. When you finish, check your essay to be sure you hit all the major points.
◆ **For essay and short-answer questions,** if you have time at the end, come back to these questions and ask yourself, What else can I say? or What did I miss?

10. **Let your instructor know if you don't understand a question.** You may not be allowed to ask questions during the test, but consider writing something like, "I wasn't sure what you meant so I'm

Box 4-8   GUIDELINES FOR MAKING EDUCATED GUESSES*

Definition of Educated Guesses: Knowing how to apply test-taking strategies to choose a right answer when you're unsure from content alone (when none of the options seem to jump out at you).

1. Be clear about directions.
2. Find out whether you're penalized for guessing.
3. Read the question *carefully*. Look at all the response choices.
   ◆ Eliminate answers you know are outright wrong.
   ◆ Look for answers that are wrong based on the directions.
   ◆ Look for clues in the questions or answers that might help you narrow it down further to the most likely best answer (see strategies 4 and 5 below).
4. When reading test questions, ask yourself four questions:
   ◆ Who is the client? (age, sex, role, etc.)
   ◆ What is the problem? (diagnosis, signs, symptoms, behavior, etc.)
   ◆ What specifically is asked about the problem? (e.g., to prevent respiratory complications … Because the cast is damp …)
   ◆ What time frame is being addressed? (e.g., immediately before surgery, on the day of admission, when?)
5. Use the following rules *together with your knowledge* to make educated guesses:
   ◆ **Initial = Assessment.** The word *initial* used in a question usually requires an assessment answer. (What would you assess?)
   ◆ **Essential = Safety.** The word *essential* used in a question usually requires a safety answer. (What's required for safety?) **Remember:** "Keep them breathing, keep them safe."
   ◆ **Law of opposites.** If you have two answers that are opposite to one another, the answer is usually one of these two opposites. *Example:* The correct answer is likely to be *a* or *c* below because they're opposites.
      a. Turn the client on to the right side.   c. Turn the client on to the left side.
      b. Encourage fluids.   d. Ambulate the client.
   ◆ **Odd man wins.** The option that's most different in length, style, or content is usually the right answer. The right answer is often the longest one or the shortest one. *Example:* The correct answer below is likely to be *b* because it's the "odd man."
      a. Decreased temperature   c. Decreased respirations
      b. Rapid pulse   d. Decreased blood pressure
   ◆ **Same answer.** If two responses say the same thing in different words, they can't both be right, so neither one is right. *Example: Tachycardia* and *rapid heart beat* as two answer options.
   ◆ **Repeated words.** If the answer contains the same word (or a synonym) that appears in the question, it's more likely to be a correct response. *Example:* The word *hypotension* in question, the word *hypotension* or *shock* in answer.
   ◆ **Absolutely not.** Answers that use "absolutes" are usually not the right response. *Example: always, never, all, none.*
   ◆ **Generally so.** Answers that use qualifiers that make the response more "generally so" tend to signify right answers. *Example: usually, frequently, often.*

* Strategies provided in consultation with Judith C. Miller, MS RN, President, Nursing Tutorial and Consulting Services, Clifton, VA 20124; 1-800-US-TUTOR, E-mail: jmillntc@aol.com.

answering the question assuming you meant. ..." If allowed, write this on your answer sheet.

11. **When in doubt, don't change answers.** Studies show your first response is more likely to be correct.

12. **For case history questions, read questions about the case history first.** Then read the histories with the intent of looking for the answers.

13. **When you're struggling to answer, consider whether sketching a picture, mind map, or diagram will help you conceptualize the answer.**

14. **Watch your time and note how the questions are weighted.** For example, if a question is worth 50% of your grade, you might want to save 50% of your time to work on that question.

15. **If you do poorly, don't think it's the end of the world.** Even the brightest, most knowledgeable minds have been known to fail tests (for example, Einstein flunked algebra; Edison was considered unteachable). Instead, do something. Explain your difficulty to your instructor; ask if there's some way you can prepare better or if you can do extra credit work; determine resources that can help you; practice, practice, practice.

To complete this section, review Box 4-9, Teaching Ourselves and Test-Taking: 10 Key Questions.

 Other Perspectives

A Tip for State Board Exams

"I teach students to remember Maslow's hierarchy.... 'Keep them breathing, keep them safe.' I had a student who called me to tell me he passed NCLEX. He said what got him through was 'Keep them breathing, keep them safe.'"[10]

—Judith Miller, MS, RN, Nursing Tutorial and Consulting Services

Box 4-9   TEACHING OURSELVES AND TEST-TAKING: 10 KEY QUESTIONS

1. **What major outcomes (observable results) do I plan to achieve?** I will demonstrate mastery of the required information by passing the appropriate tests or demonstrating competency in real situations. Or, I will get a (specify grade) on the test, or I will demonstrate competency in the required nursing skills.

2. **What problems, issues, or risks *must* be addressed to achieve the major outcomes?** Identify (1) what content and skills will be tested or required, (2) what type of test this will be, and (3) what's the best way for you to prepare for this particular test or situation. For clinical competency tests, what risks are there for the patient?

3. **What are the circumstances (what's the context)?** How important is it for you to get your desired score? Will you be tested in real or simulated situations? Do you get a second chance? Are you penalized for guessing?

4. **What knowledge is required?** Required knowledge includes knowledge of yourself (e.g., your preferred learning styles, what time of day is your peak learning time, your motivations), as well as knowledge of key learning skills (how to promote retention of key facts in long-term memory, how to use different approaches such as mind mapping) to gain understanding. For test-taking, you also need to know the test plan, content to be tested, and how to make an educated guess (see Box 4-8).

5. **How much room is there for error?** For clinical competency, risks to the patient dictate how much room there is for error. For example, in which situation below do you think you have more room for error?
   a. You need to prepare for an open-book exam on nursing care for respiratory problems.
   b. You need to master respiratory assessment and tracheal suctioning before you take care of someone with a tracheotomy tomorrow.

   If you said *a*, you're correct. The risk of harm to your patient leaves little room for error.

   For test-taking, room for error also varies according to the type of test to be taken, whether or not you're penalized for guessing, and the consequences if you don't pass the test.

6. **How much time do I have?** Time frame to prepare varies, as we all know!

7. **Who or what resources can help me?** Human resources include professionals specializing in learning and test taking and peers. Other resources include librarians, clinical specialists, texts, Internet Web sites and articles on test taking and review books (see Bibliography, page 286).

8. **What perspectives must be considered?** For clinical competency tests, your own perspective and that of the patient must be considered. For test taking, think about the perspective of whomever constructed the test. It's important to realize that the person who is testing you wants you to do well but needs to feel comfortable that you've mastered the required content or skills.

9. **What's influencing thinking?** A major influencing factor is whether you think you can pass the test (this can be a self-fulfilling prophecy). Thinking may also be influenced by any of the factors listed in Table 2-1, Factors Influencing Critical Thinking Ability (page 30).

Continued

Box 4-9 TEACHING OURSELVES AND TEST-TAKING: 10 KEY
QUESTIONS–cont'd

---

10. **What must we do to prevent, manage, or eliminate the problems, risks, or issues identified in Question 2?** Clarify exactly what content or skills are required to pass the test or demonstrate competency. Tackle learning by using your own preferred learning styles. For clinical competency tests, practice in simulated situations, mastering manual skills. For test-taking, practice taking the type of test that will be given. For example, if you're going to take the test on a computer, practice similar tests on the computer.

KEY POINTS

Seven principles guide ethical decision making: autonomy, beneficence, justice, fidelity, veracity, confidentiality, and accountability. Practice standards, ethics codes, and bills of rights also guide ethical conduct. The following are common values addressed in ethical codes and standards: maintaining client confidentiality; acting as client advocate; delivering care in a nonjudgmental and nondiscriminatory manner; being sensitive to client diversity and culture; promoting client autonomy, dignity, and rights; and seeking resources for solving ethical dilemmas. Pages 108-109 give steps for moral and ethical reasoning. Advance directives help us make decisions about cardiac resuscitation and other end-of-life treatments.

Conducting research is one of the most rigorous and disciplined examples of critical thinking in nursing. Research generates knowledge that provides a scientific basis for planning, predicting, and controlling the outcomes of nursing practice. Staff nurses have four main responsibilities in relation to nursing research: (1) to think analytically about the situations they encounter and to seek out research results that might improve nursing care, (2) to raise questions about their practice that might prompt a researcher to formulate a question to guide a study, (3) to help researchers collect data, and (4) to continue to acquire and share knowledge related to research. Before you can use research results, you must decide whether the study is valid and reliable (whether it was conducted in such a way that you can trust that the results are accurate). Quality improvement (QI), a responsibility of all nurses, is essential to attaining high standards of care.

Because people today are discharged sicker and quicker than in the past, we must be able to clearly identify what *must* be learned and then initiate a timely teaching plan that draws on client strengths. To survive today, you must have excellent independent learning skills. Successful test-taking requires that you know yourself, the test format, test-taking skills, and how to make an educated guess (see Box 4-8).

CRITICAL THINKING EXERCISES

Note: Exercises followed by asterisks have example responses listed in the Response Key at the back of the book beginning on page 246.

Teaching Others, Teaching Ourselves, Test-Taking

1. Explain why knowing how to teach others efficiently is essential to meeting nursing outcomes.*
2. Describe five strategies that can help you memorize more effectively.
3. If you don't know your preferred learning style, study page 24, and decide how you best learn.
4. Respond to the following from the prechapter self-test.
   a. Use critical thinking to create a teaching plan. To show that you can achieve this outcome, ask a fellow student something he or she would like to learn and develop a teaching plan using the approaches suggested in this chapter.
   b. Address the roles of memorizing and reasoning in teaching ourselves.*
   c. Describe five strategies that can help you improve your test scores.

References

1. E-mail communication. (April 2002).
2. American Association of Critical-Care Nurses. (n.d.) Retrieved May 29, 2002 from http://www.aacn.org.
3. Summarized from American Nurses Association. (1998). *Standards of clinical nursing practice.* Washington, DC: Author.
4. Taylor, C., Lillis, C., & Lamone, P. (2001). *Fundamentals of nursing: The art and science of nursing care* (4th ed.). Philadelphia: Lippincott-Raven.
5. Burns, N., and Groves, S. (2001). *The practice of nursing research: Conduct, critique, and utilization* (4th ed.). Philadelphia: W.B. Saunders Co.
6. Dierdorf, B., Elgin, K., & Rea, K. (2001). Examining large bore central line use in acute care settings. *MEDSURG Nursing, 10*(6),313–314.

7. Wyoming hospital maps out a better way to care for dying patients. (February, 1996). *AACN News*, 5.
8. Rogers. P., & Bocchino, N. (1999). Is it possible? *American Journal of Nursing*, 99(10),27–34.
9. Paul, R. (1993). *Critical thinking: How to prepare students for a rapidly changing world*. Santa Rosa, CA: Foundation for Critical Thinking.
10. E-mail communication. (May 2002).

See comprehensive bibliography beginning on page 286.

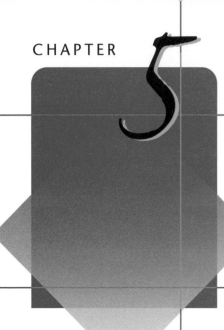

Practicing Clinical Judgment Skills: Up Close and Clinical

THIS CHAPTER at a Glance ...

1. Identifying Assumptions (page 138)
2. Assessing Systematically and Comprehensively (page 142)
3. Checking Accuracy and Reliability (Validating Data) (page 146)
4. Distinguishing Normal from Abnormal/Identifying Signs and Symptoms (page 148)
5. Making Inferences (Drawing Valid Conclusions) (page 149)
6. Clustering Related Cues (Data) (page 151)
7. Distinguishing Relevant from Irrelevant (page 153)
8. Recognizing Inconsistencies (page 155)
9. Identifying Patterns (page 156)
10. Identifying Missing Information (page 158)
11. Promoting Health by Identifying and Managing Risk Factors* (page 159)
12. Diagnosing Actual and Potential (Risk) Problems (page 161)
13. Setting Priorities (page 167)
14. Determining Client-Centered (Patient-Centered) Expected Outcomes (page 171)
15. Determining Specific Interventions (page 175)
16. Evaluating and Correcting Thinking (Self-Regulating) (page 178)
17. Determining a Comprehensive Plan/Evaluating and Updating the Plan (page 180)

---

*This skill deals with identifying risk factors in healthy people. The next skill, *Diagnosing Actual and Potential (Risk) Problems,* deals with risk factors in the context of people with existing health problems.

Read the following outcomes and decide whether you can readily achieve each one. If you can, skip this chapter. If you can achieve only some of the outcomes, complete only the sections you need to practice.

Learning Outcomes

After studying this chapter, you should be able to:

◆ Explain why each skill in this section promotes clinical judgment.

◆ Explain how to accomplish each skill in this section.

◆ Be explicit about your thinking in various simulated clinical situations (clearly express how you came to a conclusion or made a decision).

◆ Develop a comprehensive plan of care.

This chapter gives opportunities to practice clinical reasoning skills in simulated nursing situations based on real experiences (the names and some facts have been changed to ensure anonymity). Organized in logical progression according to how the skills might be used in the nursing process, each skill is presented in the following format: (1) Name of the skill, (2) definition of the skill, (3) why the skill promotes clinical judgment, (4) how to accomplish the skill, and (5) practice exercises.

CLINICAL JUDGMENT (CLINICAL REASONING) SKILLS: DYNAMIC AND INTERRELATED

Each skill in this section is presented as a *separate* skill. However, these skills aren't usually used *separately* or necessarily at any one particular point in thinking. Your mind thinks in a much more dynamic and rapid way than I can describe in a book—you often combine skills and move back and forth between them before coming to a conclusion.

Often these skills depend on and facilitate one another. ***Example:*** As you provide nursing care, you *recognize inconsistencies* (skill 8) in how the person is responding. This triggers you to wonder, *Have I identified assumptions?* (skill 1).

WHAT'S THE POINT?

Just as tennis players study interrelated tennis skills (foot placement, ball placement, swing, etc.) to analyze and improve their games *as a whole*, this section helps you practice interrelated *intellectual skills* to help you analyze and improve your thinking *as a whole*.

To keep the length of this chapter manageable, this section focuses mainly on clinical reasoning in the context of *problems*. However, keep in mind that using clinical reasoning also requires you to look for ways to improve areas that *are satisfactory* but could be better.

GENERAL INSTRUCTIONS

1. **To get the most out of these exercises, don't try to do too many at once.** Some of these exercises, as in real life, are quite time-consuming. The purpose of the exercises isn't to do them as quickly as possible. Rather, take your time and get in touch with your thinking. If possible, get at least one other person to complete the exercises with you. You learn more by discussing the skills with others.

2. **Your brain is a tricky thing—describing what goes on in someone's head to complete these skills is difficult.** If you have trouble with a section, read on and come back to it later.

Subsequent sections and skills are likely to help you clarify questions. Doing the practice exercises will also help you clarify the skill.

3. **If you encounter diseases or drugs you don't know, look them up.** As stated earlier, clinical reasoning requires knowledge of problem-specific facts (see Box 3-9, page 92). Looking up diseases or drugs and *applying* the information to the exercise will help you build your own mental storehouse of problem-specific facts. You remember best information that you *use*.

4. **Before starting this section, be sure you master the following vocabulary.** These terms are listed in order of how you can best learn them (you need to know the first term to understand the second term, and so on).

REQUIRED VOCABULARY FOR COMPLETING THIS CHAPTER

Definitive Diagnosis. The most *specific*, most correct diagnosis. For example, someone is admitted with an initial diagnosis of respiratory distress. Then, after studies are completed, the definitive diagnosis is *congestive heart failure*. To identify the *best treatment*, you must determine the *most specific diagnosis*.

Causative Factor. Something known to create or contribute to a problem. For example, dizziness is known to cause falls.

Risk Factor. Something known to cause, or be associated with, a specific problem. For example, smoking is a *risk factor* for cancer; having a family history of breast cancer is a *risk factor* for breast cancer.

Related Factor. Sometimes used interchangeably with *Risk Factor*.

Potential Problem or Risk Diagnosis. A problem or diagnosis that may occur because of certain risk factors present. For example, someone who's on prolonged bed rest has a potential or risk for *Impaired Skin Integrity*. Often used interchangeably with *high-risk problem or diagnosis*.

Data. Pieces of information about health status. For example, vital signs.

Objective Data. Information that you can clearly observe or measure. For example, a pulse of 140 beats per minute. To remember this term, remember:

O-O = **O**bjective data are **O**bserved.

Subjective Data. Information the patient states or communicates. These are the patient's *perceptions*. For example, "My heart feels like it's racing." To remember this term, remember:

S-S = **S**ubjective data are **S**tated (or written or signed in sign language).

Signs and Symptoms. Abnormal data that prompt you to suspect a health problem. *Signs* refer to objective data. *Symptoms* refer to subjective data. For example, fever is a sign of infection; chest pain is a symptom of heart disease.

Cues. Data that trigger you to think about a certain aspect of someone's health. Often used interchangeably with *signs and symptoms*.

Defining Characteristics. Signs and symptoms usually present with a diagnosis.

Baseline Data. Data collected before treatment begins.

Database Assessment. Comprehensive data collection performed to gain complete information about all aspects of health status (e.g., respiratory status, neurologic status, circulatory status).

Focus Assessment. Data collection that aims to gain specific (focused) information about only *one* aspect of health status (e.g., neurologic status).

Infer. To suspect something or to attach meaning to a cue. For example, if an infant doesn't stop crying, no matter what's done for him, you might infer that *he's in pain*.

Inference. Something we suspect to be true, based on a logical conclusion. For example, the italicized words in the preceding definition.

1. IDENTIFYING ASSUMPTIONS

Definition

Recognizing information taken for granted or presented as fact without evidence. For example, you might assume a woman on a maternity unit has just had a baby.

Why This Skill Promotes Clinical Judgment

Clinical reasoning requires that you make judgments based on the best available evidence. If you don't recognize what you assume, your thinking is likely to be flawed. By identifying assumptions, we can overcome our natural tendency to take things for granted, and can get the *facts* we need, before going on to identify problems and make decisions.

Guidelines: How to Identify Assumptions

The best way to identify assumptions is to *look* for them by asking questions like, What's being taken for granted here? and How do I know that I've got the facts right? You'll get opportunities to practice other ways of identifying assumptions as you go through some of the other skills here, like *recognizing inconsistencies, checking accuracy and reliability, identifying patterns,* and *recognizing missing information.*

Remember the following rule, which is also addressed in Chapter 3 because of its importance.

> *Rule:* Identifying assumptions requires doing a comprehensive assessment, which includes getting information from patient records, other caregivers, significant others, and applicable literature (e.g., information from a drug manual about medications being taken). **But always consider your *direct assessment of the patient* to be the primary source of information.**

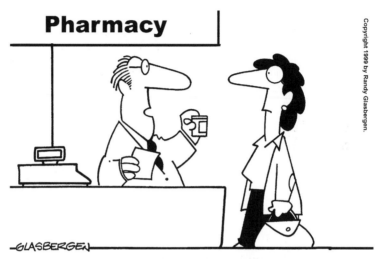

"It relieves watery eyes, runny nose, aching head, and scratchy throat. Side effects include runny eyes, watery nose, aching throat, and scratchy head."

Cartoon by Randy Glasbergen, Copyright 1999. Reprinted with special permission from www.glasbergen.com

Practice Exercises: Identifying Assumptions

Example responses are on page 250.

1. Explain why the following statement is an assumption: *We need to teach this patient how to stick to a low-salt diet because he eats whatever he wants even though his doctor told him not to eat salt.*

2. What could happen if you planned nursing care based on the preceding assumption?

3. Read the following scenarios, then answer the questions that follow them.

Scenario one   Anita plans to teach Jeff about diabetes today. She's well prepared and decides she'll create a positive attitude for Jeff by telling him about all the advances in diabetic care. She doesn't have much time, so she introduces herself and starts telling him how much easier it is to manage diabetes than it used to be. She goes on to explain how easy it can be to learn the required diet, monitor blood sugar at home, and take insulin. Jeff listens to all Anita has to say, asks a few questions, then leaves with his wife. As they drive off, he says to his wife in a discouraged tone, "She sure is a know-it-all, isn't she?"

a. Based on the information provided, what assumption does it seem Anita made about creating a positive attitude?

b. What key thing did Anita forget to do that might have helped her avoid making this assumption?

c. Why do you think Jeff said Anita is a know-it-all? ◆

Scenario two   Four-year-old Bobby is in the emergency department with his mother. He fell off his bike and had an initial period of unconsciousness lasting about a minute. He's been examined, has no skull fracture, and is now awake and alert, and ready to go home with his mother. The nurse gives his mother a computer printout of instructions for checking Bobby's neurologic status at home and says, "Let me know if you have questions."

a. What assumption does it seem the nurse has made?

b. What might happen if the nurse's assumption is incorrect? ◆

Scenario three   A friend told me this story:

I was working evenings in the emergency department of a seaside hospital. We admitted a 54-year-old man, whom I'll call Mr. Schmidt. He told me, "I just got here for vacation, and I'm not feeling so great. I had pneumonia at home, got treated, and thought I was better. Now my breathing feels lousy again." A check of his vital signs while he was sitting quietly revealed the following: T 99 P 138 R 36 BP 168/80.

As I helped him to the stretcher, he became significantly more short of breath. I checked his lung sounds and heard a lot of congestion. I notified the physician and voiced my concern that Mr. Schmidt seemed quite ill. The doctor immediately examined him and ordered an EKG and chest x-ray.

During this time we got very busy. I was helping another patient when the physician came to me and said, "I want you to give Mr. Schmidt 80 mg of furosemide (a diuretic) IV now and discharge him."

I looked at him skeptically and said, "*Discharge* him?"

He said, "Yes. I'm sure the diuretic will help him get rid of this fluid."

Being new and not really knowing this physician, I tried to tactfully voice my concern about this idea. "Can we give him some time to see how he responds?"

The physician responded: "Nope. This place is wild. I'm sending him home. He's going to a private physician in the morning. He'll be fine once he gets rid of some fluid. Discharge him with instructions to call if he doesn't feel better." Reluctantly, I went to give Mr. Schmidt the furosemide. I still had trouble with the idea of sending this man home before knowing his response to the IV diuretic.

Then I decided to use my own clout as a nurse: I had established a rapport with the Schmidts, and they trusted me. Before I gave the drug, I said, "I realize the doctor has discharged you, but I'd be interested to see if there's any change in blood pressure after you get rid of some fluid. How would you feel about sitting in the waiting room, and I'll check your blood pressure in an hour?" Both the Schmidts thought this was a good idea and went off to the waiting room. Only 45 minutes had passed when there was a shout for help. I ran to the waiting room and found Mr. Schmidt on the floor having a grand mal seizure. He then stopped breathing.

We were able to resuscitate Mr. Schmidt, and he was admitted to the hospital, diagnosed with electrolyte imbalance and heart failure, and discharged a week later.

a. What assumption does it seem the physician made about Mr. Schmidt's response to the furosemide?
b. Why do you think the nurse was so concerned about the assumption the physician made?
c. What assumption does it seem the nurse made about how the physician would respond to her if she cautioned him about discharging Mr. Schmidt?◆

 Other Perspectives

AVOIDING MAKING ASSUMPTIONS
"Heightened awareness often precedes a change in behavior. For example, once you know you tend to make assumptions, you soon begin to double-check your thinking."[1]

—*Carol Matz, RN, MSN*

2. ASSESSING SYSTEMATICALLY AND COMPREHENSIVELY

Definition

Choosing an organized, systematic approach that enhances your ability to discover all the information needed to fully understand someone's health status.

Why This Skill Promotes Clinical Judgment

One of the leading causes of clinical reasoning errors is making judgments or decisions based on incomplete information. Having an organized approach to assessment prevents you from forgetting something. For example, if you're interrupted while doing a physical assessment and you always use the same approach, you know exactly where you left off and where to continue. If you consistently use the same organized approach, you form habits that help you be systematic and complete.

Guidelines: How to Assess Systematically and Comprehensively

How you organize your assessment depends on the patient's health status and your own preference.

◆ **If the person is acutely ill**, set immediate priorities (see Setting Priorities, page 167), and tend to urgent problems first.
◆ **If the person has a specific problem**, begin by assessing that problem first, then go on to complete the assessment in the same way you would if the person were healthy.
◆ **If the person is generally healthy**, choose any method you find convenient. For example, use the head-to-toe approach, the body systems approach (Fig. 3-3, page 82), the functional health patterns approach (Box 3-7, page 82), or follow a preprinted assessment tool (see example, Fig. 5-1, page 183).

CLINICAL JUDGMENT AND PRE-ESTABLISHED ASSESSMENT TOOLS. Most places develop their own assessment tools that nurses are required to complete for each patient. Some of these tools are designed for *data base assessment* (see example, Fig. 5-1, page 183), and others are designed for *focus assessment* (see Neurologic Focus Assessment Guide, beginning on page 145).

While preestablished assessment tools help you develop habits that promote an organized and comprehensive approach to assessment, you must use these guides appropriately:

◆ Before using a tool, determine why the information the tool guides you to collect is relevant. For example, suppose you use a neurologic focus assessment tool, and it says to collect data about how the pupils react to light. Finding out *why the pupils respond to light* is relevant to determining neurologic status. To move more quickly toward an expert level of thinking, make the connection between *what* information is requested on the tool and *why* it's relevant.

◆ Remember the importance of gathering both subjective data (patient's perceptions) and objective data (your observations).

◆ Keep in mind that assessment tools don't prompt you to use all your resources. After you interview and examine your patient, ask, What other resources might provide additional information about this person's health status (medical and nursing records, significant others, other health care professionals)?

To become skilled at identifying an organized and comprehensive approach to assessment:

1. Choose a method of assessment and use it consistently.

2. Locate assessment tools that are designed for your patient's specific situation, practice using them, and be sure you understand why you collect each piece of data.

3. Keep in mind that a body systems approach to assessment helps you collect data about medical problems. Nursing frameworks, such as functional health patterns, help you collect data about human function and responses (nursing diagnoses).

Practice Exercises: Assessing Systematically and Comprehensively

Example responses are on pages 251-253.

1. You're working as a school nurse and have been asked to do physical exams to screen students for possible medical problems. Identify an organized, comprehensive approach to assessing for signs and symptoms of a medical problem.

2. You're making a home visit to Mrs. Sossa, who has a newborn child and seven other children younger than 12 years old. Both the baby and the mother are healthy. Identify an organized and comprehensive approach to assessing for problems with human function and responses (nursing diagnoses).

3. Read the following scenarios, then answer the questions that follow.

Scenario one   Pearl, an 89-year-old grandmother, is admitted overnight after fracturing her left ankle. She had surgery and a cast applied today. The cast goes from her toes to below the knee. Her toes are visible, and she can wiggle them freely. A small window has been cut in the cast over the dorsalis pedis pulse. Routine hospital protocols state that anyone with a new cast must have neurovascular checks every 2 hours for the first day of hospitalization. You know the following acrostic (memory jog) helps you remember the things you need to check when performing a neurovascular assessment for someone with a cast:

Maggie Chewed Nuts Every Place She Went stands for:
Movement, Color, Numbness, Edema, Pulses, Sensation, Warmth

a. Using the preceding acrostic to help you assess systematically, how would you assess to determine the neurovascular status of Pearl's injured leg?
b. Why is it necessary to monitor each of the assessment parameters listed in the acrostic to determine neurovascular status?
c. What would you do if Pearl told you her toes felt numb and cold?◆

Scenario two   You're about to give Mr. Wu digoxin by mouth. You know that the mnemonic TACT helps you remember what you need to monitor responses to medications:

T = **Therapeutic effect** (Is there a *therapeutic effect?*)
A = **Adverse reactions** (Are there signs of *adverse reactions?*)
C = **Contraindications** (Are there any *contraindications* to giving this drug?)
T = **Toxicity/overdose** (Are there signs of *toxicity or overdose?*)

Using **TACT** to focus your assessment to systematically gather information about how Mr. Wu is responding to the digoxin:

a. What, specifically, would you assess to decide whether to give the digoxin?
b. Why is it important to determine all of the things listed in the mnemonic TACT?◆

Scenario three   You just admitted Gerome, who fell off his bike, hit his head, and had a short period of unconsciousness. He is now awake and alert but is admitted for 24 hours of neurologic monitoring. The physician orders neurologic assessments every hour.

Respond to the questions that follow, using the neurologic focus assessment guide that follows the questions.

a. How would you assess Gerome to determine the status of each of the neurologic assessment parameters addressed in the guide?
b. Why is each piece of data on the focus assessment guide relevant to determining neurologic status?
c. What would you do if, on admission, Gerome demonstrates normal neurologic assessment findings but 2 hours later demonstrates extreme drowsiness (he awakens only if you shake him and call his name)?

d. What would you do if one pupil started to become more sluggish in its response to light than the other?

e. What would you do if you noted a general pattern of the pulse getting slower than baseline pulse?◆

Neurologic Focus Assessment Guide

VITAL SIGNS Temp.＿＿＿ Pulse＿＿＿ Resp.＿＿＿ BP＿＿＿

(Place a check mark in front of words that apply)

EYE OPENING
☐Spontaneous   ☐To command   ☐To pain   ☐No response

BEST MOTOR RESPONSE
☐ Obeys commands   ☐ Localizes pain   ☐ Flexion withdrawal
☐ Abnormal flexion   ☐ Abnormal extension   ☐ No response

BEST VERBAL RESPONSE
☐ Oriented   ☐Confused   ☐Inappropriate words
☐ Incomprehensible words ☐No response

PUPIL REACTION
☐ **Right eye:** ＿＿＿Size of pupil ＿＿＿Reaction to light (brisk, sluggish)
☐ **Left eye:** ＿＿＿Size of pupil ＿＿＿Reaction to light (brisk, sluggish)

PURPOSEFUL LIMB MOVEMENT

Right arm
☐ Spontaneous   ☐ To command   ☐Paralysis
☐ Visible muscle contraction but no movement
☐ Weak contraction; not enough to overcome gravity
☐ Moves against gravity, not to external resistance
☐ Normal range of motion; can be overcome by increased gravity
☐ Normal muscle strength

Right leg
☐ Spontaneous   ☐ To command   ☐ Paralysis
☐ Visible muscle contraction but no movement
☐ Weak contraction; not enough to overcome gravity
☐ Moves against gravity, not to external resistance
☐ Normal range of motion; can be overcome by increased gravity
☐ Normal muscle strength

Left arm
☐ Spontaneous   ☐ To command   ☐ Paralysis
☐ Visible muscle contraction but no movement

☐ Weak contraction; not enough to overcome gravity
☐ Moves against gravity, not to external resistance
☐ Normal range of motion; can be overcome by increased gravity
☐ Normal muscle strength

Left leg
☐ Spontaneous   ☐ To command   ☐ Paralysis
☐ Visible muscle contraction but no movement
☐ Weak contraction; not enough to overcome gravity
☐ Moves against gravity, not to external resistance
☐ Normal range of motion; can be overcome by increased gravity
☐ Normal muscle strength

Limb Sensation (prick limb with sterile needle)
Right arm: ☐ Normal   ☐ Decreased   ☐ Absent
Right leg: ☐ Normal   ☐ Decreased   ☐ Absent
Left arm: ☐ Normal   ☐ Decreased   ☐ Absent
Left leg: ☐ Normal   ☐ Decreased   ☐ Absent
Seizure Activity: Describe in nurse's notes.
Gag Reflex: ☐ Present   ☐ Absent

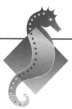

Critical Moments

PAIN AND COUGH—THE FIFTH AND SIXTH VITAL SIGNS
A key part of assessing systematically and comprehensively is taking four routine vital signs (temperature, pulse, respirations, and blood pressure). But consider pain and cough to be fifth and sixth vital signs. Ask about the presence of pain or discomfort and assess closely as indicated. Also ask the person to cough. Although asking the person to cough doesn't replace a thorough lung assessment, you can learn a lot from brief encounters even if you have only a few minutes. You can say something like, "Can you cough for me, so I can hear how it sounds?" The person's ability (or inability) to comply with this request gives you a lot of information (for example, whether the person has pain with coughing, whether there's congestion, or whether the person coughs well enough to clear the airway). These brief encounters can flag patients that need more in-depth monitoring and assessment.

3. CHECKING ACCURACY AND RELIABILITY (VALIDATING DATA)

Definition
Collecting more data to verify whether information you gathered is correct.

Why This Skill Promotes Clinical Judgment

Clinical judgments must be based on evidence. Verifying that your information is accurate, factual, and complete helps you avoid making decisions based on incorrect or incomplete data. Checking accuracy and reliability also promotes comprehensive data collection because it requires you to gather more data to double-check whether you've been correct.

Guidelines: How to Check Accuracy and Reliability

Review the data you gathered and ask questions like:
◆ Do the objective data (what you observe) support the subjective data (what the patient states)?
◆ How do I know this information is reliable?
◆ Does this information make sense in the context of this situation?
◆ How can I double-check this information by comparing it with data collected in a different way, or another time?

Next, focus your assessment to gain more information about whether your data are correct. For example, an elderly person may have told you that she took her medicine. To verify this, interview significant others or caregivers, check pill containers to see if pills are gone, and ask whether there is any record kept when pills are taken. Remember the following rule.

Rule: Remember, "more than one source, more likely of course." The more information you have coming from different resources, indicating the same thing, the more likely it is that your information is valid and reliable. For example, you may verify what your patient says by checking with family members and patient records.

Practice Exercises: Checking Accuracy and Reliability (Validating Data)

Example responses are on page 253.

For each of the following, determine how you would validate whether the data are accurate and reliable:

1. The off-going nurse tells you that Mrs. Molinas is depressed and angry about being in the hospital.

2. Mr. Nola tells you he thinks his blood sugar was about 104 when he tested it an hour ago.

3. You take a blood pressure from the left arm and find it to be abnormally high.

4. Mr. McGwire's care plan states that he has *Deficient Knowledge**: *Diabetic foot care as evidenced by statements that he doesn't know why he keeps getting skin breakdown on his feet.*

4. DISTINGUISHING NORMAL FROM ABNORMAL/IDENTIFYING SIGNS AND SYMPTOMS

Definition

Determining what patient data are within normal range and what data are outside the usual range for normalcy, then deciding what data may signify the presence of a problem. (Abnormal data that signify a problem are considered signs, symptoms, or cues).

Example: If a 62-year-old man who takes no medications has a pulse of 38 beats per minute, you know that this is *abnormal*. It may be a sign of a medical problem because a normal pulse rate rarely drops below 55 to 60 beats per minute in someone this age who takes no medications (some cardiac medications lower the heart rate).

Why This Skill Promotes Clinical Judgment

Recognizing abnormal data (signs and symptoms) is the first step to problem identification: Signs and symptoms are like red flags that prompt you to suspect a health problem. If you miss red flags, you miss recognizing problems and opportunities for early intervention.

Guidelines: How to Distinguish Normal from Abnormal/Identify Signs and Symptoms

Identifying signs and symptoms requires you to apply knowledge of what are considered normal findings. If you encounter data that are outside the normal range, then you have identified a possible sign or symptom. You must use all your senses (sight, hearing, touch, and smell) to gain all the relevant information. For example, if you *see* cloudy urine, *smell* it to check its odor.

Ask the following questions:

1. **How does my patient's information compare with accepted standards for normal for someone of this age, culture, disease process, and lifestyle?** If the patient's information isn't within normal accepted standards, they are a possible sign or symptom of a problem.

2. **Is my patient taking any medications that change normal function?** For example, someone may be taking a heart medication

---

*This is the latest NANDA terminology for Knowledge Deficit.

that lowers heart rate, in which case an abnormally low heart rate is *normal*. Check action and side effects of all medications.

3. **How does my patient's current information compare with the previously collected data?** This question is especially helpful in situations where the patient has chronic signs and symptoms and you're trying to decide whether the signs and symptoms are getting *worse*. For example, an asthmatic may always be slightly wheezy. However, if this same person is now wheezier than before, consider this increased wheeziness to be a sign of increasing problems.

Practice Exercises: Distinguishing Normal from Abnormal/Identifying Signs and Symptoms

Example responses are on page 254.

1. Place an "S" next to the data below that are signs or symptoms of a possible problem or signs or symptoms of a problem that's getting *worse*. Place an "O" if it's neither a sign nor a symptom. Place a question mark if you need more information to decide.
   a. ___ Temperature of 99.6° F.
   b. ___ Bilateral pulmonary rales.
   c. ___ Someone tells you she rarely sleeps more than 3 hours at a time.
   d. ___ Someone's nasogastric drainage has turned from brown to red.
   e. ___ Someone's abdominal incision is slightly red around the sutures.
   f. ___ A 2-year-old is inconsolable when his mother leaves the room.
   g. ___ Someone with no health problems has developed ankle edema.
   h. ___ Someone tells you he bathes every other week.
   i. ___ Someone on kidney dialysis never urinates.
   j. ___ Pulse of 54 per minute.
2. For each question mark you placed above, explain *what else* you want to know before you decide whether the information is abnormal (therefore a sign or a symptom).

5. MAKING INFERENCES (DRAWING VALID CONCLUSIONS)

Definition

Making deductions or forming opinions that follow logically by interpreting subjective and objective data. For example, note the data on the left below with the corresponding inferences on the right.

Data (Cues)	Corresponding Inference
Frowning	Seems worried
White blood cell count = 14,000	Probable infection
Deaf	Has communication problems

Why This Skill Promotes Clinical Judgment

Your ability to interpret data and draw valid conclusions (make inferences) is essential to determining health status. If you draw incorrect conclusions, your judgment will be flawed.

Making correct inferences helps you focus your assessment to look for *other information*. For example, if you infer that an elevated white blood cell count may indicate an infection, you know to look for signs and symptoms of infection.

Guidelines: How to Make Inferences (Draw Valid Conclusions)

Making correct inferences requires knowledge of common health problems, knowledge of human behavior, and knowledge of cultural and spiritual influences. For example, to make the inference of *probable infection*, you need to know the signs and symptoms of infection. Your knowledge of human behavior and spiritual and cultural influences is essential to making inferences about psychosocial data. For example, you may infer that someone's lack of eye contact indicates that he is mistrustful if you aren't aware that in his culture, lack of eye contact indicates respect.

It's important to remember the following rule.

Rule: **MORE THAN ONE CUE, MORE LIKELY IT'S TRUE**

More than one source, more likely of course
- ◆ Avoid making inferences based on only one cue (the more facts and sources you have to support your inference, the more likely it is that your inference is correct).
- ◆ Once you make an inference, verify whether it's correct by gathering more information and looking for additional cues.

To avoid jumping to conclusions, begin your statements about inferences by saying, *I suspect this information indicates. ...* Using this phrase reinforces that you to need to collect more data to decide if your suspicions are correct. Once you have enough evidence to support your inference, you can begin to view it as fact.

Practice Exercises: Making Inferences (Drawing Valid Conclusions)

Example responses are on page 254.
Make an inference about each of the following data (begin your inference by writing, *I suspect this information indicates ...*).

1. Temperature of 102° F for 3 days.

2. A mother tells you she can't afford prenatal care.

3. A diabetic is 100 pounds overweight and says his blood sugar is always out of control, even though he watches his food intake and takes his insulin regularly.

4. A 5-year-old child whose mother told you he broke his leg falling down the stairs keeps looking at his mother before answering any of your questions.

5. A grandmother who is usually alert and active in her church presents with an unkempt appearance and seems a bit confused.

6. CLUSTERING RELATED CUES (DATA)

Definition

Grouping data together in such a way that it helps you see relationships among the data. *Example:* Suppose you grouped the following cues together: 2 years old; temperature 100° F; pulse 150 per minute; rash all over trunk; recent measles exposure; never had measles; screaming that he wants his mother. If you consider the relationship among this data, you should suspect that the child's rapid pulse is related to his screaming and elevated temperature rather than a sign of cardiac problems. If you consider all of the above data, you'll probably suspect these symptoms indicate the child may have measles.

Why This Skill Promotes Clinical Judgment

Grouping information applies the scientific principle of classifying information to enhance ability to see relationships between and among data. It helps you get a beginning picture of patterns of health or illness. A good way to remember the importance of clustering related data is what I call "the puzzle analogy." When you put together a puzzle, you often begin by putting all the edges of the picture in one pile, all the pieces of a certain color in another pile, and so on. Putting the pieces in piles helps you begin to see patterns. The same principle applies to health assessment data; only in health care, you cluster *signs and symptoms.*

Guidelines: How to Cluster Related Cues (Data)

1. How you cluster data depends on your purpose:
   ◆ If you're trying to determine the status of medical problems or physiologic responses, cluster the data according to body systems (see Fig. 3-3, page 82).
   ◆ If you're trying to determine the status of nursing problems, cluster the data according to a nursing framework (for example, see Box 3-7, page 82).

2. Mind mapping, or concept mapping (see pages 266-269), is especially helpful for identifying relationships.

Practice Exercises: Clustering Related Cues (Data)

Example responses are on page 255.

Read the following scenarios, and then answer the questions that follow.

Scenario one

The 16-year-old baby-sitter next door calls and tells you that Jackson, the 7-year-old she's watching, was stung by a bee on the ear an hour ago. She tells you the ear is swollen and asks you to come and check him. You go over and examine the child. He asks you if he might die "like the kid on TV did." The baby-sitter tells you she's afraid because she doesn't know where the mother is. You check the ear and find it red, swollen, and free of the stinger. When asked, Jackson tells you he was stung before but that wasn't as scary. Jackson has no rash and no wheezing. He asks if he could have a Popsicle and watch TV. His pulse and respirations are normal.

a. Cluster the information that will help you determine Jackson's physical health status.

b. Cluster the information that will help you determine Jackson's human responses.

c. Cluster the information that will help you determine the baby-sitter's learning needs.◆

Scenario two

It's 11 AM and you just admitted Mr. Nelson, a 41-year-old businessman who has acute abdominal pain. He's never been in the hospital and tells you he hates everything about hospitals. He's been vomiting for 2 days and unable to keep any food down. His abdomen is distended and he has no bowel sounds. He is scheduled to go to the operating room at 2 PM for emergency exploratory surgery. He tells you he's worried because his brother died in the hospital after a car accident. Suddenly he doubles over and says, "Oh God, this is really getting worse!" You take his vital signs, and they are as follows: T 101 P 132 R 32 BP 140/80. These signs are the same as those taken an hour ago, except that before, his pulse was 104.

a. Cluster the information that will help you determine Mr. Nelson's physical status.

b. Cluster the information that will help you determine Mr. Nelson's human responses.◆

---

7. DISTINGUISHING RELEVANT FROM IRRELEVANT

Definition

Deciding what information is pertinent to understanding the situations at hand and what information is immaterial.

Why This Skill Promotes Clinical Judgment

When faced with a lot of information, narrowing it down to *only the pertinent facts* prevents your brain from being cluttered with *unnecessary* facts. Deciding what's relevant is also an example of one of the principles of the scientific method: classifying or categorizing information into groups of related (relevant) information.

Guidelines: How to Distinguish Relevant from Irrelevant

This skill is closely related to the previous skill, *clustering related cues*. However, we're looking at this skill a little differently. In *clustering related cues*, we simply put related information together (for example, you put all the respiratory data in one place, all the nutritional data in another, and so on). In this skill we analyze the data we put together and decide what information is relevant to a specific health concern. For example, if you suspect *constipation*, study the data and decide whether any of it is relevant to constipation. If you note that the person has a sedentary life and drinks very little fluid, it's likely that this is relevant to the *constipation*.

Distinguishing relevant from irrelevant is especially difficult for novices. They tend to find themselves asking, How can I decide what's relevant if I don't know very much about the *problems* yet? Being able to decide what's relevant *does* depend on having problem-specific knowledge and experience. For instance, if you have a patient with a heart problem, you need to know the common causes and usual progression of heart problems to decide what information is relevant. If you know that *ankle edema* is an early sign of congestive heart failure, you recognize it as being a *relevant* sign to consider when determining cardiac status.

Here are some strategies that can help you determine what's relevant, even with limited knowledge:

1. List the abnormal data collected.

2. Then ask yourself, Could there be any connection between this (abnormal data) and that (abnormal data)?

3. As appropriate, ask the person or significant others, Do you think there's any relationship between this (abnormal data) and that (abnormal data)?

4. Data that might be connected to other data are likely to be relevant.
5. To decide specifically if a piece of information is relevant to a problem, compare the person's signs, symptoms, and risk factors with the signs, symptoms, and risk factors of the problem you suspect. For example, if the person has no support system and you suspect *Ineffective Coping*, consider "no support system" as being relevant because lack of support systems is a risk factor for *Ineffective Coping*.

Practice Exercises: Distinguishing Relevant from Irrelevant

Example responses are on page 255.
Consider the following scenarios, then answer the questions that follow.

Scenario one	You work in community health and make a visit to Mrs. Blondell, who is 80 years old and had a cerebrovascular accident (CVA) a month ago. Today you notice she seems to be increasingly confused: She knows where she is but forgets what day it is and doesn't seem to remember her daily routine.
	You know that confusion in the elderly can be caused by any of the following: medications, infection, decreased oxygen to the brain, electrolyte imbalance, and brain pathology. You assess Mrs. Blondell and gather the data listed below. Consider the following data, decide its possible relevance to the problem of confusion, and mark whether you think it's relevant and why. a. Recently started taking buspirone hydrochloride for anxiety b. Temperature: 100° F orally c. History of a myocardial infarction 5 years ago d. Seems dehydrated e. Has no allergies f. Regular diet◆
Scenario two	You assess Mrs. Clark, a 32-year-old diabetic who is in for a routine visit. When you ask how the new diet is going, she breaks down into tears, saying, "I'm *never* going to be able to do this!"
	Consider the following data, decide its possible relevance to the problem with sticking to the diabetic diet, and mark whether you think it's relevant and why. a. Diagnosed with diabetes 2 months ago b. Vital signs within normal limits c. Complains of constipation

d. Married with three school-age children
e. Loves to cook
f. Has always been 50 pounds overweight
g. Allergic to aspirin◆

8. RECOGNIZING INCONSISTENCIES

Definition

Realizing when there is conflicting information. For example, suppose you have someone who tells you he has no pain after chest surgery. However, he moves very little, guards his chest carefully, and barely breathes when you ask him to take a deep breath. The way this person is moving is *inconsistent* with his statements of being pain free.

Why This Skill Promotes Clinical Judgment

Recognizing inconsistencies prompts you to investigate issues more closely. It sends up a red flag that indicates you must probe more deeply to get the facts. It also helps you focus your assessment to clarify the issues. For example, in the above case, you might say, "It seems to me that you aren't moving very well. I suspect you're having more pain than you admit. I want you to be comfortable, so that you move well and are able to take deep breaths to clear your lungs. Are you sure there isn't a particular spot that's causing you discomfort?"

Guidelines: How to Recognize Inconsistencies

One way to recognize inconsistencies is to compare what the patient states (subjective data) with what you observe (objective data). If what the person *states* isn't supported by what you *observe*, as in the preceding example, you have inconsistent information and need to investigate further.

Recognizing inconsistencies also requires a problem-specific knowledge. For example, suppose your neighbor tells you, "I've been staying in bed because I strained my back. My right side is killing me." On further questioning, she says she also has a fever and cloudy urine. What would you suspect? If you know how back injuries usually present, you know that the symptoms are *inconsistent* with a back injury and more consistent with a urinary tract infection.

To recognize inconsistencies with limited knowledge:

1. Determine the signs and symptoms of the problem you suspect by looking up the problem in a reference. For example, if you suspect pneumonia, look up the signs and symptoms of pneumonia in a textbook.

2. Compare the information in the reference with your patient's data. If your patient's signs and symptoms are different from those listed in the reference, you have inconsistencies and must investigate further: Assess the person more closely and consider other problems that the signs and symptoms might represent.

Practice Exercises: Recognizing Inconsistencies

Example responses are on page 255.
Read the following scenarios; then answer the questions that follow.

Scenario one   You're interviewing Cathy in the prenatal clinic 2 weeks before delivery. You ask her how she feels about the baby coming. She tells you she's happy that she'll get to see the baby in only 2 weeks. When you ask her if she has any questions about the delivery, she tells you she's been going to birthing classes with her boyfriend and feels like she knows what to expect.

You review her records and notice that her first clinic visit was 2 weeks ago, when she came with her mother.
a. Identify inconsistencies in the above scenario.
b. Explain what you might do to clarify the inconsistencies you identified above.◆

Scenario two   You're in the grocery store and a woman who appears to be about 20 years old comes up to you and says, "Please help me! I can't breathe, and my heart is racing. I think I'm having a heart attack!" You help her sit down, then take her pulse, and find it to be 100 per minute, regular, and strong. Her respirations are 32 per minute. She tells you she has no pain but asks the store manager to call an ambulance. As you wait for the ambulance, she tells you this has happened to her several times before and that she has had an electrocardiogram, which showed normal cardiac function. Then she says, "But I *know* I'm having a heart attack! I'm so scared!"

How consistent are this woman's signs, symptoms, and risk factors with those of a cardiac problem?◆

---

9. IDENTIFYING PATTERNS

Definition

Clustering related cues together and deciding what they indicate about a general picture of functioning. For example, you cluster cues of *chronic productive cough, wheezing, and exercise intolerance* together and decide that they indicate a pattern of possible decreased respiratory function.

Why This Skill Promotes Clinical Judgment

Identifying patterns helps you get a *beginning picture* of problems and to recognize gaps in data collection. Once you recognize gaps in data collection, you can decide how to focus your assessment to gain that missing information.

Here's an example of how identifying patterns helps you discover missing pieces of information. Suppose you clustered together the following cues:

◆ No bowel movement in 3 days
◆ Abdominal fullness
◆ States he's been "constipated off and on for the past month"

You may decide that these cues represent a pattern of *Altered Bowel Elimination.* Having recognized this pattern, you know to focus your assessment to gain more information and decide *exactly* what the problem with bowel elimination is. For example, you ask, "What does *off and on* mean?" The person responds, "I get so constipated I have to take laxatives, and then I get diarrhea." This added information is likely to make you suspect that the bowel elimination problem is being caused in part by laxative abuse. You can then explore his knowledge of problems caused by laxative use.

Guidelines: How to Identify Patterns

Identifying patterns requires knowledge of usual function and *risk factors* for abnormal function. For example, to recognize abnormal coping patterns, you need to know normal coping patterns; to recognize potential (risk) for abnormal coping patterns, you need to know the risk factors for abnormal coping patterns (e.g., social isolation, mental illness).

To identify patterns:

1. Analyze the cues you clustered together and decide which of the following categories they represent:

◆ **Normal pattern of function:** You identified no signs and symptoms.
◆ **Potential (risk) for abnormal pattern of function:** You identified *risk factors* but no signs and symptoms. For example, if your patient has little fiber intake, minimal exercise, and takes frequent laxatives, he has a potential (risk) for *Altered Bowel Elimination,* even if today he had a normal bowel movement.
◆ **Abnormal pattern of function:** You identified *signs and symptoms.* For example, your patient complains of constipation and hasn't had a bowel movement in three days.

2. Once you have a beginning idea of the patterns, ask, What *other* information might help me clarify my understanding of this pattern? Then try to find out the answers through more assessment.

Practice Exercises: Identifying Patterns

Example responses are on page 256.

Consider the data listed for each letter *a* to *e* below. Then choose which one of the following patterns best describes the cluster of data and explain why.

◆ **Potential (Risk) for Impaired Bowel Elimination Pattern**
◆ **Potential (Risk) for Ineffective Sexual-Reproductive Pattern**
◆ **Probably Normal Sleep-Rest Pattern**
◆ **Impaired Respiratory Function Pattern**
◆ **Probably Normal Coping Pattern**

a. Bilateral rales; respirations increased to 34 per minute; coughing up thick, white mucus.

b. States, "I can cope with my illness, so long as I have help from my husband." Manages daily self-care; has husband cook all meals; passes the time by knitting blankets for the homeless.

c. Eats little roughage; just started taking codeine every 4 hours; drinks about three glasses of water daily; spends most of her time in bed; normal bowel function.

d. Works nights; sleeps 4 hours in the morning and 3 hours just before going to work at night.

e. Has just been diagnosed with genital herpes; single; worried about transmitting herpes to future sex partners and future children (during delivery).

10. IDENTIFYING MISSING INFORMATION

Definition

Recognizing gaps in data collection and searching for information to fill in the gaps.

Why This Skill Promotes Clinical Judgment

Recognizing gaps in information and filling in those gaps prevents you from making one of the most common clinical reasoning errors: making judgments based on incomplete information. It also helps you clarify your understanding of the situations at hand.

Guidelines: How to Identify Missing Information

1. One of the best ways to identify missing information is to analyze your written information and ask, What's missing here? When you have

all the information on paper, your brain can more readily recognize what's missing than when going over the information mentally.

2. Other strategies for recognizing missing information include accomplishing all of the following clinical judgment skills:

◆ Identifying assumptions
◆ Checking accuracy and reliability of data
◆ Clustering related cues
◆ Recognizing inconsistencies
◆ Identifying patterns
◆ Evaluating and correcting thinking

Practice Exercises: Identifying Missing Information

Example responses are on page 256.

Go back to the practice exercises for the previous skill, *identifying patterns*. For each pattern represented by the information listed in *a* to *e*, decide what information might be missing that could add to your understanding of the pattern.

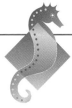

Critical Moments

ASKING, "WHAT DIFFERENCE DOES IT MAKE?" SIMPLIFIES ASSESSMENT

When trying to decide if the data you're missing are really needed, ask questions like, What difference will it make? or How will knowing this information change the approach to treatment? For example, suppose you're trying to decide whether someone needs more diagnostic studies. If you decide that doing more studies won't change treatment, then it's likely that the studies aren't necessary.

11. PROMOTING HEALTH BY IDENTIFYING AND MANAGING RISK FACTORS*

Definition

Preventing health problems by early detection and treatment of factors that cause–or put someone at risk–for decreased well-being.

Why This Skill Promotes Clinical Judgment

Critical thinking is proactive. We don't wait for problems to appear to put a plan into action. By identifying risk factors, we use the proactive

---

*This skill deals with identifying risk factors in *healthy people*. The next skill, *Diagnosing Actual and Potential (Risk) Problems*, deals with risk factors in the context of people with *existing health problems*.

Predict, Prevent, Manage, Promote (PPMP) approach, rather than the reactive Diagnose and Treat (DT) approach (see pages 164-167).

Guidelines: How to Identify and Manage Risk Factors

1. Assess the person's awareness of and motivation for identifying and managing risk factors. For example, determine whether they know what's required for adequate nutrition, rest, exercise, and spiritual and psychological well-being and whether they're willing to do what's needed. Not knowing about risk factors and not wanting to do something about them are risk factors in themselves.

2. Keep growth and development in mind. For example:
   ◆ A woman who is pregnant or planning on becoming pregnant must consider risk factors for both herself *and* the fetus when taking medications. She should be aware that inadequate intake of folic acid increases risk of spontaneous abortion and other problems such as infant neural tube defects.[2]
   ◆ After menopause, women should know that they are at risk for calcium loss and decreased bone density.

3. Look for risk factors that are known to put people at risk for a variety of common problems. Some common examples:
   ◆ Obesity, poor diet, high cholesterol, tobacco use, immobility, sedentary life, stressful life, poor sleeping habits, allergies, chronic illness, extremes of age (very young or old), low socioeconomic status, illiteracy, sun exposure, excessive use of medications, alcohol, or illicit drugs.

4. Also assess for:
   ◆ Genetic, cultural, or biological factors (e.g., race, family history, and personal history predisposing one to health problems)
   ◆ Behavioral factors (e.g., problems with anger management, attention deficit disorders)
   ◆ Psychosocial/economic factors (e.g., lack of significant others, poverty)
   ◆ Environmental factors (e.g., air quality)
   ◆ Age-related factors (e.g., women after menopause are at risk for osteoporosis; infants are at risk for ear infection)
   ◆ Sexual pattern factors (e.g., whether one is sexually active and with whom)
   ◆ Safety-related factors (e.g., whether seat belts are worn, whether the home environment is safe for children)
   ◆ Disease-related factors (e.g., someone with chronic lung disease is at risk for pneumonia; someone with diabetes is at risk for skin problems)
   ◆ Treatment-related factors (e.g., complicated medication or treatment regimen)

5. Teach the importance of managing risk factors to prevent costly, debilitating illnesses in the future.

Want to know more about risk management?

Go to the Harvard Center For Risk Analysis at http://www.hcra.harvard.edu/, which is dedicated to promoting reasoned public responses to health, safety, and environmental hazards. It also addresses statistics and approaches for problems like stroke, heart disease, suicide, cancer, and drowning and other accidents. The Centers for Disease Control and Prevention Web page (http://www.cdc.gov/) also has a wealth of information on disease and disability prevention. Also, look up "Risk Factors" in the index of any up-to-date fundamentals or medical-surgical nursing textbook. Usually you can find excellent tables on common diseases and risk factors that present information in an easy-to-understand format.

Practice Exercises: Promoting Health by Identifying and Managing Risk Factors

Example responses are on page 257.

1. You assess a 25-year-old man and determine that he is healthy. What questions might you ask to identify risk factors for possible problems?

2. You assess a 72-year-old woman and find that she is healthy, but she says "I tend to be little clumsy—I lose my balance." In relation to normally encountered risk factors for a woman of this age, why should you be concerned about this?

3. You're at a barbecue talking casually with a 50-year-old man. He says, "You know I guess I'm getting to the age where I should be doing more to look after myself. How can I find out my risk factors?" What's your response?

---

12. DIAGNOSING ACTUAL AND POTENTIAL (RISK) PROBLEMS

Definition

Naming the problems that are present or may become present based on evidence from the health assessment. This skill includes choosing a diagnostic label that best describes the problem, determining the cause(s) or related factors of the problems, and providing the evidence that leads you to believe the diagnosis is present.

Why This Skill Promotes Clinical Judgment

Keeping in mind the predict, prevent, manage, promote (PPMP) approach to delivering health care, this skill is important for several reasons:

1. Making definitive diagnoses (the most specific, correct diagnoses) is key to being able to determine specific actions designed to prevent, manage, or resolve them.

2. You don't fully understand the problem(s) or know what to do about them until you clearly identify what's causing or contributing to them.

3. Predicting potential problems helps you:
   ◆ Know what signs and symptoms to look for
   ◆ Think about what could happen if things get worse (therefore allowing you to plan ahead to be prepared)

4. Providing the supporting evidence that led you to conclude exactly what the actual and potential problems are helps you and others evaluate thinking. For example, consider the two problem statements below. Which one helps you better evaluate the thinking that led to the conclusion that there is a potential for violence?
   ◆ Potential for Violence
   ◆ Potential for Violence related to a history of combative behavior and failure to attend anger management courses

To grasp the importance of being able to accurately diagnose actual and potential problems, think about what can happen when you make a diagnostic error.

Rule: **Diagnostic errors (missing problems, being too vague about the problems, or naming them incorrectly) can cause you to:**
   ◆ **Initiate actions that aggravate the problems or waste time.**
   ◆ **Omit essential actions required to prevent and manage the problems.**
   ◆ **Allow problems to go untreated.**
   ◆ **Influence others to believe the problems exist as described incorrectly.**

Guidelines: How to Diagnose Actual and Potential Problems

The ability to identify and predict problems depends on knowledge and clinical expertise. Experts can usually identify problems much more quickly than novices because they've "seen it all before." They generate better hypotheses (they have better hunches about what the problems are), and they move through the steps of problem identification in a very dynamic way.

If your knowledge and expertise are limited, you have an increased risk of making any one of the following mistakes.

◆ Overvaluing the probability of one diagnosis
◆ Not considering all the relevant data because of a narrow focus
◆ Failing to recognize personal biases or assumptions
◆ Making a diagnosis that's too general
◆ Overanalyzing ("analysis paralysis") and delaying taking action

Being aware that beginning nurses are at risk for the above errors can help them and more experienced nurses to look for these types of errors so that they can be corrected early.

IDENTIFYING ACTUAL PROBLEMS

1. Verify that your information is correct and complete.

2. Avoid drawing conclusions or identifying problems based on only one cue. The more cues and sources you have to support your conclusions, the more likely it is that your conclusions are valid.

3. Cluster abnormal data (signs and symptoms): Cluster according to body systems to identify medical problems and a nursing framework to identify nursing problems.

4. Consider the signs and symptoms and ask yourself what information you could have missed.

5. Create a list of suspected problems that may be suggested by the signs and symptoms (Box 5-1 on page 164 gives a helpful checklist to consider possible problems). Remember the following rule.

Rule: If you're not sure where to start when trying to create a suspected problem list, report *signs and symptoms* to speed up problem identification.

6. After you complete your list of suspected problems, compare your patient's signs and symptoms with the signs and symptoms or defining characteristics of the problems you listed. Some look at this phase as testing hypotheses (testing your hunches about what the problems may be).

7. Name the problems by choosing the diagnoses that *most closely resemble* your patient's signs and symptoms.

8. Determine what's *causing* or *contributing to* the problems:

◆ Always ask yourself whether it's possible that medications, allergies, or untreated (or inadequately treated) medical problems are causing the problems. If so, initiate a medical consultation immediately.
◆ Ask the person and significant others if they can identify factors that are contributing to the problems.

Box 5-1   CHECKLIST FOR IDENTIFYING ACTUAL AND POTENTIAL PROBLEMS

1. List current medications (include over-the-counter and herbal drugs). Ask yourself whether any of the patient's problems could be related to any of the medications (remember **SODA**).
   Side effect?
   Overdose?
   Drug interaction?
   Allergy/Adverse reaction?
2. List any history of allergies, disease, surgery, or trauma.

3. Consider whether any of the patient's current problems are related to Questions 1 or 2 above.
4. Complete the following checklist: (Circle those that apply)

Is there a problem with breathing?	Yes	No	AR[1] Pos[2]
Is there a problem with circulation?	Yes	No	AR Pos
Is there a problem with comfort?	Yes	No	AR Pos
Is there a problem with nutrition?	Yes	No	AR Pos
Is there a problem with urinary or bowel elimination?	Yes	No	AR Pos
Is there a problem with fluid or electrolyte balance?	Yes	No	AR Pos
Is there a problem with ability to think or perceive environment?	Yes	No	AR Pos
Is there a problem with communication?	Yes	No	AR Pos
Is there a problem with safety (risk for injury or falls)?	Yes	No	AR Pos
Is there a problem with sleeping or exercising?	Yes	No	AR Pos
Is there a risk for infection (self or transmission to others)?	Yes	No	AR Pos
Is there risk for impaired skin integrity?	Yes	No	AR Pos
Is there a problem with coping or stress?	Yes	No	AR Pos
Is there a psychological, developmental, self-esteem problem?	Yes	No	AR Pos
Is there a sociocultural problem?	Yes	No	AR Pos
Is there a problem with roles, relationships, or sexuality?	Yes	No	AR Pos
Does the person have a problem with taking medications?	Yes	No	AR Pos
Does the patient require teaching?	Yes	No	AR Pos
Is there a problem with health maintenance at home?	Yes	No	AR Pos
Is this admission going to cause difficulties at home?	Yes	No	AR Pos
Is there a problem with personal or religious beliefs?	Yes	No	AR Pos
Is there a problem with coping or managing stress?	Yes	No	AR Pos
Could this person be pregnant?	Yes	No	AR Pos

[1]AR = At Risk for problem (no signs and symptoms present, but risk factors are evident).
[2]Pos = Possible problem (insufficient data, but you suspect a problem).

◆ Consider whether there are factors related to age, disease process, medications, or life changes that could be contributing to the problems.

◆ Look up the diagnoses you identified and check common related or causative factors; then assess your patient to determine whether he or she exhibits any of these factors.

9. As appropriate, use the mnemonic PRE (problem, related factors, evidence) and develop a problem statement that describes the:

◆ **P**roblem

◆ **R**elated factors (cause, risk factors)

◆ **E**vidence that led you to conclude the problem exists

10. Use *related to* to link the problem and its cause. For example: *Acute pain related to left rib fracture as evidenced by statements of extreme tenderness in the left rib cage area.*

PREDICTING POTENTIAL PROBLEMS

1. *For nursing problems and diagnoses:*

◆ Cluster data that indicate risk factors for problems. For example, you may cluster the following data: immobile, elderly, fragile skin.

◆ Name the potential (risk) problem by stating the problem and the risk factors, using *related to* to link the problem and risk factors. For example: *Risk for Impaired Skin Integrity related to immobility and fragile skin.*

2. *For potential complications, consider:*

◆ Medical problems, medications, and treatments present

◆ Whether invasive monitoring or diagnostic modalities were used recently

◆ What common potential complications are associated with the above. For example, if your patient just had a myocardial infarction (MI) and has an arterial line in place, determine common potential complications of MI (e.g., congestive heart failure, arrhythmias, pericarditis, MI extension, and cardiac arrest) and of the arterial line (e.g., thrombus or emboli)

◆ Describe the potential complication by using the letters PC, followed by a colon,[3] for example,

PC: hemorrhage or PC: increased intracranial pressure

Practice Exercises: Diagnosing Actual and Potential (Risk) Problems

Example responses are on page 257.

Scenario one You just admitted Nigel to the psychiatric unit. He is agitated but won't talk to anyone. You check previous records and note that he has a history of striking caregivers.◆

Write a diagnostic statement that best describes this potential problem by stating the problem and its related factors.

Scenario two   Elaine is in the recovery room after having an emergency appendectomy under general anesthesia. She's very groggy and extremely nauseated.◆

Based on the above information, predict the potential complications Elaine might experience.

Scenario three   You clustered together the following data: Mrs. Pue has just been told she has terminal cancer. She refuses to take her medications. She sleeps most of the time and says she doesn't want to talk to anyone. Mrs. Pue states her situation is hopeless and she's going to die so she'd rather not bother talking.◆

Based on the above information write a problem statement that best describes the problem using the PRE format.

Scenario four   You're caring for a 41-year-old man who has four fractured ribs. What risk factors might you look for to determine whether he is at high risk for respiratory problems?◆

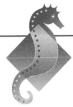

Critical Moments

TOLERATING AMBIGUITY: A GOOD THING—OR NOT
Acceptance of ambiguity is often listed as a critical thinking characteristic. Certainly there are times, as the saying goes, that there is "no black or white—only gray." But you must ask, How much ambiguity is acceptable in this particular situation? For example, if you were sick, would you be happy with an ambiguous diagnosis or would you want it to be specific? Remember that clearly and specifically defining the problem and its cause helps you identify specific interventions to resolve it.

13. SETTING PRIORITIES

Definition

Differentiating between problems needing immediate attention and those requiring subsequent action; deciding what problems to delegate and what problems *must* be addressed in the plan of care.

This skill is important for four main reasons:

1. If you don't know how to set priorities, you may contribute to life-threatening treatment delays. For example, if you don't recognize that treating congestive heart failure early is a major priority, it can progress to pulmonary edema and death.

2. If you give equal attention to major and minor problems, you won't be able to devote the time you need to resolve the *most important* problems.

3. By determining *relationships* among problems–a key part of setting priorities–you can treat the ones that are contributing to *other* problems first. You avoid "quick fixes" and develop a safe, effective plan. For example, suppose you have someone with abdominal pain and you give him pain medication without diagnosing what problem is causing it. You may resolve the pain, but allow the abdominal problem to progress undetected.

4. By deciding what you can delegate to others, you have more time for "must do" priorities.

Critical Moments

SETTING PRIORITIES: USE THE 80/20 RULE

The 80/20 Rule, developed by an economist years ago, applies to many situations. For example, some say that you wear 20% of your clothes 80% of the time. Others say you get 80% of your business from 20% of your clients. Think of the things you have to do for your patients as 100%. Then realize that you have to figure out the 20% that must *get done. This is where you need to spend 80% of your time.*

Guidelines: How to Set Priorities

This section addresses how to set priorities in the clinical setting. Pages 213-218 (Managing Your Time) provide additional important insights.

1. Identify which problems are most urgent (those requiring immediate attention, such as breathing problems). Boxes 5-2 and 5-3 provide key concepts about setting priorities. Notice that there's more than one way to set priorities. Choose the one that makes the most sense to you in context of each patient situation.

Box 5-2   SETTING PRIORITIES: PRINCIPLES AND APPROACH

Major Principles

1. Always consider the relationship between the problems: For example, if problem Y causes problem Z, problem Y takes priority over problem Z.
2. Treatment for first- and second-level priorities listed below is usually initiated in rapid succession or simultaneously. At times, the order of priority might change, depending on the seriousness and relationship of the problems. For example, if abnormal lab values are life-threatening, they are likely to be highest priority; if your patient is having trouble breathing because of acute rib pain, managing the pain might be a higher priority than dealing with a rapid pulse (first-level priority, listed below).

Approach to setting priorities:

1. First-level priority problems (immediate priorities): Remember "ABC's plus V."
   ◆ Airway problems
   ◆ Breathing problems
   ◆ Cardiac/circulation problems
   ◆ Vital signs concerns (such as high fever)
2. Second-level priority problems (immediate, after you initiate treatment for first-level priorities)
   ◆ Mental status change (e.g., confusion, decreased alertness)
   ◆ Untreated medical problems requiring immediate attention (e.g., a diabetic who hasn't had insulin)
   ◆ Acute pain
   ◆ Acute urinary elimination problems
   ◆ Abnormal lab values
   ◆ Risks of infection, safety, or security (for patient or for others)
3. Third-level priority problems (later priorities)
   ◆ Health problems that don't fit into the above categories (e.g., problems with lack of knowledge, activity, rest, family coping)

Box 5-3   SETTING PRIORITIES ACCORDING TO MASLOW'S HIERARCHY OF HUMAN NEEDS

No. 1 priorities: problems with survival needs (e.g., food, fluids, oxygen, elimination, warmth, physical comfort)

No. 2 priorities: problems with safety and security needs (e.g., risks of injury or infection, threats to feeling secure)

No. 3 priorities: problems with love and belonging (e.g., family problems, separation from loved ones)

No. 4 priorities: problems with self-esteem needs (e.g., need for privacy, respect, independence, and positive self-image)

No. 5 priorities: problems with self-actualization needs (e.g., need to grow and achieve outcomes)

Summarized from Maslow, A. (1970). *Motivation in personality.* New York: Harper & Row.

2. Decide what and how to delegate to others. This information is covered in Box 5-4.

3. Determine what problems *must* be recorded in the patient record. To do this:

◆ Determine the major expected outcome(s). For example, *Mrs. Marrero will return home able to manage diabetic regimen independently.* (How to determine expected outcomes is addressed in the next skill. To help you complete this section, outcomes are provided for you.)

Box 5-4 **DELEGATING IN THE CLINICAL SETTING***

WHEN IS IT SAFE TO DELEGATE?

Delegate When:
◆ The patient is stable.
◆ The task is within the worker's job description and capabilities.
◆ The amount of RN time with the patient isn't significantly reduced.

Don't Delegate When:
◆ Complex assessment, thinking, and judgment are required.
◆ The outcome of the task is unpredictable.
◆ There's increased risk of harm (e.g., arterial puncture can cause more severe complications than venous puncture).
◆ Problem solving and creativity are required.

KEY POINTS ON DELEGATION

Delegation defined: Transferring to a competent individual the authority to perform a selected task in a selected situation, while retaining accountability for results.

1. Remember the "five rights of delegation." Delegate:
◆ **The right task**–one that doesn't fall under nursing's practice scope only.
◆ **To the right person**–someone qualified and competent to do the job. Keep costs in mind (e.g., a dietician may cost more than a nurse to do diet teaching in the home).
◆ **In the right situation**–see left column (When Is It Safe to Delegate?)
◆ **With the right communication**–be clear and concise when describing the task, the goal, and what you want reported.
◆ **With the right supervision, evaluation, and feedback**– timely evaluation of patients' responses and worker's performance is key. Let the caregiver know what he/she's doing well and give tips for improvement.

2. Delegate with full knowledge of:
◆ Your state practice act, and applicable standards, policies, and procedures (e.g., what you're allowed to delegate and to whom may vary from state to state and facility to facility).
◆ The person's specific job description and competencies.

3. When delegating to patients or family caregivers, learn whether they have the required knowledge and skills.

Source: R. Alfaro-LeFevre workshop handouts © 2001. All rights reserved.
Recommended Reading:
Alfaro-LeFevre, R. (2001). *Applying Nursing Process: Promoting Collaborative Care* (5th ed.). Philadelphia: Lippincott Williams and Wilkins. Fisher, M. *Do Your Nurses Delegate Effectively?* Retrieved April 29, 2001 from http://www.springnet.com/ce/m905a.htm
Hansten, R., & Washburn, M. (2001). *Delegating to UAPs.* Retrieved May 17, 2002 from http://www.nurseweek.com/ce/ce1680a.html and
National Council of State Boards of Nursing (NCSBN) (1995). Delegation: Concepts and Decision-Making Process. *Issues* (December) 1–4.

◆ List the problems and their causes (or contributing factors). Decide what problems *must* be addressed in order to achieve the overall outcomes. For example in the case of Mrs. Marrero, she may have the following two problems:

1. Deficient Knowledge: Insulin administration
2. Ineffective Coping related to marital problems

Only the first problem above relates to the overall outcome, so that's the problem you must address in the plan of care.

◆ Assign a high priority to recording an individualized plan of care for the following problems:

1. Those not covered by facility standard plans, protocols, or physician's orders
2. Those that may jeopardize achieving the major expected outcomes of the plan of care.

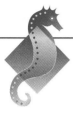

Critical Moments

REMEMBER THE CHAIN OF COMMAND, AVOID MALPRACTICE SUITS

Too many nurses have tunnel vision, focusing only on what they can do to resolve a problem. This can create delays in crucial treatment, causing patient harm. Always ask yourself, Could any of these signs and symptoms be due to a medication, allergy, or a problem that requires medical management? If the answer is yes, an immediate priority is to notify the appropriate person in the chain of command. For example, you may have to notify an instructor or supervisor before calling the doctor. Problems with nurses not initiating the chain of command early are key contributing factors to adverse outcomes (and malpractice suits).

Practice Exercises: Setting Priorities

Example responses are on page 258.

1. If the expected outcome is *will be discharged home by in 5 days able to manage colostomy care*, which of the following problems *must* be addressed in the plan of care?

   a. Anxiety related to inability to return to work for 6 weeks
   b. Deficient Knowledge: colostomy care
   c. Risk for Impaired Skin Integrity related to colostomy drainage

2. Read the following scenarios; then answer the questions that follow.

Scenario one   Mr. Santos, a 64-year-old migrant worker, is admitted with a right calf thrombophlebitis. He is on bed rest, warm soaks, and anticoagulants. His knowledge of English is minimal. You try to teach him how to give himself anticoagulant injections. You have problems communicating, so you decide to contact social services to get a translator to attend the teaching sessions. Mr. Santos conveys to you that his leg is still painful and that he's also been getting pains in his chest.◆

Based on the above information, what's your most *immediate* priority?

Scenario two You're caring for Neil, a 16-year-old football player who had surgery for a ruptured spleen 10 hours earlier. He is alert, his vital signs are stable, and his abdominal dressing is clean and dry. He has some incisional discomfort and hasn't been medicated for pain since surgery. He is also uncomfortable because he hasn't been able to void since surgery. He says, "I feel so lousy, I wish my mother could stay with me." When you offer to call her, he replies, "No, she's dying of cancer. I don't know what I'm going to do without her. Would you call my aunt?"◆

1. You've identified the following nursing concerns. Using Box 5-1 as a guide, decide how you would prioritize the needs/problems below: Place a "1" (for first priority), "2" (second priority), or "3" (third priority) in the appropriate blank.
   a. _____Wants his aunt to come in
   b. _____Hasn't voided
   c. _____Has incisional pain
2. Explain why you chose the order of priorities you listed above.
3. The expected outcome for Neil is, *Will be discharged home after 3 days, able to change dry sterile dressings.* Neil demonstrates dressing changes the day after surgery and relates the importance of impeccable wound care. He is ambulatory and voiding well. Which of the following is not likely to be addressed on the care plan and why?
   a. Risk for infection related to incision
   b. Anticipatory grieving related to loss of his mother as evidenced by statements that mother has terminal cancer and he wishes she could be with him
   c. Deficient Knowledge: dressing changes

14. DETERMINING CLIENT-CENTERED (PATIENT-CENTERED) EXPECTED OUTCOMES

Definition

Describing exactly what results will be observed *in the patient or client* to show the expected benefits of the plan of care at a certain point in time. ***Example:*** Twenty-four hours after intubation for open-heart surgery, the patient will be able to breathe independently. Pages 69-71 provide additional definitions for various kinds of outcomes (clinical, functional, and other outcomes). If you're not familiar with these definitions, read those pages before going on to complete this section.

Why This Skill Promotes Clinical Judgment

Clearly describing what beneficial results you expect to observe in the patient or client, and at what point you expect to see the results helps you:

◆ Explain why nursing care is worthwhile.

◆ Keep the focus on *how the person is responding to care,* the most important measure of how well the plan is working.

◆ Determine priorities. You need to know exactly what you aim to do before you can decide what's most important and what needs to be done first.

◆ Get everyone motivated (knowing the benefits and time frame for outcome achievement motivates clients and caregivers to initiate actions in a timely fashion).

◆ Determine specific interventions designed to achieve the outcomes. As the saying goes, If you don't know where you're going, it's hard to figure out how to get there.

Guidelines: How to Determine Client-Centered (Patient-Centered) Expected Outcomes

1. Be sure you clearly understand principles of client-centered (patient-centered) expected outcomes (see Box 5-5).

2. Find out whether there are standard plans that address the expected outcomes for your patient's particular problems. For example, if your patient has pneumonia, is there a critical path that addresses outcomes for patients with pneumonia? If there are standard plans that address outcomes, determine whether the outcomes are appropriate for your patient's particular situation.

3. Partner with the patient, significant others, and key caregivers to develop outcomes together. If outcomes are predetermined by standard plans, get agreement that the outcomes are attainable. Remember the following rule.

Rule: If you haven't given enough thought to exactly what end results (expected outcomes) you need, and what will be assessed to determine if the results have been met, you aren't thinking critically. Example expected outcome: After daily dressing changes the skin around the abdominal incision will be clean, dry, and free from signs of infection (redness, pain, swelling, heat).

Box 5-5 **PRINCIPLES OF CLIENT-CENTERED (PATIENT-CENTERED) EXPECTED OUTCOMES**

1. Expected outcomes reflect the benefits expected to be observed after nursing care.
2. Be sure you understand the difference between clinical, functional, quality of life, and other outcomes as discussed in pages 69-71.
3. Expected outcomes may be written from a problem or intervention perspective.
   - Outcomes written for problems describe exactly what will be observed in the client to show that the problems are resolved (or managed).
   - Outcomes written for interventions describe the expected observable response to the intervention.
4. Simply put, determining expected outcomes requires you to *reverse the problem* (state what happens when the person doesn't have the problem) or state the *desired response to the intervention* as noted in the following examples.

EXAMPLE PROBLEM	CORRESPONDING EXPECTED OUTCOME
Pain	Using a numerical or pictorial pain scale will relate being pain free or that pain level doesn't interfere with daily activities or sleep

EXAMPLE INTERVENTION	CORRESPONDING EXPECTED OUTCOME
Nasogastric irrigation	Nasogastric tube will be patent and patient non-distended

5. Expected outcomes should have the following components:
   - **Subject:** Who is expected to achieve the outcome? Or, what part of the patient will be observed to demonstrate the expected benefit?
   - **Verb:** What will the person do (or what will be observed) to demonstrate outcome achievement?
   - **Condition:** Under what circumstances will the person do it?
   - **Performance Criteria:** How well will the person do it?
   - **Target Time:** By when will the person be able to do it?

   Examples: "By Friday, Jim will walk with a walker to the end of the hall." Or "By Friday, the skin on the bottom of the heel will be intact, free from signs of irritation."
6. Use verbs that are observable and measurable (actions you can clearly see or hear).
   - Use verbs like *explain, describe, state, list, demonstrate, show, communicate, express, walk, gain, lose.*
   - Don't use verbs like *know, understand, appreciate, feel* (these aren't measurable because no one can read someone else's mind to find out if they know, understand, appreciate, etc.).
7. Use *as evidenced by* to describe exactly what behaviors will indicate that the outcome has been met. *Example:* The client will demonstrate diabetes management as evidenced by ability to state how insulin works, perform glucose monitoring, adjust insulin dose according to blood sugar level, and use sterile injection technique.

Continued

Box 5-5   PRINCIPLES OF CLIENT-CENTERED
(PATIENT-CENTERED) EXPECTED OUTCOMES–cont'd

8. Be realistic, considering:
   ◆ Physical health state, overall prognosis
   ◆ Expected length of stay
   ◆ Growth and development
   ◆ Available human and material resources
   ◆ Other planned therapies for the client
9. In complex cases, develop both short-and long-term outcomes, using short-term outcomes as stepping stones to the long-term outcomes. **Example:** (Short term) "After 1 week, Al will be able to bathe and dress himself with assistance." (Long-term) "After 4 weeks, Al will be totally independent performing his morning care."

4. To determine daily outcomes, ask, What will be observed in this particular person at the end of today after care has been delivered? What will be the status of the problems and what will be the responses to the interventions?

Want to know more about research on nursing outcomes?

Find a comprehensive discussion of research on nursing outcomes in *Nursing Outcomes Classification (NOC)*, edited by M. Johnson and M. Maas, St. Louis: Mosby, 2000. See page 81 for related Websites.

Practice Exercises: Determining Client-Centered (Patient-Centered) Expected Outcomes

Example responses are on page 258.

For each problem or intervention below, determine the most specific, client-centered outcome.

1. Risk For Impaired Skin Integrity related to age, obesity, and prolonged bed rest

2. Suction patient prn (as needed)

3. Powerlessness related to quadriplegia as evidenced by statements such as "I have no choices"

4. Irrigate Foley catheter every 4 hours

5. Endotracheal intubation

6. Activity Intolerance related to muscle weakness secondary to prolonged bed rest as evidenced by inability to walk the length of the hall without assistance

15. DETERMINING SPECIFIC INTERVENTIONS

Definition

Identifying nursing actions designed to: (1) prevent, manage, or resolve problems and risk factors, and (2) achieve outcomes by predicting responses, weighing risks and benefits, and tailoring actions to make them specific to the patient.

Why This Skill Promotes Clinical Judgment

Identifying specific interventions designed to achieve the outcomes, manage the problems, and decrease the likelihood of harm is the key to developing a safe and efficient plan. Predicting the responses to interventions helps you be proactive: You can test interventions mentally before putting the plan into action. By anticipating possible responses (both desired and untoward) you can be more prepared. For example, you may ask yourself questions like, How likely am I to get the desired response? What happens if this person gets dizzy when I get him up? How likely is this to happen? and, What can I do to make sure he doesn't fall?

Weighing risks against benefits helps you determine harmful interventions—you can decide whether your actions have a greater likelihood of causing harm than good. For example, in the previous case, you may decide not to get the person out of bed at all if you don't have a second person there to help you.

Describing very specific interventions increases the likelihood that the actions will be carried out as specified. Notice how vague *a* is compared with *b*:

a. Monitor breath sounds and have the person cough and breathe deeply.

b. Monitor breath sounds, splint front left lower ribs, and have the person cough and deep breathe every 4 hours during waking hours

Guidelines: How to Determine Specific Interventions

1. Whether dealing with standard plans or developing your own plans, remember the following rule.

Rule: **To determine specific nursing interventions, consider the problems, their causes (or related factors), and the expected outcomes.**

◆ **Consider each problem and ask, What can be done about the problem, and what can be done about the problem's cause or related factors?**

◆ **Consider the outcomes and ask, How can we tailor the interventions to achieve these specific outcomes and reduce the risk of harm?**

2. Apply the PPMP (Predict, Prevent, Manage, Promote) approach. Determine specific actions to:

◆ Detect, prevent, manage, or remove the cause (risk factors) of the problem(s). For example, if a person is spending a lot of time in bed, get him out of bed as much as possible, changing his position frequently.

◆ Detect, prevent, manage, or remove the problem(s). Sometimes you can't do much about the *cause* of the problems, but you can manage the symptoms or potential complications of the problems. For example, if someone has his jaws wired shut, you can't do much about it, but you better be prepared to handle the potential complication of aspiration (e.g., have wire cutters and suction equipment nearby).

◆ Promote optimum function and well-being. For instance, in both the preceding examples, you could talk with the patient about his feelings and concerns about being incapacitated and identify ways to allay his concerns.

3. Include patients and significant others in tailoring interventions. They know themselves best.

4. Predict responses to your interventions; weigh the risks of harm against the likelihood of getting the desired response.

5. Fine-tune interventions to include ways of increasing the likelihood of beneficial responses and decreasing the risk of harm.

6. Remember the words *see, do, teach,* and *record.* Consider what you'd see (assess), what you'd do, what you'd teach, and what you'd record. For example:

◆ See (assess). Assess ability to walk with walker in the room before allowing him to go out in the hall alone.

◆ Do. Have him walk the length of the hall three times a day.

◆ Teach. Reinforce that sticking to the plan will increase muscle strength and reduce fatigue.

◆ Record. Record pulse and blood pressure before and after walking at least once a day.

7. Keep in mind both direct-care interventions (things you do directly for or with the patient, such as helping someone get out of bed) and indirect-care interventions (things you do away from the patient, such as monitoring lab results).

Want to know more about research on nursing interventions?

Find a comprehensive discussion of research on nursing interventions affecting patient care in *Nursing Intervention Classification (NIC)* (3rd ed.) by J. McCloskey and G. Bulechek, St. Louis: Mosby. See page 81 for related Web sites.

Practice Exercises: Determining Specific Interventions

Example responses are on page 258.

1. Determine specific interventions for each of the following problems and corresponding outcomes.

Problems	Corresponding Expected Outcomes
a. Risk for Fluid Volume Deficit related to diarrhea and insufficient fluid intake.	Will maintain adequate hydration as evdienced by drinking at least 4 quarts of clear liquids per 24-hour period.
b. Anxiety related to insufficient knowledge of hospital procedures.	By the end of today, the person will relate knowledge of hospital procedures and express that anxiety is reduced.
c. *Chronic Pain* related to arthritic joints as evidenced by statements of pain with range of motion for the past 20 years.	After application of heat and assistance with range of motion, the person will express that joint pain is manageable.

2. Consider the following scenario; then respond to the questions that follow.

Scenario

You make a home visit to the Supopoffs, Russian immigrants who live in the suburbs in a church-sponsored house. The family has three children ages 5, 7, and 10. Their home is adjacent to a tall grassy area, which is full of deer ticks. Mrs. Supopoff is upset because she keeps finding deer ticks on the children, and she knows Lyme disease comes from deer tick bites. Even though she's told the children not to go into the grassy area, she suspects they disregard her instructions. Mrs. Supopoff is considering punishing the children when she finds a tick on them, hoping this will make them more careful.

You look up Lyme disease and learn that the best treatment is *prevention* of tick bites.◆

You identify the following problem and expected outcome:

Problem: Risk for Infection related to tick bites.

Expected outcome: The children will have a decreased risk of tick bites and infection as evidenced by wearing insect repellent when outside, avoidance of tall grassy areas, and monitoring themselves and each other for ticks.

a. Consider the risks and benefits of the following actions:
   1. What might happen if the children are punished when a tick is found on them?
   2. What might happen if you reward the children for finding ticks?
b. What interventions might safely motivate the children to participate in spotting ticks? Write specific interventions to achieve the expected outcome listed for this situation.

16. EVALUATING AND CORRECTING THINKING (SELF-REGULATING)

Definition

Paying attention to how you are thinking (for example, looking for flaws, deciding whether your thinking is focused, clear, and in enough depth) then making necessary corrections.

Why This Skill Promotes Clinical Judgment

Developing clinical judgment skills requires you to self-regulate, which means you must constantly reflect on your thinking, asking yourself questions like, Am I clear about what's going on here? What am I missing? How can I be more sure that my reasoning is sound? Am I holding myself to high standards? Do I know what I'll do if things go wrong? and What creative approaches might work here?

Critical Moments

AVOID JUDGMENT ERRORS—THINK ABOUT ALTERNATIVE EXPLANATIONS, PROBLEMS, OR SOLUTIONS

A key part of self-regulating is considering alternative problems, explanations, and solutions. Successful nurses aren't successful because they can come up with one right answer or explanation—they come up with many, *and then choose the best one.*

Guidelines: How to Evaluate and Correct Thinking (Self-Regulate)

As discussed in previous skills, evaluating and correcting thinking is an ongoing process. Box 5-6 shows the types of questions you should

Box 5-6   **EXAMPLE QUESTIONS ASKED TO EVALUATE AND CORRECT THINKING AT VARIOUS STAGES OF THE NURSING PROCESS**

1. **Assessment**
   - ◆ What assumptions could I have made?
   - ◆ How complete is data collection?
   - ◆ How accurate and reliable is my information?
   - ◆ How well do I understand my patient's perceptions?
   - ◆ How sure am I of the conclusions I've drawn (inferences I've made)?
   - ◆ Have I considered what data I need from both nursing and medical perspectives?

2. **Diagnosis**
   - ◆ How well does the evidence support that the problems I identified are correct?
   - ◆ Have I missed any other problems that could be indicated by the evidence?
   - ◆ Am I clear about the underlying causes?
   - ◆ How clearly and specifically are the problems stated?
   - ◆ Am I clear about the definitive diagnoses?
   - ◆ Have I identified both nursing problems and problems requiring a multi-disciplinary approach?
   - ◆ Were client strengths and resources identified?

3. **Planning**
   - ◆ What immediate priorities could have been missed?
   - ◆ Did I remember to include the patient and significant others in setting priorities?
   - ◆ Have I missed any problems that must be addressed on the plan of care?
   - ◆ How well do the outcomes reflect the benefits I expect to see?
   - ◆ Are the outcomes realistic, clear, and client-centered?
   - ◆ Did I consider both the problems and the outcomes when identifying interventions?
   - ◆ Did I consider client preferences when developing the plan, and did I take advantage of client strengths and resources?

4. **Implementation**
   - ◆ Are the problems still the same?
   - ◆ Am I missing any new problems?
   - ◆ Am I keeping the focus on client responses?
   - ◆ Should I be doing anything differently? Are the interventions still appropriate?

5. **Evaluation**
   - ◆ How accurately and completely have I completed each of the previous steps?
   - ◆ What could I be doing differently/better?

ask at various points in the nursing process to evaluate and correct thinking.

There are no practice exercises for this skill, as opportunities for evaluating and correcting thinking have been provided throughout the other skills.

17. DETERMINING A COMPREHENSIVE PLAN/EVALUATING AND UPDATING THE PLAN

Definition

Ensuring that all major actual and potential problems and corresponding outcomes and interventions are recorded; keeping the plan up to date.

Why This Skill Promotes Clinical Judgment

Developing a comprehensive plan and ensuring that the major care plan components are recorded:

◆ Forces you to think about the most important aspects of giving care
◆ Promotes communication between caregivers (therefore improving thinking of the health care team)
◆ Provides data for evaluation, research, legal, and insurance purposes. Remember the first letters of the word EASE to jog your mind about the key care plan components that must be recorded on a comprehensive plan:

Expected outcomes

Actual and potential problems (those that must be addressed to reach the overall outcomes)

Specific interventions designed to achieve the outcomes

Evaluation statements (progress notes)

Continually thinking about how the plan is working and what changes must be made *early* is essential to reaching outcomes efficiently.

Guidelines: How to Develop a Comprehensive Plan/ Update the Plan

1. Being able to determine a comprehensive plan requires all of the skills listed in this section and knowing the purpose and components of the recorded plan (see Box 5-7).

2. Identify the major problems and interventions yourself. Then:

◆ Check the patient record to see whether the problems and interventions are addressed by pre-established plans, policies, or doctor's orders.
◆ Compare your patient's situation with the interventions on pre-established plans. Modify or add interventions if needed.

3. To evaluate and update the plan, compare what's *supposed* to happen (or what you're supposed to find) as described in the standard plan with what you *actually* find when you assess the patient.

◆ Determine progress toward expected outcomes. For example, if the expected outcome states *will be free of signs of infection around incision*, assess the incision for signs of infection (e.g., redness, drainage, heat, and tenderness).

Box 5-7 PURPOSE AND COMPONENTS OF THE RECORDED
PLAN OF CARE

Purpose of Recorded Plan
◆ Promotes communication between caregivers
◆ Directs care, interventions, and documentation
◆ Creates a record that can later be used for evaluation, research, legal and insurance purposes

Components of Recorded Plan (Use memory jog EASE)
◆ **E**xpected outcomes
◆ **A**ctual and potential problems that must be addressed to achieve the major outcomes of care
◆ **S**pecific interventions designed to control or resolve the problems and achieve the outcomes
◆ **E**valuation statements (progress notes)

◆ Monitor problems closely; watch closely for new risk factors or problems. If risk factors or problems change, be sure the plan of care reflects this.
◆ Monitor outcomes of interventions after each intervention. If you aren't seeing the expected results, start thinking about what you could change to improve the results.
◆ Modify interventions as needed, changing the record as needed.
4. Remember the following rule.

Rule: An essential daily nursing responsibility is looking for care variances (instances when patients haven't achieved activities or outcomes by the time frame noted on a critical path). If you identify a care variance, ask, What additional assessment do I need to do to determine whether this delay is justified? and What can I do to improve this person's likelihood of achieving the outcome? Think in terms of, What resources and multidisciplinary approaches might help? Then take appropriate action.

Practice Exercises: Determining a Comprehensive Plan/Updating the Plan

Example responses are on page 259.
1. Consider each of the expected outcomes and corresponding patient data and decide whether the outcome has been achieved, partially achieved, or not achieved.
   a. **Expected outcome:** Will be ready for discharge by day three after surgery as evidenced by ability to relate how to manage wound

packing. **Data:** Patient says that managing wound packing shouldn't be his concern and feels he's incapable of doing so.

b. **Expected outcome:** Will drink at least 4 quarts of fluid as evidenced by keeping a written record of fluid intake. **Data:** Patient's record indicates 5 quarts of fluid intake daily.

c. **Expected outcome:** The baby will be discharged home with parents able to perform CPR. **Data:** Father demonstrates CPR well. Mother has trouble establishing airway.

2. Develop a comprehensive plan, identifying two priority diagnoses for the following scenario. Include an overall expected discharge outcome, outcomes for each diagnosis, and specific interventions.

Scenario

It's Monday. You admit Mrs. Edmunds, who has just suffered anaphylactic shock after a bee sting. She is expected to be discharged by Wednesday, June 29. The doctor gives Mrs. Edmunds an emergency epinephrine injection kit and tells her, "The nurse will teach you how to use it." Mrs. Edmunds still has hives all over her body and says her itching feet are driving her crazy. You find that placing her feet in cool water every so often helps her discomfort. She is still slightly wheezy from the bee sting reaction.

When you ask her about using the injection kit, she replies, "No way!" Her husband, who is retired, says, "I'll be glad to learn." It's decided that it's satisfactory to discharge Mrs. Edmunds on June 29, with her husband able to demonstrate how to give epinephrine in an emergency. ◆

3. Suppose you're using the critical path on page 266. Today is your patient's first postoperative day. You assess the patient and find out that she is voiding frequently in small amounts. What should you do and why?

4. Suppose you're reviewing someone's chart to determine if a comprehensive plan of care is present. What four care plan components will you be looking for?

5. Get an actual patient chart. Determine whether the four components of the plan of care are recorded (no response for this one).

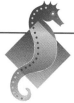

Critical Moments

JUST WHO IS AN EXPERT ANYWAY?

If a little knowledge is dangerous, there are a lot of dangerous people walking around out there. Don't just assume others know more than you do, even if they sound knowledgeable: Ask questions, seek clarification, and think independently (e.g., ask, Where might I find a reference to add to my knowledge of this?)

COMPLETE THIS SECTION FOR ALL PATIENTS
UNLESS SPECIFIC ASSESSMENT IS WARRANTED

Patient Name: _____

CULTURE/RELIGIOUS/SPIRITUAL	ACTION TAKEN
Religious Preference: ☐None ☐Catholic ☐Protestant ☐Jewish ☐Other_____	☐ Refer to Chaplain
Any special cultural, spiritual or religious needs while in the hospital? ☐No ☐Yes Specify: _____	☐ Other Referral _____
Would like to see the hospital Chaplain/Other _____ ☐No ☐Yes	

SOCIAL/DISCHARGE PLANNING	ACTION TAKEN
☐Lives Alone ☐ Stairs ☐ Bathroom on same level as living quarters ☐Lives with spouse/significant other/family/caretaker ☐Lives in nursing home/assisted living ❶ ☐Compromised in ADLs and /or lack of support network ❶ ☐Special discharge needs ❶_____ ☐Insurance concerns ☐Received supports prior to admission: ☐unknown ☐home care ☐med equip ❶ ☐Patient plans to be discharged to: _____ ☐Discharge Transportation (Name) _____ (Phone#)_____ ☐Unable to return to previous living arrangement ❷ ☐Financial concerns ❷ ☐Evidence of physical/emotional abuse or neglect or domestic violence ❷ ☐Current substance abuse ❷ **☐No discharge planning needs identified**	☐Assist with ADLs ☐Patient Education ❶☐ Refer to Case Manager Referral ❷☐ Refer to Social Work Referral

EDUCATION NEEDS ASSESSMENT

Learning Readiness: ☐Willing to Learn ☐Unable to Learn
Barriers to Learning: ☐No Barriers ☐Cognitive ☐Cultural ☐Educational ☐Emotional
☐Language ☐Motivational ☐Financial ☐Physical ☐Religious ☐Refuses at this time
☐Comments/Other_____

Plans to Overcome Barriers to Education: ☐Family involvement ☐Reinforcement ☐Written Materials
☐Audiovisual Aids ☐Interpreter ☐Other_____

Specific Educational Needs: ☐Disease Process ☐Activity Level ☐Diet ☐Procedures ☐Hygiene
☐Medications (including Drug and Food Interactions) ☐Medical Equipment/Assistive Devices
☐Skin/Ostomy (Certified wound Ostomy Continence notified)
☐Other _____

Teaching to be directed primarily to: ☐Patient ☐Family ☐Other_____

Patient Folder Given? ☐Yes ☐No

Clinical Pathway Initiated? ☐ Yes ☐ See Flowsheet/ Progress Note

Correct ID band in place ☐ Yes
☐ Patient Handbook/Patient's Rights and Responsibilities reviewed.
☐ Patient/family oriented to room

Completed by RN:_____ Date: _____ Time:_____

Reviewed by RN:_____ Date:_____ Time:_____

Figure 5-1 ◆ Example pre-printed assessment tool. Source: Health, Jefferson System, Philadelphia.

Main Line Health

❼ Jefferson Health System

☐ Paoli Hospital   ☐ Lankenau Hospital
☐ Bryn Mawr Hospital

INITIAL PATIENT ASSESSMENT

Complete shaded area   **OR**   ☐ See 24 Hour Flow Sheet   ☐ See E.D. Triage Sheet
☐ See Critical Care Pathway

Date:	Time:	Height:	Weight:	Language spoken other than English:

Primary Care Physician: _____   Specialist: _____

Vital Signs Temp _____ P _____ RR _____ BP _____
O2 Sat _____ O2 _____ RA _____

Reason for procedure/hospitalization: _____

Procedure: _____

Allergies: Drug/Food/Latex/Tape/Dyes   ☐ None Known

ALLERGIES	REACTION	ALLERGIES	REACTION	ALLERGIES	REACTION

ALL MEDICATIONS ☐SENT HOME ☐TO PHARMACY (include over-the-counter drugs, vitamins, diet pills, and herbals currently being taken)	Dose	Route	Frequency	Last Taken	Reason for Taking/Comments
1.					
2.					
3.					
4.					
5.					
6.					
7.					
8.					
9.					
10.					
11.					

Recent Aspirin/ Ibuprofen/ Anti-inflammatory/ Vitamin E/ Blood Thinner: _____

| PAST SURGICAL HISTORY |

Past surgical History: _____

Previous anesthesia: ☐ General   ☐ Spinal   ☐ Other _____

Problems with Anesthesia? _____

Blood Donations- This Admission   ☐ Autologous   ☐ Direct Donor   ☐ None

MLH 900-177 (1/01)

Figure 5-1 ◆ Cont'd

Patient Name: _____   MR #: _____

HEALTH HISTORY	Check Applicable Boxes Only

NEUROLOGIC
- ☐CVA/TIA
- ☐Speech Difficulty
- ☐Swallowing/Choking
- ☐Blackouts/Fainting/Vertigo
- ☐Seizures
- ☐Migraine/Headaches
- ☐Numbness/Tingling
- ☐Confusion
- ☐Memory Changes
- ☐Head Injury
- ☐Other_____
- ☐**No identified problems**

CARDIOVASCULAR
- ☐High Blood Pressure/Low Blood Pressure
- ☐Aneurysm
- ☐Heart Attack
- ☐Heart Failure
- ☐Murmur
- ☐Chest Pain/Angina
- ☐Irregular Pulse
- ☐Circulation Problem
- ☐Phlebitis/Clots
- ☐Pacemaker/Defib.
- ☐High Cholesterol
- ☐Other_____
- ☐**No identified problems**

RESPIRATORY
- ☐Emphysema/Bronchitis
- ☐Asthma
- ☐Shortness of breath
- ☐TB
- ☐Pneumonia
- ☐Seasonal/Environmental
  Allergies
- ☐Snoring/Apnea
- ☐Breathing Devices:_____
- ☐Other_____
- ☐**No identified problems**

GASTROINTESTINAL
- ☐Hiatal Hernia/Reflux
- ☐Hepatitis
- ☐Ulcers
- ☐Crohn's/Colitis
- ☐Gall Bladder Disease
- ☐Irritable Bowels
- ☐Diverticular Disease
- ☐Ostomy _____
- ☐Recent change in bowel habits
- ☐Blood in stool
- ☐Last B.M. _____
- ☐Other_____
- ☐**No identified problems**

Comments: _____

MUSCULOSKELETAL
- ☐Arthritis
- ☐Muscle Weakness
- ☐Joint Replacement _____
- ☐Spinal Problems
- ☐Other _____
- ☐**No identified problems**

METABOLIC
- ☐Diabetes Type: _____
- ☐Thyroid
- ☐Hypoglycemia
- ☐Anemia
- ☐Other_____
- ☐**No identified problems**

GENITOURINARY
- ☐Kidney Stones
- ☐Prostate Problems
- ☐Ostomy
- ☐Burning/Urgency Frequency
- ☐Blood in Urine
- ☐Kidney Failure
- ☐Dialysis
- ☐Breast Masses/
  Tenderness/Discharge
- ☐LMP _____
- ☐Possibility of Pregnancy
- ☐Breast Feeding
- ☐Other_____
- ☐**No identified problems**

PSYCHOSOCIAL
- ☐Alcohol use _____
- ☐Drug use _____
- ☐Panic/Anxiety Attacks
- ☐Depression
- ☐Physical/ Psychological Abuse
- ☐Tobacco use _____
- ☐Claustrophobia
- ☐ADD
- ☐Growth and Development
  not appropiate for age
- ☐Bereavement
- ☐Other_____
- ☐**No identified problems**

MISCELLANEOUS
- ☐Vision Changes
- ☐Hearing Deficit
- ☐Glaucoma/Cataracts
- ☐Blood/Bleeding Disorders
- ☐CA _____
- ☐Skin Problems
- ☐Hearing Deficit
- ☐Infectious Disease/STD
- ☐Head Circumference _____
  (if appropriate)
- ☐Immunizations up to date ($< \, > = 18$ yrs)
- ☐Other_____
- ☐**No identified problems**

Comments: _____

Needs Assessment

☐ Orthodontic appliance	☐ Prosthesis	☐ Religious Items
☐ Dentures _____	☐ Glasses/Contacts	☐ Crutches/Walker/Cane/Wheelchair
☐ Hearing Aid	☐ Hairpiece	☐ Other _____

CURRENT PAIN	CARE OR LEARNING NEED
☐ Denies Pain Duration of Pain? _____ What Controls the Pain:_____ _____ What is the Impact on ADL's? _____ _____ X = Pain O = Wound	☐ Pain Management ☐ Patient Education Indicate in the diagram where pain is located and label the intensity 1-10, with "1" meaning minimal pain to "10" being the worst pain. **INTEGUMENTARY** ☐ Skin problems ☐ Old scars ☐ Rash ☐ Ecchymosis ☐ Tatoos ☐ Dry skin ☐ Pressure Ulcers ☐ Lower leg/foot wounds **☐ No identified problems**

Advance Directives	☐ NA (Patient < 18 years old) ☐ Unable to Assess	
Does the patient have an advance directive?	☐ Yes	☐ No ☐ Information Given ☐ Information Declined

If "Yes" copy in current chart?
   ☐ Obtain from previous chart
	☐ Yes	☐ No Follow-up action:
		   ☐ Family to obtain copy for record
		   ☐ Patient to formulate another advance directive
		   (sample in "It's Up To You")
		   ☐ Substance as stated by patient: _____
		   _____
		   ☐ Patient declines stating content
		   ☐ Patient/family declines to bring, and/or complete advance directive information

If "No" does the patient wish to make an advance directive?	☐ Yes- Refer to Social Work	☐ No

Figure 5-1 ◆ Cont'd

COMPLETE THIS SECTION FOR INPATIENTS ONLY
UNLESS SPECIFIC ASSESSMENT IS WARRANTED

Patient Name: _____   MR #: _____

NUTRITIONAL STATUS □ No Identified Problems	ACTION/TAKEN
If any of the following are present, send computer order to Nutrition Services □ Any Specific diet and/or restrictions ❶ □ Unintentional Weight Loss/Gain ≥10 lbs in the Last 6 Months ❶ □ Vomiting /Diarrhea for the Last 3 Days or Longer ❶ □ Poor Appetite for the Last 5 Days or Longer ❶ □ Swallowing Difficulties resulting in inadequate intake ❶ □ Newly Diagnosed Pt with Diabetes Need for Education ❶,❷ □ Pressure Ulcer Stage II or greater ❶,❸ □ Dialysis ❶ □ New to modified Diet and Needs Education ❶	❶ □ Nutrition Referral ❷ □ Diabetes Educator Referral ❸ □ Certified Wound Ostomy Continence Nurse Referral

RESPIRATORY ASSESSMENT □ No Identified Problems	ACTION TAKEN
□ Patient is pre-op for upper abdominal or thoracic surgery <u>and</u> has a history of Emphysema, Bronchitis, Asthma, or Pulmonary Fibrosis	□ Respiratory Care Referred

FUNCTIONAL STATUS ASSESSMENT	Independent	Some Assist	Total Assist	ACTION TAKEN
Feeding				□ Assist with ADL's
Bathing				
Dressing				
Toileting				
Transfers(bed to chair, to/from toilet)				□ Patient / Family Education
Walking/ Use of Wheelchair				

If any of the following are present, refer as follows:

□ Physician Order Requested For:

OCCUPATIONAL THERAPY   □ No Needs Identified
□ Condition Resulted in difficulty in use of one or both arms.
□ Decreased Ability for Self-Care That Could Be Helped With Therapy.
□ Physically Unable To Feed Self

     ❏ OCCUPATIONAL THERAPY

PHYSICAL THERAPY   □ No Needs Identified
□ Condition has Resulted in Walking, and Transfer That Could Be Resolved with Therapy.
□ Condition has Resulted in Decreased Strength and/or Range of Motion of arms and legs.
□ Condition has Resulted in Acute Increase in Muscle or Back Pain.

     ❏ PHYSICAL THERAPY

SPEECH THERAPY   □ No Needs Identified
□ Difficulty Swallowing or Signs of Choking While Drinking/Eating.
□ Diagnosis of Stroke, Myasthenia Gravis and Multiple Intubations.
□ Unable to Follow Simple Instructions for Daily Care and/or Unable to Communicate Wants and Needs.

     ❏ SPEECH/LANGUAGE PATHOLOGY

FALL RISK ASSESSMENT* Low Risk 0-20 Moderate Risk 25-60 High Risk 65-100 *See Patient Safety: Fall Safety Program		
Fall Assessment Indicators	**Weight Score**	**Assessment Score**
Admission or transfer	5	
History of falls	20	
Recent change in functional mobility	20	
Alteration in elimination	20	
Diagnosis/Medication which effects cognition/mobility/balance	10	
Confusion/impairment of judgement/forgetful/agitated and/or non-compliant	20	
Sensory/Visual/Perceptual impairment (unrelated to above)	5	
TOTAL SCORE	100	

Figure 5-1 ◆ Cont'd

References

1. E-mail communication. (June 2002).
2. Ladewig, P., London, M., Moberly, S., & Olds, S. (2001). *Contemporary maternal-newborn nursing care* (5th ed.). Upper Saddle River, NJ: Prentice Hall.
3. Carpenito, L. (2002). *Nursing diagnosis: Application to clinical practice* (9th ed.). Philadelphia: Lippincott Williams & Wilkins.

See comprehensive bibliography beginning on page 286.

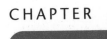

Applied Critical Thinking: Mastering Common Workplace Skills

THIS CHAPTER at a Glance ...

1. Navigating and Facilitating Change (page 190)
2. Communicating Bad News (page 194)
3. Dealing with Complaints Constructively (page 196)
4. Developing Empowered Partnerships (page 199)
5. Giving and Taking Feedback (page 204)
6. Managing Conflict Constructively (page 207)
7. Managing Your Time (page 213)
8. Preventing and Dealing with Mistakes Constructively (page 218)
9. Transforming a Group into a Team (page 227)
10. Accessing and Using Information Effectively (page 233)
11. Outcome-Focused Writing (Writing to Get Results) (page 238)

Read the Learning Outcomes listed at the beginning of each skill in this section. If you can readily achieve them, skip that particular skill. If you can achieve them all, skip this chapter.

How to Best Use This Chapter

This chapter helps you gain key intellectual skills that are required when working in any position that's highly relational (any position that demands a lot of interaction with others). When you know how to build positive relationships with patients and other professionals, you spend less time getting sidetracked by interpersonal and "human nature" problems—and more time fully engaged in progress.

Each skill is presented in the following format: (1) Name of the Skill, (2) Definition of the Skill, (3) Learning Outcomes, (4) Thinking Critically about the Skill, (5) How to Accomplish the Skill, and (6) Critical Thinking Exercises. To complete many of the critical thinking exercises, you should partner with at least one other person. Content is presented in a way that can help you plan a seminar for each skill to promote in-depth discussion and thought. As part of the seminar requirements, each participant should read at least two up-to-date articles on the topic. **Note:** Because the Critical Thinking exercises are intended to be done in groups, there are no example responses in the Response Key in the back of the book.

1. NAVIGATING AND FACILITATING CHANGE

Definition

Knowing how to chart a course to make necessary changes, and helping others to do the same.

Learning Outcomes

After you study this information and complete the accompanying exercises you should be able to:
◆ Explain your reaction when faced with change.
◆ Identify strategies to help you navigate change.
◆ Describe how to facilitate change in others.

Thinking Critically about Change

I can't think of a saying that describes the need for change better than this one: Even if you're on the right track, you still get hit by the train if you don't keep moving. Knowing how to plot a course through the many changes we face on a daily basis is essential to thriving in this rapidly changing world. When you know how to navigate change–and how to help others do the same–you can move more quickly from the commonly associated feelings of disruption and frustration to a point where you feel a sense of progress and accomplishment.

How to Navigate and Facilitate Change

This section first addresses navigating change, and then it addresses facilitating change.

NAVIGATING CHANGE

◆ When first faced with change, suspend judgment and fairly explore reasons for the required change. Navigating change doesn't mean embracing change uncritically–it means clarifying the pros and cons and making a conscious, reasoned decision about whether change is worthwhile.
◆ Curb the tendency to be influenced by the natural desire to keep the status quo because it's easy and comfortable.
◆ Make sure you understand why the change is being made and how you feel about it. If you can get something out of the change, it will help you accept it. If you have strong feelings against making the change, you need to explore and work through them.
◆ Identify barriers to making the change and find ways to deal with them. For example, if you must start using new equipment, making yourself a "cheat sheet" can help you remember key information.

- Ask for help. If you express the problems you're having, others may be able to help and you may also identify common concerns that are bothering everyone.
- Expect the following natural sequence of events commonly associated with adapting to change:
  - **Losing focus.** Expect some confusion, disorientation, and forgetfulness at first. You may be unsure about boundaries and responsibilities. Ask for clarification, keep notes, and use to-do lists.
  - **Denial.** You may want to minimize or deny the effect the change has on you. However, connecting with and dealing with your feelings will help you move forward. Acknowledge how you feel about what you lose and gain by making the change.
  - **Anger/Depression.** If you feel angry, discouraged, or frustrated:
    - Vent your anger in a safe place. Be careful with *whom, how,* and *where* you ventilate. Your words can come back to haunt you. Find someone who'll listen empathetically without being affected by your feelings (e.g., someone who has gone through the change you're experiencing, not someone who also is struggling and who may be pulled down by your negativity).
    - Use stress management strategies (e.g., exercise helps diffuse anger and frustration).
    - Keep away from negative people because their thoughts might influence you.
  - **Acceptance.** Stay focused on what you'll gain from making the change. Be patient with yourself, let go of the past, and take it one step at a time. Make a conscious effort to think critically and not emotionally.
  - **Moving forward.** Seek opportunities to use the new skills and procedures you've learned. Celebrate small successes, recognizing how far you've come and what you learned along the way. Share your experience with those who may not have come as far as you have.
- Remember to represent your organization positively in public, even if you don't feel that way at the moment.

FACILITATING CHANGE IN OTHERS

- Including key stakeholders, determine how the change will impact those involved. Be clear about the positives and negatives from their perspectives.
- Clearly articulate both the required changes and the expected benefits.
- Clarify changes in roles and responsibilities.
- Get the backing of formal and informal group leaders and try to win them toward the change (they can help deter the process).

◆ Allow people to explore how the change will affect their daily lives. Encourage their involvement in finding ways to make the change easier.

◆ Convey an understanding of negative feelings and extra work associated with having to make a change. Provide necessary resources and support (for example, technical and decision support) until the change has been fully implemented.

◆ Ask for ownership of responsibility for change (both leaders and subordinates own some of the work).

◆ Involving key players, identify barriers to making the change and find ways to deal with them. For example, if the staff is expected to take time to practice using a new computer system, provide extra personnel to do ordinary chores.

◆ Be clear about time lines: Key players must know exactly what change is expected to occur and by when.

◆ Be patient. Going through the stages of adapting to change takes time.

Other Perspectives

HOW TO CHANGE THE WORLD
"We must be the change we wish to see in the world."

—Mohandas Ghandi

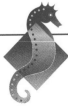

Critical Moments

TRANSFORM RATHER THAN CONFORM
When facilitating change, aim to transform rather than conform. Inspire, show benefits, encourage, and support. When people are transformed, they change because they want to.

CRITICAL THINKING EXERCISES

In a group or in a journal entry:
1. Share your best and worst experiences with navigating and facilitating change and what factors made them your best and worst experiences.
2. Describe a personal or work change that you experienced that wasn't of your choice (for example, moving, changing job description).
   ◆ Think about how you felt at the time and the effect it had on your ability to make the change.
   ◆ Identify some things you could have done to make the change easier.

CRITICAL THINKING EXERCISES—cont'd

3. Share a time you tried to help someone else change.
   ◆ How successful were you?
   ◆ What, if anything, would you do differently?
4. Study Box 6-1 (Four Ways We Change). Explain why paradigm change facilitates critical thinking.
5. Explain the difference between change that transforms and change that conforms.
6. Determine whether you can achieve the Learning Outcomes at the beginning of this skill.

Box 6-1 **FOUR WAYS WE CHANGE***

Four Ways We Change
1. Pendulum change: I was wrong before, but now I'm right.
2. Change by exception: I'm right, except for ... .
3. Incremental change: I was almost right before, but now I'm right.
4. Paradigm change: What I knew before was partially right. What I know now is more right but only part of what I'll know tomorrow.

Paradigm Change Is Transformational
Paradigm change combines what's useful about old ways with what's useful about new ways and keeps us open to looking for even better ways.
We realize:
◆ Our previous views were only part of the picture.
◆ What we now know is only part of what we'll know later.
◆ Change is no longer threatening: It enlarges and enriches.
◆ The unknown can then be friendly and interesting.
◆ Each insight smooths the road, making the change process easier.

*Adapted and summarized from Ferguson, M. (1980). *Aquarian conspiracy: Personal and social transformation in our time.* New York: G. P. Putnam's Sons.

Recommended Reading

American Association of Critical Care Nurses. *Influencing practice: understand the change process.* Retrieved May 31, 2002 from http://www.aacn.org/AACN/aacnnews.nsf/ ff1487bfe89b77df882565a6006cfc3f/8423a3efbe82646588256a930054d4d6?OpenDocument# influence.

Briles, J. (1998). To embrace or not to embrace change. *The Journal of Nurse Empowerment,* Spring, 43–46.

Harrington, S. (2002). How RNs can meet the challenge of self-change. Retrieved May 31, 2002 from http://community.nursingspectrum.com/MagazineArticles/article.cfm?AID=5928.

Johnson, S., & Blanchard, K. (1998). *Who moved my cheese?* New York: Putnam Publishing Group.

Menix, K. (2000). Educating to manage the accelerated change environment effectively: Part 1. *Journal for Nurses in Staff Development,* 16(6),282–288.

2. COMMUNICATING BAD NEWS

Definition

Knowing how to convey honesty, empathy, and responsibility when giving someone information that will have a negative impact on them.

Learning Outcomes

After you study this information and complete the accompanying exercises you should be able to:

◆ Explain what can happen when you avoid giving bad news.
◆ Identify strategies to minimize the impact of bad news.
◆ Determine how you can reduce your stress when faced with giving bad news.

Thinking Critically about Bad News

No one likes having to be the messenger with bad news. All too often people who have bad news tend to avoid this unpleasant chore altogether, making things worse. When you communicate bad news at an appropriate time, in an appropriate place, and with honesty, empathy, and responsibility, you can soften the blow by minimizing the common feelings of anger, disappointment, and betrayal.

How you handle giving bad news can make the difference between escalating an already difficult situation and building positive relationships in spite of adversity. Using the following strategies can help reduce your stress and give you more brain power to focus on achieving a positive outcome.

How to Communicate Bad News

Steps	Example
1. Give the bad news in a timely way. Offer an apology and don't try to obscure the situation.	I'm sorry to tell you we won't be able to do your x-ray today.
2. Showing concern, explain what happened and why.	Somehow you were scheduled in our book for next week, but your appointment card says today. I'm not sure how this happened, but I'll find out.
3. Present alternative solutions and give pros and cons of each.	I could schedule the x-ray for later today, but we get better pictures if you fast for 12 hours before the x-ray. I realize you'd have to go home and come back, and that you'd like

Continued

How to Communicate Bad News (cont'd)

Steps	Example
	to get it over with. I think it's worth waiting to be sure we get a good quality x-ray.
4. Recommend a course of action. Include: (a) How the plan addresses the problem, and (b) How the plan addresses hardships resulting from what happened.	I think the best solution is to schedule the x-ray as soon as possible. Since you've already had enough problems, I'll do my best to schedule you whenever it's convenient for you. I'll also find out who made this mistake and see what we can do to prevent this from happening again.
5. Reaffirm your goals and vision for the future. Include: (a) Key points that give confidence to those involved, and (b) Time frame for expected results.	We're here to serve you the best way we can. Soon we'll have a system that allows you to confirm appointments over the phone. We hope to have the system in place by May. Everyone will be encouraged to call and confirm their appointments when they get home.
6. Follow up to see if results were satisfactory.	I'll send your name to our community relations department. They will call you to see if everything was resolved to your satisfaction. Please feel free to call and discuss anything you'd like with them as well. We want you to feel satisfied with your experience with us. Please let me know if you still have problems.

CRITICAL THINKING EXERCISES

Instructions: In a group, in a personal journal, or both:

1. Describe:
   ◆ Your best and worst experiences with how someone gave you bad news.
   ◆ The emotions you feel when giving bad news.
   ◆ How people you know have responded to bad news situations and why you think they responded that way.

CRITICAL THINKING EXERCISES—cont'd

2. Imagine you and five classmates or colleagues are responsible for making a presentation. The night before the presentation, your computer crashes and you lose your part of the presentation. How will you tell the group this?
3. On a computer that has Microsoft PowerPoint software, write a letter communicating imaginary bad news using the "Communicating Bad News" wizard.
4. Determine whether you can achieve the Learning Outcomes at the beginning of this skill.

Recommended Reading

Goleman, D. (2000). *Working with emotional intelligence.* New York: Bantam Doubleday Dell Publishing Group.

Rager, P. (1998). Emotional intelligence and the management edge. *Nursing Spectrum (FL ED),* 8(3),3.

Lusardi, P. *Research Corner: Communication: What Is the Patient's Reality?* Retrieved July 2, 2002 from: http://www.aacn.org/AACN/aacnnews.nsf/ff1487bfe89b77df882565a6006cfc3f/4b21707cd865d06d88256a15007947e1?OpenDocument#research.

Martin, B. *Social Skills Training Part 1: Empathy* Retrieved July 2, 2002 from: http://www.onlinece.net/courses.asp?course=106&action=view.

Weisinger, H. (1998). *Emotional intelligence at work.* San Francisco: Jossey-Bass.

3. DEALING WITH COMPLAINTS CONSTRUCTIVELY

Definition

Using complaints as an opportunity to improve customer satisfaction.

Learning Outcomes

After you study this information and complete the accompanying exercises you should be able to:
◆ Explain the value of complaints.
◆ Express more confidence about dealing with complaints.
◆ Deal with complaints more confidently and competently.

Thinking Critically about Complaints

Thinking about dealing with complaints makes most of us squirm. However, if we recognize that complaints are useful, maybe we can change our attitude and greet this challenge in more positive ways. Think about the last time you complained about service. Was it just because you wanted your situation corrected, or did you think it might help them improve their service for others? Listen to complaints because they're valuable and can help you:

◆ Correct problems before they become worse or happen to someone else.

◆ Identify trends in unmet needs of consumers.

◆ Find out about complaints before people start complaining to others.

Like all businesses, health care organizations thrive when consumers are happy. Satisfied consumers tell others about their experience and return as needed. The opposite is also true: If your consumers are unhappy, they tell others and they take their business elsewhere.

When someone complains, take time to listen and do something about it.

Other Perspectives

Do You Listen Well Enough?

"… patient-driven data indicate that the most effective communication focuses on a patient's self-focused needs, worries, and concerns. In fact, in a series of studies, between 13% and 100% of patients worried about an inability to communicate their concerns. The ability not only to interact but also to be understood appears to be key to a patient's contentment[†] and confidence. … Patients emphasize that being understood and having their needs met are the most crucial element for patient satisfaction and security. …"[*]

—Paula Lusardi, RN, PhD, CCNS, CCRN, Member,
American Association of Critical Care Nurses
Research Work Group

How to Deal with Complaints

◆ **Start off on the right foot.** Don't take things personally. Assume there's a very good reason for the complaints (although these reasons may be unclear at first).

---

[*]Lusardi, P. Research corner: communication: What is the patient's reality? *AACN News, 18*(3)3,5,12. Retrieved July 2, 2002 from http://www.aacn.org/AACN/aacnnews.nsf/ff1487bfe89b77df882565a6006cfc3f/4b21707cd8 65d06d88256a15007947e1?OpenDocument#research.

◆ **Take a deep breath and remain calm in the face of anger.** People requiring health care often have extenuating circumstances that cause them to have a "short fuse." Some examples:
  ● Previous bad experience with health care providers or treatment plans.
  ● Effects of illness or disability on self, family, and work.
  ● Problems of being in limbo (the patient may not be responding as quickly or favorably as expected).
  ● Family reaction to illness or disability.
◆ **Listen actively** to figure out what the person really values and needs.
  ● Give the person your full attention.
  ● Repeat what you hear to be sure that you're clear on the issues.
  ● Aim to give the person what he needs or values if at all possible (this requires that you get a clear understanding from your boss about what rules you can bend or break to immediately resolve issues).
  ● If you come in late to the situation, remain quiet, listen, and ask to verify your understanding of the problem.
◆ **Focus on the issues** and try to learn from them.
◆ **Swallow your pride**, offer an apology, and avoid weak excuses (e.g., we're shorthanded, nobody's perfect). You'll move more quickly to a solution.
◆ **Involve the person** in problem solving (ask for solutions).
◆ **Take an immediate step to resolve the problem.** Explain what you're going to do and let her feel like they're winning in some way.
◆ **Keep the person informed** (e.g., I promise to let you know the minute I know more about this).
◆ **Report and record special needs.** Let your supervisor know about all major complaints or incidents.
◆ **Follow up** to see if solutions are working.
◆ **If anger explodes**:
  ● Keep your own anger in check.
  ● Don't defend yourself. Listen completely; focus keenly on what is being said.
  ● Keep in mind that some people cope in ways you consider negative (abrasive, manipulative).
  ● Think about whether having your manager come and talk with the person would help.

Related Skills: Communicating Bad News, Managing Conflicts Constructively, Giving and Taking Feedback, Developing Partnerships.

CRITICAL THINKING EXERCISES

In a group or in a journal entry:

1. Address the feelings associated with making complaints (e.g., anger, guilt, frustration).
2. Give an example of a time when you thought about complaining but decided it just wasn't worth it. How did this make you feel, and whom do you think lost in this situation?
3. Describe your best and worst experience with making a complaint.
4. Explain how you usually deal with other people's complaints, and then think of some ways you could improve your response.
5. Discuss the implications of the following Other Perspectives.

 Other Perspectives

GIVE FIVE-STAR SERVICE

"Treat every patient or customer as though they were your favorite celebrity, hero, friend, neighbor, or your grandma."

—Author Unknown

6. Determine whether you can achieve the Learning Outcomes at the beginning of this skill.

Recommended Reading

Adams, J. (2002). Exceeding customer expectations. *Advance for Nurses (2FL)24*, 27–28.

Goleman, D. (2000). *Working with emotional intelligence.* New York: Bantam Doubleday Dell Publishing Group.

Weisinger, H. (1998). *Emotional intelligence at work.* San Francisco: Jossey-Bass.

Wetter, D. *Service through the customer's eyes.* Retrieved from http://www.corexcel.com/Customer_Service_Web_Handout.doc.

Wolf, Z., Brennan, R., Ferchau, L., Magee, M., et al. (1997). Creating and implementing guidelines on caring for difficult patients: A research utilization project. *MEDSURG NURSING,* 6(3), 137–147.

4. DEVELOPING EMPOWERED PARTNERSHIPS

Definition

Building mutually beneficial relationships based on the belief that people have the right and responsibility to make their own choices and grow in their own way.[1]

Learning Outcomes

After you study this information and complete the accompanying exercises you should be able to:

◆ Compare and contrast a Parental Model* and an Empowered Partnership Model.

◆ Explain the benefits of empowered partnerships.

◆ Begin to build empowered partnerships.

Thinking Critically about Empowered Partnerships

Developing empowered partnerships with peers, colleagues, and patients requires a shift in thinking from a Parental Model (*I'll take care of you*) to an Empowered Partnership Model (*It's your life—you have rights and responsibilities as well as I do, and we both should grow and learn from our experience together*). Table 6-1 lists phrases that exemplify these two models.

Many nurses with excellent intentions still function in a parental way. They haven't made the shift in thinking to an empowered partnership, which is the key to achieving quality outcomes and satisfaction. As nurses, we must encourage and empower peers, coworkers, patients, and families to take as much responsibility as possible for managing their own lives. This is when true growth happens.

How to Develop Empowered Partnerships

1. **Be sure you can explain the concept of an empowered partnership.** Although you can't completely balance power in all relationships, the aim of an empowered partnership is to balance the power as much as possible.

   Examples of Empowered Partnerships

Nurse–patient/client	Staff nurse–nurse manager
Teacher–student	Nurse–pharmacist
Nurse–unlicensed workers	Nurse–employer
Nurse–nurse	Nurse–physician

2. To establish a partnership the partners must agree to the following statements:

   ◆ We're both clear about our joint purpose, and we're both responsible.†

---

*Some people call this a Paternal Model. "Parental" is used to avoid sexism.

†In the context of the nurse-patient relationship, these statements aren't always so: Nurses are often held more accountable than patients. Nurses don't have the right to say no if it jeopardizes patients' health (they must find a replacement). Patients often have few choices about where they are.

Table 6-1 PARENTAL VERSUS EMPOWERED PARTNERSHIP MODEL

Phrases Exemplifying Parental	Phrases Exemplifying Empowered Partnership
◆ I want to look after you.	◆ How can I empower you to be able to be independent?
◆ I know what's best for you.	◆ You know yourself best. Tell me what you'd like to see happen, what's most important to you.
◆ You should do as I say.	◆ I want you to be able to make informed choices.
◆ I'm responsible for you.	◆ We share a common purpose and we're both responsible for what happens.

◆ I can be trusted; I promise to be honest.
◆ We're each responsible for our own emotional well-being (if I feel bad about something, it's my responsibility to do something about it).[†]
◆ We should make decisions together as much as possible.
◆ We both have the right to say no, so long as no harm is done.[†]
◆ We'll both agree to rules for resolving conflict between us.
◆ We both can expect to grow and learn from our experience.
◆ I choose to be here, so nobody's to blame.[†]
◆ We're both responsible for the outcomes (consequences) of our actions.[†]
◆ If one of us sees the other engage in unsafe or unethical conduct, we have the responsibility to address it appropriately.

3. An empowered partnership requires choosing to:
   ◆ Rise to the challenge of taking charge over the comfort of remaining dependent
   ◆ Give up some of the power; take calculated, thoughtful risks; and be willing to do the work needed to be independent
4. An empowered partnership also requires:[2]
   ◆ Nonjudgmental acceptance
   ◆ Space for self-expression
   ◆ Structure for conflict resolution
   ◆ Respect for each other's boundaries

[†]See previous page for footnote.

- ◆ Support and encouragement for growth in the areas where one is limited
- ◆ Coaching skills that transform (coaching that truly affects the learner's attitudes and skills)
- ◆ Growth of partners

5. Many people are uncomfortable in an empowered partnership for the following reasons:
   - ◆ They are used to being taken care of and aren't accustomed to taking responsibility.
   - ◆ They are unwilling to accept the responsibility that comes with power.
   - ◆ They are unwilling to give up some of the power they're accustomed to having.
   - ◆ They haven't made the required shift in thinking (they don't truly believe in the benefits of partnership).

6. Gently coach those who aren't accustomed to the roles and responsibilities of being in a partnership. Change takes time.

Other Perspectives

PATIENTS AS PARTNERS

"Patients have to be partners, equally responsible for treatment."

–Tommy LaSorda, former Los Angeles Dodgers manager

TEACHER-STUDENT PARTNERSHIPS

"(Many students believe) 'teacher knows what's best for me.' We think that the task of these leaders is to create an environment where we can live a life of safety and predictability. Dependency also holds those above us responsible for how we feel about ourselves (we want that positive feedback)."[3]

–Peter Block, Author and Consultant

NOT WHAT YOU KNOW, WHAT YOU SHARE

"What matters most to students is not how much you know, but rather how much you are willing to share. Your simplest actions and smallest words have the potential to influence their world forever. ... with very little effort, you can be viewed as a 'superstar' to a nursing student. They admire someone who loves being a nurse, cares about their patients, and is willing to share their experiences. We work every day with wonderful

Continued

nurses who want to dispel the myth that 'nurses eat their young.' No act of kindness will be forgotten. Remember, it takes a team to make a nurse."[4]

–Elizabeth Henneman, RN, PhD, CCNS, and Joan Roche, APRN, MS, CCRN

Related Skills: Giving and Taking Feedback, Managing Conflicts Constructively.

CRITICAL THINKING EXERCISES

Instructions: In a group, in a personal journal, or both:

1. Discuss how establishing partnerships with peers is different from establishing partnerships with patients.
2. Address how establishing an empowered partnership is affected by:
   ◆ The length of contact you have with a patient.
   ◆ The patient's health state.
   ◆ Growth and development (e.g., How do you partner with a child or an elderly person?)
3. Explain what is meant by the following statement: Partnership is an attitude as much as a model for relationships.
4. Ask a peer to partner with you in completing a course or accomplishing a goal. Agree from the beginning to follow the strategies listed in this section.
5. Determine whether you can achieve the Learning Outcomes at the beginning of this skill.

Recommended Reading

Austin, K., & Jurkovich, T. Forging partnerships in critical care. Retrieved July 1, 2002 from http://community.nursingspectrum.com/MagazineArticles/article.cfm?AID=284.

Block, P. (1996). *Stewardship: Choosing service over self-interest.* San Francisco: Berrett-Koehler.

Johnson. L. A partnership approach to the OR nursing shortage. Retrieved from http://community.nursingspectrum.com/MagazineArticles/article.cfm?AID=1987

Hansten, R., & Washburn, M. (1999). Outcome-based care: An alternative to extensive redesign. *ADVISOR for nurse executives, 15*(2), 12.

Paul, S. (1998). The advanced practice/staff nurse partnership: Building a winning team. *Critical Care Nurse, 18*(2), 92–97.

Tarapchak, P. (2002). Breath of fresh air. *Advance For Nurses, 3*(FL11), 21–22, 27.

5. GIVING AND TAKING FEEDBACK

Definition

Being able to give (and respond to) constructive criticism appropriately.

Learning Outcomes

After you study this information and complete the accompanying exercises you should be able to:
◆ Discuss the effect of emotional responses to criticism.
◆ Determine how you can improve your response to criticism.
◆ Identify strategies for giving constructive criticism.

Thinking Critically about Giving and Taking Feedback

How we think and behave is an extremely complex issue that's closely linked to self-esteem. Being told we could be better thinkers, improve in some way, or approach things differently often brings up intensely uncomfortable feelings of being wrong or not good enough. These gut reactions cloud key issues and paralyze our ability to be objective. Knowing how to provide constructive criticism in a supportive way can make the difference between alienating others and motivating them to improve. Knowing how to respond to criticism—to be objective and work through the negative aspects of criticism—reduces our stress and helps us grow.

Other Perspectives

IS IT CRITICISM OR ADVICE? WORDS MATTER!

"Replace the term constructive criticism *with words that express the intent to* help. *For example, say something like, 'May I give you some practical advice?' instead of 'May I give you some constructive criticism?' Try to replace* constructive *with* practical, helpful, *or* useful. *Try to replace* criticism *with* advice, recommendation, suggestion, observation, *or* opinion.*"

—Suggestions from My Workshop Participants

How to Give and Take Feedback*

GIVING FEEDBACK
◆ Be sensitive to personality differences (personalities of both the giver and the receiver greatly affect feedback).

---

*Strategies developed with the help of Barbara A. Musinski, RNC, BS, Independent Nursing Consultant, West Palm Beach, FL.

◆ Keep in mind that without mutual trust, feedback is unlikely to be viewed constructively.

◆ Give feedback frequently and in a timely way (this way it's viewed as being more sincere).

◆ Separate negative and positive feedback as much as possible. When you sandwich positive and negative in one statement, it dilutes the effects of both.

◆ Start with what's being done right (for example, Here are the things I see you do right). Next, focus on what could be improved (rather than on what's *wrong*).

◆ Remain fully engaged in the communication; listen actively to avoid misunderstandings and making false assumptions.

◆ Give positive feedback often to reward growth (for example, "catch" people being effective and surprise them with positive feedback).

◆ Be aware that constant negative feedback can hinder progress by making the person afraid of failure.

◆ Learn how to be assertive without being aggressive (see Box 6-2).

TAKING FEEDBACK

◆ Pay attention to how your emotions affect your ability to use the feedback in a positive way. For example, say to yourself, I'm getting upset. I'd better take a deep breath, calm down, and listen. If I work to be objective and not take things personally, I might learn something when I think about this later when I'm less stressed. Befriend criticism, evaluating it objectively. Someone wanted you to succeed or would not have bothered to share their thoughts.

◆ Ask yourself, Have I heard this same criticism from other people? If so, it's most likely true.

◆ Keep in mind that not all criticism is given constructively, but try to focus on what you can learn.

◆ If you agree with the criticism, acknowledge that the critic is right and begin to think about what you can do about it.

◆ Don't make excuses for yourself, don't be defensive, and sincerely try to see the benefits of the criticism.

◆ Practice personal feedback by monitoring your own behavior and paying attention to how others respond to you.

◆ Don't let false pride, rationalization, or other negative factors get in the way of your growth.

◆ Remember that no one's perfect, but we can all improve. Be prepared to expend some physical and emotional energy to change.

Box 6-2 BEING ASSERTIVE WITHOUT BEING AGGRESSIVE*

Assertive Behavior Means:
◆ Expressing your feelings, ideas, and needs calmly and openly
◆ Standing up for your own rights while showing respect for the rights of others
◆ Confronting fairly, being sensitive to when others feel threatened
◆ Valuing yourself, acting with confidence
◆ Owning responsibility and speaking with authority
◆ Building equal relationships and finding common goals

Using Assertive Behavior:
1. Accept the anger or discomfort you may have as your own. Do not blame others. You own the problem!
   ◆ Identify the key components of the situation and how you feel about them.
   ◆ How do you think others who are involved feel about the issue?
   ◆ Decide which of your needs were not met.
2. Be cognizant of your own behavior. Keep a lid on your emotions (no easy task!)
3. Meet privately with the person(s). Listen before you speak.
4. Use assertive listening (this is an intellectual function that requires patience, hard work, and practice).
   ◆ Actively commit to the other person; concentrate your attention so you accurately hear feelings, opinions, and wishes.
   ◆ Try to understand completely before responding.
   ◆ Paraphrase what the other person(s) have said to be sure you understand.
5. State your own feelings, thoughts, and needs clearly, in a nonthreatening way.
   ◆ Use eye contact, a direct body posture, and a controlled voice volume and tone.
   ◆ Using "I" messages, be clear about behavior that disturbs you and how you feel (for example, I was very embarrassed and hurt when I saw you walk away from our conversation. Rather than, You made me feel like such a jerk when ...).

*Developed with the help of Barbara A. Musinski, RN, C. BS, Independent Nursing Consultant, West Palm Beach, FL.

Other Perspectives

FEEDBACK: DEAL WITH IT

"Feedback is important. It helps us stay focused and on course. We all need to know how to give it, take it, deal with it, and accept it."[5]

−Barbara A. Musinski, RNC, BS

Related Skills: Managing Conflict Constructively (page 207).

CRITICAL THINKING EXERCISES—cont'd

Instructions: In a group, in a personal journal, or both:

1. Think about a time you tried to give feedback to someone to help him improve. Describe what happened and how you felt at the time. What, if anything, would you do differently if you had to do it again?

2. Think about a time someone gave you feedback. Explain what happened and how you felt at the time. Then follow up with your thoughts on the matter today. For example, what made things easier or harder? What did you learn in the long run?

3. Think about the following statement and decide what you would do if you had to give feedback to someone you don't get along with.

   Without mutual trust, feedback is unlikely to be viewed constructively.

4. Study the Other Perspectives on page 204. Practice using some other phrases for "I want to give you some constructive criticism."

5. Determine whether you can achieve the Learning Outcomes at the beginning of this skill.

Recommended Reading

Cadwell, C. (1995). *Powerful performance appraisals.* Franklin Lakes, NJ: Career Press.

Rager, P. (1998). Emotional intelligence and the management edge. *Nursing Spectrum (FL ED)*, *8*(3),3.

Weisinger, H. (1998). *Emotional intelligence at work.* San Francisco: Jossey-Bass.

Zurlinden, J. Preparing for a performance review. Retrieved July 1, 2002 from http://community.nursingspectrum.com/MagazineArticles/article.cfm?AID=5672.

6. MANAGING CONFLICT CONSTRUCTIVELY

Definition

Being able to make conflict work in positive ways (e.g., learning, growth, improvement).

Learning Outcomes

After you study this information and complete the accompanying exercises you should be able to:

♦ Identify your usual approach to dealing with conflict.

♦ Determine ways to improve your ability to make conflict work in positive ways.

Thinking Critically about Conflict

Conflict is a basic human instinct. From the beginning of mankind, when survival of the fittest reigned, humans instinctually looked for differences in those around them. To survive, they knew the importance

Table 6-2   OUTCOMES OF CONFLICT

Negative Outcomes of Conflict	Positive Outcomes of Managing Conflict Constructively
Increased stress	Reduced stress
Decreased productivity	Increased harmony and productivity
Poor relationships/feelings of isolation	Better relationships/more interaction
Wasted time and energy	Better understanding of others involved
Frustration, anger, hopelessness	Improved ability to clarify main issues/find creative solutions
Lack of growth	Improved self-esteem
Poor self-esteem	Opportunity to improve bothersome things

of being suspicious when they came in contact with humans who appeared different than what they expected.

Today, we still notice differences almost immediately, though often subconsciously. Conflict can be mild, taking the form of subtle opposition to an idea or action, or it can be severe, taking the form of sharp disagreement and fighting. For many, the word "conflict" has negative connotations, bringing feelings of discomfort and dread. Most of us deeply want to live in a world where everyone gets along and everything goes smoothly. Critical thinking requires being able to understand and exchange different viewpoints, wants, and needs and to come to a sincere agreement about what's most important. Knowing how to make conflict work in positive ways helps you seize opportunities for growth and achieve realistic outcomes. When you're comfortable and skilled in recognizing and managing conflict, you have more brainpower to focus on making real progress—you reduce the amount of time and energy spent dealing with the negative outcomes of conflict (see Table 6-2).

How to Manage Conflict Constructively

You can manage conflict constructively by following five key steps:

1. **Gain insight into your natural style of dealing with conflict (Box 6-3).** Make a commitment to consciously draw upon strengths and work on weaknesses in an objective, purposeful manner.
2. **Learn how to recognize patterns and appearances of conflict early.** Become cognizant of verbal and nonverbal behaviors that signal conflict may be developing (for example, withdrawal, verbalization of problems with current state of affairs).

Box 6-3 MANAGING CONFLICT: WHAT'S YOUR STYLE?

AVOIDERS pull away. They ignore issues or withdraw from people they feel are causing conflict. Avoiders often get along well with others because they focus on promoting peace and harmony. However, they tend to allow problems to persist and place little importance on their own needs. As a result, they miss opportunities to make improvements and tend to "explode" when things finally get to be too much, even though the trigger issue may be minor.

ACCOMMODATORS/SMOOTHERS give up their own needs and try to make others feel better. This group often struggles with inner conflicts because they secretly wish to speak their minds. They, too, can explode, damaging relationships because of failure to honestly confront issues that are important to them.

FORCERS try to get THEIR way even if it means others have to give up what they want or need. They're minimally interested in or aware of what others need and don't really care if they are liked.

COMPROMISERS give up part of their wants and needs and persuade others to give up part of their wants and needs. They think they get win-win solutions but may be settling for minimally acceptable solutions that continue the conflict (because they assume everyone has to lose something in negotiations rather than persisting to find answers that fully satisfy everyone involved).

COLLABORATIVE PROBLEM SOLVERS make it a rule to fairly face issues together. This group has equal concern for both the issues and the relationship. They see conflict as a means of improving relationships by gaining understanding and reducing tension. They look for solutions that allow everyone to win by identifying areas of agreement and differences, evaluating alternatives, and choosing solutions that have the full support of the key parties involved.

Summary

Collaborating = win-win.

Compromising = win a little, lose a little (sometimes unavoidable).

Avoiding = lose-lose (sometimes may be used purposely to buy time, which is an appropriate use of this strategy).

Accommodating = one side consistently loses so the other has its way.

Forcing = one side consistently wins, while the other loses.

3. **Practice using conflict management strategies (Box 6-4).**
4. **Develop skills you need to function more comfortably when faced with conflict (e.g., being assertive without being aggressive; see Box 6-2).**
5. **Use a comprehensive approach to assessing and managing conflict:**
   - ◆ Hold opinions until you're sure of all the facts.
   - ◆ Choose an appropriate time and place to open discussion (ensure privacy and find a convenient time for those involved).
   - ◆ Be willing to persevere until you clearly understand the issues, values, and goals of the key players involved.
   - ◆ Foster an atmosphere of trust and sincere desire to face issues fairly together; encourage free exchange of ideas, feelings, and attitudes.

Box 6-4   MAD ABOUT YOU: MANAGING CONFLICT
CONSTRUCTIVELY

- **Listen with the intent to understand** the other parties' points of view before presenting your own.
- **Keep a lid on your emotions.** It's hard to think clearly when your adrenaline is flowing.
- **Using "I" messages** and a nonthreatening tone of voice, clearly explain how the problem is affecting you and what you'd like to happen.
  - "I feel (name the feeling)."
  - "When I see/hear (state the problem)."
  - "I would like (state the change you want to happen)."
- **Ask yourself, What can I find in this situation that I'm doing to contribute to the problem?** You have more control over things that you're doing to contribute to the problem than over things that others are doing to contribute to the problem.
- **Get rid of old baggage** (feelings and preconceptions you have because of things that have happened in the past). For example, thinking, I'm just not the type of person who can handle conflict, so she knows she can get her way.
- **Look for deep issues.** For example, say, "Tell me what's really bothering you" (keep repeating this if the answer is "I don't know").
- **Be willing to hear things you don't like to hear.** You need honest feedback to work through the issues.
- **Ask for help from those involved.** For example, "Can we agree to not be so hard on one another?"
- **Change your approach** to managing conflict depending on the situation rather than using the style you're most comfortable with. For example, studies indicate that nurses use *avoidance* as the main approach to resolving conflicts.[*] The most frequently used styles are compromise and accommodation. All three styles may involve more losing than necessary.
  - **Use collaborative problem solving** as the overall, optimum way to manage conflict. Because this approach takes more time than you may have at the moment, initially you may need to use one of the following approaches. You also may need to use all the methods below as stepping stones to collaborative problem solving.
  - **Use avoidance** only when trying to delay confrontation until a more appropriate time, when time-out is required, or when issues are of minor importance in relation to overall goal.
  - **Use accommodation/smoothing** when the goal is to preserve relationships or encourage the others to express themselves.
  - **Use compromise** when time is too limited for a full collaborative approach and there are two equally empowered sides that must maintain a positive relationship yet reach agreement. Find a common ground to achieve temporary settlement that at least satisfies each side's main objectives.
  - **Use forcing** only when there isn't time for discussion (for example, in an emergency), when you must implement unpopular changes, or when all other strategies have failed and the change is required.

*Eason, F., & Brown, S. (1999). Conflict management: Assessing educational needs. *Journal for Nurses in Staff Development, 15*(3), 95.

- ◆ Stay focused on common values and goals; look for win-win solutions (some compromising may be needed).
- ◆ Look for several solutions to the problems, evaluating each solution with the key players involved.
- ◆ Make a conscious effort to stay calm, help others stay calm, and keep the focus on the positive outcomes of resolving the conflict.
- ◆ Take a break or get help from outside sources as needed. Allow for time out but keep interacting until all parties agree to the solution.
- ◆ Set up a time to revisit issues to see if the solutions are actually being carried out and helping reduce the problem.

6. **Apply principles of negotiation (Box 6-5).**

Other Perspectives

IT TAKES COURAGE TO CONFRONT

"Confrontation takes considerable courage, and many people would rather take the course of least resistance (belittling and criticizing, betraying confidences, or participating in gossip about others behind their backs.) But in the long run, people will trust and respect you if you are honest and open and kind with them. You care enough to confront."[6]

—Author and Leadership Coach, Stephen Covey

Box 6-5 **HOW TO NEGOTIATE***

Negotiation Requires:
- ◆ Being clear about what results you want to achieve.
- ◆ Building and maintaining a communication climate that supports problem solving under stress.
- ◆ Letting other parties know your interests and actively working to discover theirs.
- ◆ Being willing to explore the needs of all parties and use problem-solving skills to find mutually agreeable solutions.
- ◆ Determining common interests as well as conflicting needs and desires.
- ◆ Being willing to think about various proposals and making a decision about whether to reject, reframe, or accept them.
- ◆ Knowing your BATNA (**B**est **A**lternative **T**o a **N**egotiated **A**greement). A BATNA is like a worst-case scenario. It's the lowest level of what you're willing to accept. Reject any offer that falls below this level. Consider and discuss any offer that's less than you'd like but better than your BATNA.

*Data from Glaser, R. (1994). *Building negotiating power.* King of Prussia, PA: Organization Design and Development.

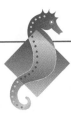

Critical Moments

ADRENALINE RUSH CLOUDS YOUR THINKING

Ever notice how hard it is to stay calm and objective when faced with conflict? The fight or flight response easily initiated by threats to self causes our adrenal glands to inject adrenaline into the blood stream, bringing a rush of emotion and excitement that makes it harder to think clearly. When faced with conflict, give yourself and others time to calm down and think things through.

Related Skills: Communicating Bad News, Giving and Taking Feedback.

CRITICAL THINKING EXERCISES

1. **Gain insight into how you tend to respond to conflict and how you feel about others' styles for resolving conflict.** In a group, in a personal journal, or both:
   a. List three or four conflicts that you can remember in some detail.
   b. Review the styles in Box 6-3 and honestly consider what styles you used while in conflict. Once you've considered your own style, think about what styles the other person(s) used and how they affected you.
   c. How could you have handled the situation differently (what style[s] may have achieved a better outcome?)

2. **Choose one or two of the preceding situations and share them with a partner or in a group,** asking for a different viewpoint on what was going on in the conflict and what styles and strategies might have been helpful.

3. **Practice using "I" messages.** Change the following statements to ones that send "I" messages.
   a. You never listen to me.
   b. I wish you wouldn't be so sloppy all the time.
   c. You make me feel like I'm the one who causes all the problems.
   d. You make me feel insignificant when you ignore me like that.
   e. Why are you always attacking me?

4. **Imagine this: Someone tells you one of your patients has numerous complaints.** You go directly to the room, introduce yourself, and inquire about the problem. The patient's wife immediately becomes hostile and tells you to "just get out." What do you do? Explain your rationale.

5. **Use role playing to practice assertive communication and conflict resolution.** Get a partner. Have one of you be the manager in the following situation and the other,

Continued

CRITICAL THINKING EXERCISES—cont'd

the staff nurse. Here's the situation:

A staff nurse is angry because he didn't get a specific day off, even though he had put in a written request well ahead of time. He needs the weekend off for his daughter's birthday. The manager spent hours trying to find proper coverage but couldn't honor his request because two other nurses also needed to be off and had been turned down for their requests the previous month.

6. **Evaluate whether you can achieve the Learning Outcomes at the beginning of this section.**

Recommended Reading

Bartol, G., Parrish, R., & McSweeney, M. (2001). Effective conflict management begins with knowing your style. *Journal for Nurses in Staff Development, 17*(1), 34–37.

Eason, F., & Brown, S. (1999). Conflict management: Assessing educational needs. *Journal for Nurses in Staff Development, 15*(3), 92–96.

Glaser, R. (1994). *Building negotiating power.* King of Prussia, PA: Organization Design and Development.

Leadership Development Work Group. Influencing practice: Managing conflict essential in today's critical care world. Retrieved July 2, 2002 from http://www.aacn.org/AACN/aacnnews.nsf/ff1487bfe89b77df882565a6006cfc3f/518cdc35386d9d7e88256a96000061a8?OpenDocument#conflict.

Martin, B. Social skills training–Part 2: Anger management. Retrieved July 2, 2002 from http://www.onlinece.net/courses.asp?course=107&action=view.

McCann, J., & Spillers, G. Conflict management. Retrieved July 2, 2002 from http://www.aacn.org/AACN/freece.nsf/ff1487bfe89b77df882565a6006cfc3f/d623afb59a5c0eff882566530052e316?OpenDocument. Penny, J. Coaxing a pest to bug off–Assertive Communication Skills. Retrieved July 2, 2002 from http://www.onlinece.net/courses.asp?course=71&action=view.

Weisinger, H. (1998). *Emotional intelligence at work.* San Francisco: Jossey-Bass.

Wolf, Z., Brennan, R., Ferchau, L., Magee, M., et al. (1997). Creating and implementing guidelines on caring for difficult patients: A research utilization project. *MEDSURG Nursing, 6*(3),137–147.

7. MANAGING YOUR TIME*

Definition

Knowing how to use time effectively through prioritization and organization.

Learning Outcomes

After you study this information and complete the accompanying exercises, you should be able to:

◆ Explain how an activity diary (or log) helps you manage your time.

---

*Contributed by Donna D. Ignatavicius, MS, RN, Cm, DI Associates, Inc, iggy@diassociates.com.

- ◆ Describe how to set priorities based on your personal and professional goals.
- ◆ Identify ways to improve how you organize your work.

Thinking Critically about Managing Your Time

You might sometimes feel that your days seem like an endless race to catch a rapidly moving train. But you need to be on that train at the controls! Otherwise, you can become frustrated, pressured, and unproductive. In contrast, managing your time–taking control–improves self-confidence, reduces stress, and promotes quality and job satisfaction.

Critical Moments

Work Smarter, Not Harder
Making the commitment to develop time management skills pays off in the end because you learn to work smarter, not harder.

HOW TO MANAGE YOUR TIME. This section is organized by the following headings: Determining What Must Be Done, Ranking Priorities, and Organizing Your Work.

DETERMINING WHAT MUST BE DONE

1. **Start by developing and writing down your personal, professional, and work goals.** Keep them in a readily accessible place. These goals serve as a guide to help you prioritize and organize.

2. **Begin an activity diary (or log).** For several consecutives days, write down everything you do. Include what you do, the amount of time you spend doing it, and the time of day you do it. It should look something like this:

Time	Activities/Tasks
8–8:30 AM	Drive to health club
8:30–9 AM	Work out
9–9:45 AM	Drive to class
10–11:15 AM	Go to class
11:15 AM –1 PM	Have lunch/Hang out with friends
1–2:15 PM	Go to class

3. **After a few days, analyze your log, and mark each of the activities/tasks according to the following categories:**
   - ◆ Must do (essential) activities/tasks
   - ◆ Should/could do (or could be delegated to someone else) activities/ tasks
   - ◆ Nice to do (if you had more time) activities
   - ◆ Not necessary (time waster) activities/tasks

4. **Arrange the activities/tasks into each of these categories.** Be sure that things under your "must do" category reflect your personal and professional/work goals. If they don't, reevaluate whether you truly must do them.

5. **Decide whether there are things missing on your "must do" list.** Add these to the list.

6. **Find ways to spend most of your time each day on the "must do" list.** Figure out how to get rid of time wasters. For example, in the activity log in number 2 of this section, you could get rid of an hour's driving by working out at home instead of the health club.

7. **Review the list of "nice to do" activities.** Ask, Are there things on this list that I could be/should be delegating to someone else? If so, who would be the best person(s) to do the tasks? and What would be the results in the long run? (Box 5-4, page 169, addresses key points on delegating in the clinical setting).

8. **Consider whether you could combine some activities.** For example, if you have specific educational goals, you might listen to educational tapes while driving.

RANKING PRIORITIES. This section addresses ranking priorities in relation to everyday life. For ranking priorities in the clinical setting, see Box 5-2, page 168.

1. **Determine the following priority needs, being clear about the rationale for your choices:**
   - First-order priority: Must do—important and urgent
   - Second-order priority: Must do—important but not urgent
   - Third-order priority: Nice to do—not as important and not urgent

2. **For each priority, consider:**
   - How much time you have
   - Whether you (and only you) can do what needs to be done, or whether you can delegate the task(s) or parts of the task(s) to others
   - Whether technology or equipment can help you be more efficient (for example, mastering computer skills)
   - Whether paying a price to get things done quicker or obtain better quality will improve either your results or the time you have to spend on major goals
   - Whether there is a cheaper way of accomplishing the task (for example, using a library computer is cheaper than hiring a typist)

ORGANIZING YOUR WORK

1. **Review your personal, professional, and work goals.** These goals serve as a guide to help you prioritize and organize.

2. **Set limits on what you agree to do,** as noted in the following Other Perspectives.

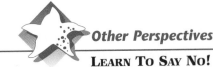

Other Perspectives

LEARN TO SAY NO!

"Learning to say "no" if the request for your time is not a "must do" or "should/could do" activity is good time management. Saying something like "I would love to help you, but I'm overloaded right now" works very well. In some cases, you may also have to say something like, "I need a bit more time if you want me to do a good job." Does this mean shirking responsibilities or procrastinating? Not at all. It means when you have a track record of showing responsibility, and want to do a good job, asking for more time or simply saying "No" may be good time management."

—Donna D. Ignatavicius, MS, RN Cm

3. **Reserve time in your daily schedule for unexpected events.** Life is unpredictable.

4. **Make a "to do" list for each day and estimate the time each activity on your list will require.** Be sure that your list includes only those activities that you *must or should* do.

5. **For long-term (or large) projects, keep a master list to refer to periodically.** For each project, map out interim target dates that ensure you will complete the project in a timely way or by the designated deadline.

6. **Don't procrastinate!** Avoid the human tendency to put off large projects, find excuses to evade things you don't enjoy. Procrastination is a major time waster.

7. **Don't expect or demand perfection.** Letting go of a task once it's done is crucial for managing time. Perfectionism can also be a time waster!

8. **Eliminate unnecessary work or steps in the work.** Look for ways to streamline work. For example:

Ways to Streamline Work in the Clinical Setting

- ◆ Plan to cluster activities before entering a room.
- ◆ Think ahead; anticipate needs, such as a need for pain medication.
- ◆ Document in one place; don't duplicate information. Focus most on charting what's *different*–for example, use charting by exception (CBE) if allowed by charting policies.
- ◆ Organize supply and medication carts so that the commonly used items are easily found.
- ◆ Label all supply shelves and cabinets clearly for easy access.
- ◆ Get to work a few minutes early to allow for planning time.
- ◆ Use a daily worksheet that is legible and organized.

9. Do tasks that require the greatest effort or concentration when you're rested. Some people find that early morning is best, and others work better late at night. When you're not feeling energetic, try to do things that require little concentration or effort like washing dishes.

10. Use technology to organize your personal and professional/student work. For example:

    ◆ Personal digital assistants (PDAs) and other electronic organizers are becoming very popular. Handheld PDAs, such as Palm Pilots and Handspring's Visors, allow you to not only keep a calendar, daily schedule, addresses, and phone numbers, but they can be loaded with software for quick reference, such as essential drug information.

    ◆ The BlackBerry©, a handheld electronic wireless device that accesses e-mail.

    ◆ A paper system, such as the Franklin-Covey planner, also works well. The advantage of a paper system is that it is usually less expensive, and doesn't require interaction with a personal computer (PC).

11. Whatever organizing system you use, keep all scheduled activities within the same organizing system, rather than keeping multiple or duplicate systems. For example, don't keep your work schedule on a PDA and your social calendar elsewhere.

Critical Moments

HELPING PEOPLE HELP THEMSELVES: GOOD TIME MANAGEMENT

If you don't have time to do something for someone, help the person figure out how to do it. I remember how thrilled we were when my friend and I were allowed to come in and wash the hair of my neighbor, who was hospitalized with a fractured hip. Often, getting these "nice to do" things done by friends and family adds significantly to patient and family satisfaction.

CRITICAL THINKING EXERCISES

1. Develop at least three personal or professional goals that you want to accomplish within the next year, and write them down.

2. Keep an activity diary for three consecutive days during the week. Be sure to include all activities for work, school, and home, if applicable. Keeping the goals you identified in the preceding exercise:

   ◆ Identify the essential or "must do" activities that will help you achieve your goals for the next year.

Continued

CRITICAL THINKING EXERCISES—cont'd

- ◆ Identify time wasters and decide how you might eliminate them.
- ◆ Rank the "must do" activities by assigning priorities (first-order, second-order, or third-order priorities).
- ◆ Ask yourself whether there are some things you should be/could be doing to achieve your personal and professional goals. Add these to the list.

3. In a group discussion or with a partner, "compare notes" on the above exercises.
4. Together with a partner, in a group, or in a personal journal, explain specific strategies you will use to organize your work. Keep organization of time and environment in mind.
5. Determine where you stand in relation to the Learning Outcomes at the beginning of this skill.
6. Go to the library or Amazon.com. Study the table of contents and sample pages of the following recommended readings. Identify common themes among the books. Or go hog-wild and make time to read one!

Recommended Reading

Allen, D. (2001). *Getting things done: The art of stress-free productivity.* New York: Viking Press.

Bryant, T. (1999). *Self-discipline in 10 days: How to go from thinking to doing.* New York: HUB Publishing.

Emmett, R. (2000). *The procrastinator's handbook: Mastering the art of doing it now.* New York: Walker & Co.

Lagatree, K. (2000). *Checklists for life:104 lists to help you get organized, save time, and unclutter your life.* New York: Random House.

Lehmkuhl, D., & Lamping, D. (1993). *Organizing for the creative person.* New York: Crown Publishers.

Morgenstern, J. (1998). *Organizing from the inside out: The foolproof system for organizing your home, your office, and your life.* New York: Owl Books.

Morgenstern, J. (2000). *Time management from the inside out: The foolproof system for taking control of your schedule and your life.* New York: Henry Holt.

8. PREVENTING AND DEALING WITH MISTAKES CONSTRUCTIVELY

Definition

Knowing how to prevent, detect, correct, and learn from errors. An error is when you do something (commit an act) or forget to do something (omit an act) resulting in a failure to achieve your intended outcome.* The following related terms are also important to understand in the context of nursing and health care.

---

*This definition and the ones that follow are adapted from: Joint Commission on Accreditation of Healthcare Organizations. *Revisions to Joint Commission Standards in Support of Patient Safety and Medical/Health Care Error Reduction.* Available at: http://www.jcaho.org./standard/fr_ptsafety.html. 6/4/2002.

◆ **Sentinel Event.** An unexpected occurrence involving death or serious physical or psychological injury or the risk thereof. Serious injury specifically includes loss of limb or function. The phrase "or risk thereof" means any variation from the usual process of care, that if it happens again, there is a significant chance of causing a serious adverse outcome. *Example:* If there is a break in procedures that caused nurses to omit checking that the correct leg is marked for amputation. Whether the wrong leg is amputated or not, a sentinel event has occurred. The term *sentinel* is used because if it's relationship to a sentinel guard—a soldier who stands guard to keep his people safe. Sentinel events are so serious that they signal the need for immediate investigation to ensure they don't happen again.

◆ **Near Miss.** Anything that happens during the process of care that didn't affect the outcome, but if it happened again, there is a significant chance of a serious adverse outcome. *Example:* If a physician almost operates on the wrong site, but this is caught just in time, it's a near miss. Near misses are considered Sentinel Events, but they may not be reviewed by the Joint Commission of Accreditation of Healthcare Organizations (JCAHO) under its Sentinel Event Policy.

◆ **Hazardous Condition.** Any set of circumstances (exclusive of the disease or condition for which the patient is being treated) that significantly increases the likelihood of a serious adverse outcome. *Example:* Nurses who have too many acutely ill patients to give appropriate care.

Learning Outcomes

After you study this information and complete the accompanying exercises you should be able to:

◆ Define the terms *error, sentinel event, near miss,* and *hazardous condition* using your own words.

◆ Explain how to determine the seriousness of a mistake.

◆ Identify circumstances that lead you to make mistakes.

◆ Develop a personal plan for preventing, detecting, correcting, and learning from mistakes.

Thinking Critically about Preventing and Dealing with Mistakes

Mistakes can be our worst nightmare, or they can be stepping-stones to learning and improvement. And sometimes, they can be both. Dealing with mistakes is a complex issue that includes considering legal consequences (in some states, it's the law that patients be informed of errors; mistakes sometimes end up in malpractice litigation). This section addresses how to know what constitutes a serious error, why errors happen, and how to prevent, detect, correct, and learn from errors.

Too many people have a one-size-fits-all mindset when it comes to dealing with mistakes. Deep down, they believe that all errors are bad; that all errors happen because of lack of knowledge or laziness, and that the best way to deal with people who make errors is to punish them. However, this approach shames those involved, doesn't examine the real causes of errors and does little to reduce the incidence of mistakes. The reality is that many mistakes happen for multiple reasons and in spite of good intentions. We must change the mindset from "mistakes shouldn't happen" to "when dealing with humans, mistakes will happen for various reasons." We must encourage health care professionals to share their mistakes freely so that we can work together to find ways to prevent future mistakes. Box 6-6 shows four common reasons medication errors happen.

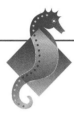

Critical Moments

FAILURE TO MONITOR AND FAILURE TO DIAGNOSE: DON'T MAKE THESE MISTAKES

Failure to monitor and failure to diagnose are common errors noted on malpractice claims (see Figure 6-1). Don't skip assessments, even if they seem routine. When you perform assessments, ask questions like, Could I be missing any problems here? Could I be seeing these problems incorrectly? Should I be getting a second opinion?

Box 6-6 FOUR REASONS WHY MEDICATION ERRORS HAPPEN

1. **Inadequate knowledge and skill**: Lack of knowledge of patient's diagnosis, and the names, purposes, and correct administration of medications.
2. **Failure to comply with policies and procedures**: Lack of attention to safeguards in medication administration procedures intended to prevent errors.
3. **Communication failure**: These include transcription errors, use of abbreviations, illegible handwriting, incorrect interpretation of physician's orders, use of verbal orders, failure to record medications given or omitted, and unclear medication administration records.
4. **Individual and system problems**: These include things like the number of years of experience of the nurse, number of consecutive hours worked, rotating shifts, workload, distractions and interruptions, floating nurses to unfamiliar units, hospital and pharmacy design features, and drug manufacturing problems (e.g., look-alike and sound-alike drug names, look-alike packaging, confusing and unclear labeling, failure to specify drug concentrations on dose-calculation charts).

Claims At A Glance

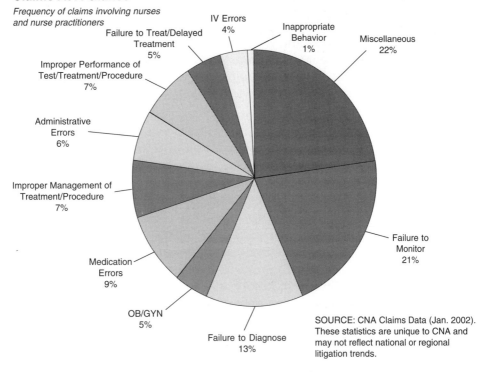

Frequency of claims involving nurses and nurse practitioners

- IV Errors 4%
- Inappropriate Behavior 1%
- Miscellaneous 22%
- Failure to Treat/Delayed Treatment 5%
- Improper Performance of Test/Treatment/Procedure 7%
- Administrative Errors 6%
- Improper Management of Treatment/Procedure 7%
- Medication Errors 9%
- OB/GYN 5%
- Failure to Diagnose 13%
- Failure to Monitor 21%

SOURCE: CNA Claims Data (Jan. 2002). These statistics are unique to CNA and may not reflect national or regional litigation trends.

Figure 6-1 ◆ Pie chart illustrating the types of mistakes commonly seen on malpractice claims. Reprinted from the *NSO Risk Advisor, 11*(1), 2 with permission from Nurses Service Organization.

How to Prevent and Deal with Mistakes Constructively

1. **All mistakes aren't created equal—in addition to knowing the difference between a Sentinel Event, Near Miss, or Hazardous Condition, know the following different types of mistakes, what things cause them, and how you can prevent them.**

- ◆ **Mental slip:** These mistakes happen when there's a lapse in your attention to what you're doing or when there's a lapse in short-term memory. *Example:* You're on the way to check an IV, but you're interrupted to help lift someone up in bed. After you finish helping, you forget that you were on the way to check the IV and go on to another task. *Prevention:* Keep a personal worksheet that prompts you to do important tasks (for example, check IV every hour). Get your charting done as soon as possible to help you notice when you've forgotten to do something. Checklists, protocols, and computerized decision aides all help reduce mental slips because they relieve you from relying on short-term memory, a part of memory that becomes most imperfect under stress or fatigue.

◆ **Interaction error:** These mistakes happen when people misunderstand each other. *Example:* You're working in the emergency department and have been talking to Dr. French about one of the patients, Mrs. Moran. A few minutes later, Dr. French comes to you and says, "Would you send her to x-ray?" nodding in the direction of another patient. You don't see him nod in the other direction and assume Dr. French is referring to Mrs. Moran. *Prevention:* Repeat what you think you hear to clarify verbal interactions (for example, you want me to send Mrs. Moran to x-ray?). Check written orders to clarify verbal orders.

◆ **Knowledge error:** These mistakes are due to insufficient knowledge. *Example:* You cause unnecessary side effects by giving an IV drug too quickly because you didn't know it should be given slowly. *Prevention:* Be sure you know the answers to who, what, why, when, and how in the context of each individual patient situation before you give any drug or perform any intervention.

◆ **Learning error:** Although these mistakes often include knowledge errors, learning errors usually are related to several different factors associated with being in a learning situation (for example, doing something for the first time, having less than astute observation skills, being stressed). *Example:* You're changing sterile dressings for the first time. You contaminate your glove by slightly touching an unsterile field. You don't notice it because you're focusing on assessing the wound. *Prevention:* A sure-fire way to avoid learning errors is not to try anything new, which makes no sense. Many students hide from new experiences because they're afraid of making mistakes, which doesn't work either because it just postpones the inevitable. The best way to avoid learning errors is to be prepared and to practice, practice, practice in as safe an environment as possible (for example, in a skills lab). In *risky* situations it's best to have a more experienced nurse guide performance, give advice, or actually handle the task at hand.

◆ **Overreliance on technology:** These mistakes happen when you rely too much on technology, without using your human capabilities. *Example:* Someone complains that a heating pad is too hot, but when you check it, you find that it's on the low setting. Rather than carefully feeling the pad yourself, you explain that it's probably okay because it's set on low. *Prevention:* Read all instruction manuals carefully. Don't trust machines more than your own knowledge and perceptions.

◆ **System error:** These mistakes are related to something wrong with the way things are accomplished within the facility as a whole. *Examples:* Drugs that aren't given because the pharmacist is overloaded and unable to dispense the drug in a timely manner; errors that happen because a policy or procedure is unclear; errors that happen because a facility uses a lot of per diem personnel who are more at risk for making mistakes. *Prevention:* Report possible system problems to the risk management or quality assurance department. Create a multidisciplinary panel to examine possible and actual system problems.

2. **Determine how serious an error is.** Serious errors need to be examined more closely, prevented more meticulously, and detected and corrected more quickly than less serious errors.

3. **Follow policies and procedures and be sure you understand the rationale behind them.** These are designed by experts to prevent, detect, and correct errors early.

4. **When using checklists, focus on each item carefully.** Checklists are supposed to jog your brain, not replace it.

5. **Involve patients and families in their own health care as much as possible.** Educate them and encourage them to become participants in preventing errors by verifying that they're getting the right treatments and medications and speaking up when they have questions (see Box 6-7).

6. **Never perform an intervention without being sure you understand why it's indicated in each particular situation.** Be careful about multitasking.

7. **Involve experts.** For example, if confused about a medication regimen, ask a pharmacist.

8. **Look after yourself.** If you're rested, you're less likely to make mistakes.

Rule: **To determine the seriousness of a mistake, decide two things:**

1. What harm could result if the error happens (primarily consider harm in terms of human morbidity, mortality, and suffering; secondarily consider harm in terms of inconvenience, cost, and lost time); if you're unable to decide what harm could result, ask for help.

2. Whether the incident should be classified as a sentinel event, near miss, or hazardous condition. **Example of a serious error:** You forget to check someone's identification bracelet before sending him to the operating room. **Example of a less serious error:** While inserting a Foley catheter, you contaminate the package and have to get a new one.

Box 6-7   IMPROVE SAFETY: URGE YOUR PATIENTS TO "SPEAK UP"

The following steps are based on research that shows patients who take part in decisions about their health care are more likely to have better outcomes.

Speak up if you have questions or concerns, and if you don't understand, ask again. It's your body and you have a right to know.

Pay attention to the care you are receiving. Make sure you're getting the right treatments and medications by the right health care professionals. Don't assume anything.

Educate yourself about your diagnosis, the medical tests you are undergoing, and your treatment plan.

Ask a trusted family member or friend to be your advocate.

Know what medications you take and why you take them. Medication errors are the most common health care errors.

Use a hospital, clinic, surgery center, or other type of health care organization that has undergone a rigorous on-site evaluation against established state-of-the-art quality and safety standards, such as that provided by the Joint Commission on Accreditation of Healthcare Organizations (JCAHO).

Participate in all decisions about your treatment. You are the center of the health care team.

Courtesy of JCAHO. For a more detailed version of the SPEAK UP approach, go to www.jcaho.org.

Rule: **WHAT TO DO WHEN MISTAKES HAPPEN**

1. Determine the seriousness of the error as soon as it's recognized, and take immediate steps to prevent or reduce harm. Get help if needed.

2. Follow policy and procedures for dealing with mistakes, including how to report and record the mistake. Standards and some state laws mandate that patients be informed when mistakes happen.

3. Chart actions taken to address the error (for example, increasing the frequency of monitoring or a transfer to another unit).

4. Curb the tendency to focus too much on guilt and not enough on what can be learned from the mistake.

5. Explore the specifics of the incident objectively, examining the procedures and circumstances leading to the errors. Consider the value of sharing the mistake with others to alert them of the possibility of its happening again. If procedures were followed and a mistake still happened, maybe the procedures should be revised to make them more error proof.

Want to know more about error prevention?

The following Web pages have excellent, helpful information.

◆ National Patient Safety Foundation
   (http://www.ama-assn.org/med-sci/npsf/main.htm)
◆ Agency For Health Care Research and Quality
   http://www.ahrq.gov/qual/errorsix.htm
◆ The Patient Safety Officer Society (www.PSOS.org)
◆ The Joint Commission on Accreditation of Healthcare Organizations
   (http://www.jcaho.org./standard/fr_ptsafety.html).
◆ The Institute of Medicine (http://www.iom.edu/iom/iomhome.nsf)

 Other Perspectives

SUPPORT FOR REPORTING ERRORS ESSENTIAL TO IMPROVING SAFETY
To make the changes needed to improve safety, we must get the commitment from the Board of Trustees of each organization to make safety a priority–to change the culture of the organization from one that is punitive when mistakes are reported to one that welcomes the reporting of errors. Only then can we all learn from what happened and find ways to change care practices to reduce future mistakes.

–Medical Error and Compliance Expert, Ann Kobs, MS, RN, Ann Kobs &
Associates, Inc., www.annkobs.com

Related Skills: Communicating Bad News.

CRITICAL THINKING EXERCISES

Instructions: In a group, in a personal journal, or both:
1. **Address the implications of the following statements.**
   a. To be ignorant doesn't merely mean not to know; it means not to know what you don't know; being educated means knowing precisely what you don't know.
   b. As a nurse it's your responsibility to be alert not only to situations that might cause you to make a mistake but also to situations that may cause others to make a mistake.
2. **Respond to the following:**
   a. How do you feel when you make a mistake?

Continued

CRITICAL THINKING EXERCISES—cont'd

b. What can you do to help someone else who has made a mistake?

c. How can you help correct systems that are error-prone and increase checks to prevent medication errors?

3. **Give an example of a Sentinel Event, Near Miss, and Hazardous Condition.**

4. **View and discuss the video *Beyond Blame*, an award-winning 10-minute documentary, which focuses on how medication errors affect both patients and staff.** (Check with your educator, librarian, or go to www.mederrors.com.)

5. **Discuss the implications of the following Critical Moments and Other Perspectives.**

Critical Moments

THREE KEY STEPS TO PREVENTING MISTAKES

We all share accountability for ensuring patient safety: (1) Pay attention to things you're doing that may create risks for errors. (2) Report systems that fail to adequately protect patients (for example, notify the risk management department if you think of a change in a policy or procedure that could be made to reduce chances for human error). (3) Empower your patients by teaching them what to expect and telling them that the main thing they can do to prevent mistakes is to become actively involved in managing their own care.

Other Perspectives

EVIDENCE-BASED PRACTICE CHALLENGES THE SAFETY OF RESTRAINTS

A study on the use of restraints found that while many nurses assume that restraining confused patients protects them from injury and prevents complications, the evidence is to the contrary.[3] The study shows that restrained patients are more likely to sustain serious injury when they fall, that they are hospitalized twice as long as those who aren't restrained, and that they are eight times more likely to die during hospitalization than non-restrained patients. It also shows that restraints contribute to depression, anger, nosocomial (hospital-acquired) infection, pressure ulcers, and deconditioning–all of which leave patients in a worse state than when they were admitted. Think twice before restraining patients.

6. **Determine whether you can achieve the Learning Outcomes at the beginning of this skill.**

Recommended Reading

Bombard, C. JCAHO shines a light on patient safety. Retrieved June 26, 2002 from
http://community.nursingspectrum.com/MagazineArticles/article.cfm?AID=4601.

JCAHO. Revisions to joint commission standards in support of patient safety and medical/health
care error reduction. Retrieved June 24, 2002 from http://nsweb.nursingspectrum.com/
ce/m32a.htm

Farella, C. Turning the table on medication errors. Retrieved June 24, 2002 from
http://community.nursingspectrum.com/MagazineArticles/article.cfm?AID=879.

Penny, J. That's *not* supposed to happen: Medical error reduction. Retrieved June 24, 2002 from
http://www.onlinece.net/courses.asp?course=153&action=view.

Savard, M. (2000). *How to save your own life: The Savard system for managing–and
controlling–your health care.* New York: Time Warner.

Wolf, Z. Preventing medication errors (parts 1 and 2). Retrieved June 24, 2002 from
http://nsweb.nursingspectrum.com/ce/m32a.htm.

Zurlinden, J. *Dangers of Multitasking.* Retrieved June 24, 2002 from
http://www.myfreece.com/Public/Course_Take.asp?CourseId=39.

9. TRANSFORMING A GROUP INTO A TEAM

Definition

Knowing how to work together to combine efforts to achieve shared outcomes within a specific time frame.

Learning Outcomes

After you study this information and complete the accompanying exercises you should be able to:

◆ Explain the common stages of team building.
◆ Describe strategies that transform groups into teams.
◆ Participate more effectively as part of a team.

Thinking Critically about Teamwork

How well a team works together determines whether you have frustrated, unhappy patients and staff; whether the atmosphere makes you dread coming into work; or whether you have great patient outcomes, job satisfaction, and sense of good will. Yet teamwork doesn't just happen. The team must be nurtured as it evolves from being a group of diverse, relatively insecure, strangers to a group that values common goals and brings together diverse talents and strengths.

True teamwork occurs when all team members are:

◆ Committed to common goals and a high level of output.
◆ Energized by their ability to work together.
◆ Concerned about how team members feel during the work process.

For example, consider the difference between what's going on in groups A and B below.

Group A consists of several nurses who have worked together for the past 6 months. They don't feel like they're working as a team and wonder what they can do to change the situation. Their manager is a busy person who happens to have a demanding boss. When the pressure is on, she barks orders and personally takes over some tasks. The staff responds by doing what they are told or lying low until things calm down. Group participation in problem solving and decision making is almost nonexistent. Most of the nurses want to perform their responsibilities in a satisfactory way. But they haven't given much thought to the need for group goals or concerted group action. Under these circumstances it seems nothing will change, morale is low, and everyone talks about how unhappy they are.

Group B consists of several nurses who also have been working together for 6 months in a situation similar to that of Group A. By contrast these nurses are energized and proud of their successes. Like Group A, their manager also is a busy person with a demanding boss. However, when the pressure is on, she stops the action and convenes a problem-solving discussion, focusing on common goals and getting input from team members. The result is that better solutions are found because the pressure is channeled into a spirit of let's fix this together. These nurses enjoy a sense of growing and improving together–work is more than just a job.*

How to Transform a Group into a Team

Communication in word and deeds, the most powerful tool for team-building, sets the tone for the relationships we need to be successful. All those involved should remember the importance of using behaviors that enhance interpersonal relationships (see Box 6-8).

Team *leaders* should:
◆ Create a shared vision of the team's mission or purpose: Everyone must be committed to reaching clearly defined outcomes.
◆ Stress that everyone is responsible for improving performance by scrutinizing practices and pointing out improvements that could be made.
◆ Turn diversity to the team's advantage (for example, assign tasks based on individual strengths and preferences as much as possible).
◆ Ask for consensus in decisions (everyone agrees to agree), rather than settling for a majority vote.
◆ Be careful not to criticize ideas.
◆ Keep team members well-informed so that everyone has a good understanding of the big picture.

---

*Adapted from *Building a Winning Team* © 1994 by Dr. Rollin Glaser and Christine Glaser with permission of Organization Design and Development Inc., King of Prussia, PA, 2.

Box 6-8 **BEHAVIORS ENHANCING AND IMPEDING INTERPERSONAL RELATIONSHIPS***

Behaviors Enhancing Interpersonal Relationships

- Conveying an attitude of openness, acceptance, and lack of prejudice
- Being honest
- Taking initiative and responsibility
- Being reliable
- Demonstrating humility
- Showing respect for what others are, have been, or may become
- Accepting accountability
- Being confident and prepared
- Showing genuine interest
- Conveying appreciation for others' time
- Accepting expression of positive and negative feelings
- Taking enough time
- Being frank and forthright
- Admitting when we've been wrong
- Apologizing if we've caused distress or inconvenience

Behaviors Inhibiting Interpersonal Relationships

- Conveying an attitude of doubt, mistrust, or negative judgment
- Giving false information
- Conveying an "it's not my job" attitude
- Not meeting commitments, only partially meeting commitments, or not being punctual
- Demonstrating self-importance
- "Talking down," or assuming familiarity
- Making excuses or placing blame where it doesn't belong
- Being unsure and trying to "wing it"
- Acting like you're only doing something because it's a job
- Assuming others have more time than we do
- Demonstrating annoyance when negative feelings are expressed
- Rushing
- Sending mixed messages, saying things just because we think it's what the other person wants to hear, or talking behind others' backs
- Denying or ignoring when we've made a mistake
- Acting like nothing happened or making excuses

*Adapted from Alfaro-LeFevre, R. (2002). *Applying nursing process: Promoting collaborative care* (5th ed.). Philadelphia: JB Lippincott.

- Recognize team members for their contributions.
- Be sure team members are familiar with the common stages of team building (see Box 6-9). Although not every group goes through every stage, and length of time for each stage varies, it helps to know that there are common struggles in every team.

Box 6-9   COMMON STAGES OF TEAM BUILDING

Forming
Group members start to get to know one another, testing each other's values, beliefs, and attitudes. Basic goals and tasks are defined, roles assigned, and ideas shared.

Storming
Conflict within begins, often because of misunderstandings or disagreement about what realistically can get done and how exactly things will get done. More testing goes on in this phase, with some people asking themselves questions like, How much am I willing to do? This is a time to maintain high standards, provide emotional support, and aim to get consensus (agreement from everyone). Beware of false consensus during this phase–some people will say they agree when they really don't (just to avoid further conflict). Because this is a stressful stage, you may need to take more breaks.

Norming
The group becomes more cohesive and really wants to work together in a positive way. Group members agree on rules–for example, when meetings will be held, who should attend, what proper lines of communication are, and how problems and disagreements will be handled. At this point the leader needs to be sensitive to group values, asking for votes to determine common needs and desires.

Performing
Team members begin to bond to one another and function well together with a good understanding of role, responsibilities, and relationships.

Team *members* should:
◆ Agree about roles, responsibilities, and proper lines of communication.
◆ Be clear on what's expected of you, work hard to be good at what you do, and deliver what you promise.
◆ Get involved and contribute to the good of the group.
◆ Stay focused on the big picture of what the team is trying to accomplish.
◆ Remember to listen actively.
◆ Make a conscious effort to overcome the human tendency to focus narrowly on self–too often team members who feel very responsible have difficulty seeing other members' struggles because they themselves are working so hard.
◆ Model behaviors that promote trust and create a caring and energized environment:
  1. Follow the Golden Rule–point out when it's not being followed (without blaming).
  2. Show enthusiasm–it's contagious and energizes others.
  3. Address and resolve conflicts early–push for high-quality communication.

4. Be aware of the group process and where the team is in relation to the stages of team building (see Box 6-9).

5. Recognize individual and team efforts; be a good sport, help new teammates make entry.

6. Support creativity and new ways of doing things.

7. Broaden your skills; offer to try new tasks or to cross train.

8. Promote group learning by collecting, sharing, and analyzing information.

9. Spend fun time together (here's where relationships grow).

Related Skills: Developing Empowered Partnerships, Managing Conflict Constructively.

Critical thinking exercises

1. **In a group, in a personal journal, or both:**

a. Think about a group you currently belong to (for example, your peers, colleagues, or another group) in relation to the stages of team building shown in Box 6-9, page 230. What stage is your group in?

b. Share your best and worst experience with being part of a team. Consider what went right and why you think it went right and what went wrong and why you think it went wrong.

c. Discuss the implications of the following Other Perspectives.

Other Perspectives

TEAMWORK REQUIRES EMPOWERMENT

"Teamwork requires empowerment, a willingness and commitment to 'let go' of self (one's own ideas, plans, strategies) to the benefit of the group. As I see it, there are five stages of empowerment:
1. *Letting go of self-promotion*
2. *Believing that others are capable and competent*
3. *Trusting others*
4. *Willingness to forgo one's own processes/plans/strategies to give others a chance*
5. *Sharing the outcomes/celebrating success."*[8]

—Sylvia Whiting, PhD, RN, CS

STEPS TO TEAM BUILDING

"… One of the first things you need to do is realize and acknowledge that you and your co-workers are all on the same team—you are there to provide the best care to your patient/clients that you can. You don't have to become best friends with your co-workers, you don't even

Continued

STEPS TO TEAM BUILDING—cont'd

have to like them. What you do need to do, is treat them with respect and work with them to accomplish what needs to be accomplished. Approach work with a positive attitude–negativity only adds to the stress and tension of your workday. Remember your coworkers are in the same situation you are. If you have a problem with a co-worker, ask to speak to them privately. … One of the most difficult tasks of collaboration, the "big picture" approach, requires repeatedly asking, "Will this help us achieve our goal?" Continual focus on the mutually agreed upon outcome is the most likely path to success, for without it the partnership is doomed."[9]

—*Nancy Dickenson-Hazard, RN, MSN, FAAN,*
Editor of *Reflections on Nursing LEADERSHIP*

FOSTERING CROSS-CULTURAL UNDERSTANDING

"Working successfully with a culturally diverse staff and patient population encompasses two sets of skills. First, nurses need the holistic skills to manage patients who are different from themselves.… However, the skill that's frequently overlooked is learning to work with diversity among staff members. Embracing cultural diversity in the workplace, as well as in the community, has to be an institutional commitment."[10]

—*Antonia Villaruel, RN, PhD, FAAN President,*
National Association of Hispanic Nurses

---

2. **Practice brainstorming as a group.** Get in a group of 6 to 10 persons. Name one person the recorder and have him use a flip chart or blackboard. Identify a problem you'd like to resolve or a situation that could be improved (for example, how you could get teenagers to come to a meeting on sex education). For 30 minutes, have group members each share ideas to be recorded by the recorder without interpretation. Once you're finished, spend 10 minutes discussing what happened (the group dynamics) as you brainstormed.

3. **Determine whether you can achieve the Learning Outcomes at the beginning of this skill.**

Recommended Reading

Dickenson-Hazard, N. (2001). Block party. *Reflections on Nursing LEADERSHIP, 27*(1), 5.

Dunbar, C. Are you a team player? Retrieved June 25 from http://community.nursing spectrum.com/MagazineArticles/article.cfm?AID=2147.

Glaser, R., & Glaser, C. (1994). *Building a winning team.* King of Prussia, PA: Organization Design and Development.

Jones, A. (1998). *104 activities that build: Self-esteem, teamwork, communication, anger management, self-discovery, and coping skills.* Richland, WA: Rec Room Publishing.

Paul, S. (1998). The advanced practice/staff nurse partnership: Building a winning team. *Critical Care Nurse, 18*(2),92–97.

Porter-O'Grady, T., & Wilson, C. (1999). *The healthcare teambook.* St. Louis: Mosby.

Wheelan, S. Take Teamwork to New Heights. *Nursing Management.* Retrieved July 2, 2002 from http://www.springnet.com/ce/m904a.htm.

Wenckus, E. Working with an interdisciplinary team. Retrieved June 25 from http://nsweb.nursingspectrum.com/ce/ce90.htm.

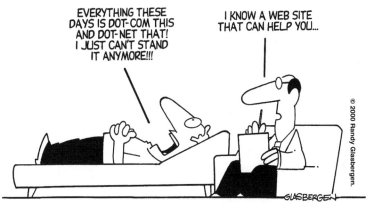

Cartoon by Randy Glasbergen, Copyright 2000. Reprinted with special permission from www.glasbergen.com

10. ACCESSING AND USING INFORMATION EFFECTIVELY

Definition

Knowing how to find relevant information, then interpret and apply it in the context of specific situations.

Learning Outcomes

After you study this section and complete the accompanying exercises you should be able to:

◆ Access information from a variety of sources.

◆ Apply information in the context of specific situations or purposes.

◆ Keep your files or notes organized for easy access.

Thinking Critically about Accessing and Using Information

Knowing how to find, interpret, and apply information is a key workplace survival skill. You can't carry all you need to know in your head. Whether or not you have the knowledge and skills needed to search for and apply data can make the difference between spending hours feeling panicky, stupid, and frustrated due to information overload—and feeling confident, interested, and in charge.

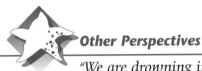 *Other Perspectives*

"We are drowning in information and starved for knowledge."

—Unknown

How to Access and Use Information Effectively

◆ **Learn how to use Internet and library resources**: indexes, catalogs, interlibrary loan services, circulation department, reference department, audiovisual services, and computer databases (recommended search engines and databases are listed in Box 6-10). Introduce yourself to the librarian and ask for help if you get stuck. Also remember that Internet search engines have Help buttons to assist you with questions.

◆ **Whether you're using a published reference or Web-based information, always determine whether the sources are**

Box 6-10 **HELPFUL SEARCH ENGINES AND HEALTH-RELATED DATABASES**

> **Alta Vista and Google**: These are general search engines but are very good for health-related information.
> **CINAHL** (Cumulative Index to Nursing and Allied Health Literature) (http://www.cinahl.com/): Has articles from more than 1,200 journals and nearly all are available by fax or mail.
> **Pub Med** (http://www.ncbi.nlm.nih.gov/entrez/query.fcgi): A service of the National Library of Medicine. Provides access to more than 11 million **MEDLINE** citations back to the mid-1960s and additional life science journals. Includes links to many sites providing full text articles and other related resources.
> **NurseLinx.com** (http://www.NurseLinx.com): Provides nurses with an easy way to access the latest advances in their field.
> **Health on the Net** (**www.hon.ch**) and **Healthfinder** (http://www.healthfinder.org/): Bypasses the all-purpose commercial search engines and goes straight to health care portals. These portals eliminate irrelevant sources for you.
> **Agency for Healthcare Research and Quality** (**www.ahrq.gov**) **and the Cochrane Library** (**http://www.cochrane.org/cochrane/cc-broch.htm#CC** and **http://www.update-software.com/cochrane/**): Best evidence-based practice (EBP) Web sites for updating practice standards.
> **BIOETHICSLINE** (http://wings.buffalo.edu/faculty/research/bioethics/bio-line.html): Provides a database of bibliographic references concerning ethical and public policy issues in health care and biomedical research.

reliable. Ask questions like, Who are the authors? Are they authorities on the subject? and What are their educational backgrounds and credentials?

◆ **Examine their reference list.** What references are they using? Are they up to date? Are journals peer reviewed or refereed?* Are publishers reputable? Do they have a vested interest (e.g., if drug information is being provided, is the drug company paying them?)?

◆ **Additional questions for Web sites:**
  ● Is it clear how to contact the Web site owner?
  ● Can you tell which organization(s) contribute funds, services, or other support to the Web site?
  ● If there is funding, is it from a reputable source?
  ● Is this site for consumers, health professionals, or another audience?
  ● When was the information last updated?
  ● Does the site display a seal of approval that signifies it maintains strict standards? Although there are good Web sites that have not applied for a seal of approval, the seals of approval listed in Box 6-11 give you added confidence.

◆ **Decide whether the information is applicable in the context of the current situation.** For example, is the information relevant to your project or to your specific client(s)' situation?

Box 6-11 WEB SITES' SEALS OF APPROVAL

The Internet is widely used for accessing health-related information. Yet anyone can set up a Web site and publish anything, making it look reliable. Although not every good Web site has applied for a seal of approval, if a seal is displayed, you can feel more confident about the information displayed. Below are three seals of approval that ensure high standards.

◆ **HON Code of Conduct (HONcode) of the Health on the Net Foundation.** For information on requirements to display this seal, go to http://www.hon.ch/HONcode/.

◆ **URAC Health Web Site Accreditation** seal helps consumers to identify health Web sites that follow rigorous standards for quality and accountability. For information on requirements to display this seal, go to http://www.urac.org/.

◆ **TRUSTe Program:** Ensures that your privacy is protected through open disclosure, empowering you to make informed choices. For information on requirements to display this seal, go to http://www.etrust.com/consumers/users_how.html.

---

*Peer-reviewed or refereed journals are those that have all manuscripts reviewed by two to three knowledgeable nurses before publication. Whether a journal is peer-reviewed or not can be found in the front of the journal, usually where you find journal specifics like address and editorial board members.

◆ If the information is questionable, compare it with at least two other reputable sources on the same topic. Remember, "more than one source, more likely of course."

◆ When getting information from newspapers or nonprofessional magazines, verify it by checking original sources. Watch for follow-up articles and read letters to the editor (often you find thoughtful and professional commentary there).

◆ When overwhelmed, ask for help. Nurse educators, pharmacists, librarians, and other professionals can point you in the right direction.

◆ Develop information processing and management skills so that you can focus on what's important and keep data available in a way that helps you access the most important information quickly

1. **Never read without taking notes**–your notes help you process the information so you understand and remember it better. Don't highlight your way through an article–it may be easier, but it doesn't help you process, unless you're picking out only a few key ideas.

2. **Make the information your own by asking yourself questions** like, How well do I understand what's known and unknown about this topic? What are the relationships between key concepts? and What questions does this information raise for me? *Think* about what you're reading!

3. **When faced with an overwhelming amount of reading, scan article titles, introductions, and summaries** of each to eliminate articles that are unlikely to be helpful. Focus on the top three to five most useful and relevant.

4. **Draw mind maps** (see page 260) to identify relationships between key data.

5. **Revise notes and mind maps at least once to force yourself to do more in-depth thinking about what's most important.** Organizing and reorganizing information to find new relationships gives you more in-depth understanding and will help you remember the content better.

6. **Get rid of irrelevant or unimportant information.**

7. **When you find a good article, summarize the information on a card or word processor,** including the bibliographic citation you might need for future purposes. Save all this until you finish the project or graduate. In the long run, this saves time.

8. **Develop a filing system either in a file cabinet, box, or on your computer.** For example, when I read an article, I make a document with the bibliographic citation and key points on my computer. Then I put the actual articles in a file cabinet in case I need to look into more detail later.

9. **Put key data into the computer whenever possible.** Project management programs can help you.

10. **Carry a little notebook or make yourself a cheat sheet with key information that you need (e.g., formulas, lab values).** Know how to access the computer at any site where you are assigned for easy access to information.

Want to Know More?

Check out *How to Conduct Web Research.* Retrieved June 27, 2002 from http://www.rscc.cc.tn.us/owl/owl.html.

Other Perspectives

INFORMATION EXPLOSION? YEAH, RIGHT

"Duh and yeah right have arisen to fill a void in language.... Few questions these days can effectively be answered with yes or no.... The information age is more complicated than yes or no. It's more subtle ... more loaded with content, hype, and media manipulation (than it used to be)."

—Courtesy of The New York Times

Critical Moments

TURNING INFORMATION INTO KNOWLEDGE

You can't equate information with knowledge. Information is simply a group of facts. Turn information into knowledge by analyzing the data, identifying patterns and relationships, and working to gain insight into what the information implies.

USE YOUR NOODLE AS WELL AS YOUR COMPUTER

Computerized information is only as good as the mind that interprets it. Computers aren't able to think. They have no common sense, and they "believe" anything anyone tells them. In fact, computers simply shuffle data around like books on a tabletop. It's up to you to discriminate and decide which "books" apply and whether they are the latest "copyright." Use your noodle (brain) to interpret the information in the context of each situation. Ask questions like, How does this information apply to this particular case? How can I be sure this information is up to date? and Does this sound reasonable?

CRITICAL THINKING EXERCISES

1. In a group, exchange information management problems and strategies you've found helpful. Choose three strategies you can use.
2. Suppose someone comes to you and says "I have to read over 150 articles for my paper in 2 weeks!" Identify some things he can do to be more realistic about the reading.
3. Together with one or two peers, pick a topic you'd like to know more about. Then using the library and the Internet and sharing what you found, choose three good articles on the topic.
   ◆ Narrow the articles down to the two that are the most relevant and usable.
   ◆ Explain how you will use the information.
4. Draw a mind map showing the relationships between the most important information presented in this section.
5. Go to the Web sites for the seals of approval listed in Box 6-11 and summarize what you'd have to do to gain their seal of approval.
6. Determine whether you can achieve the Learning Outcomes at the beginning of this skill.

Recommended Reading

Alexander, J., & Tate, M. Evaluating web resources. Retrieved June 25, 2002 from http://www2.widener.edu/Wolfgram-Memorial-Library/webevaluation/webeval.htm

Burns, N., & Groves, S. (2001). *The practice of nursing research: Conduct, critique, and utilization* (4th ed). Philadelphia: W.B. Saunders.

Haybauch, P. A nurse's guide to the net. Retrieved from http://nsweb.nursingspectrum.com/ce/ce160.htm.

Sparks, S. (1998). World wide web search tools. *Image: Journal of Nursing Scholarship, 30*(2),167–171.

Walker, A. (2002). Electronic data, the internet, and private practice. *MEDSURG Nursing, 11*(1), 8, 47–48.

11. OUTCOME-FOCUSED WRITING (WRITING TO GET RESULTS)

Definition

Knowing how to write in a way that attains the results you want.

Learning Outcomes

After you study this information and complete the accompanying exercises you should be able to:
◆ Improve the clarity of your writing by using specific strategies.
◆ Evaluate your writings to determine if they meet your intended purpose.
◆ Collaborate with others to improve writing projects.

Thinking Critically about Writing

Many of us don't feel like we're getting much done unless our pens or fingers are moving and we're seeing some of the final form of our paper. But the time you take to clearly identify what you aim to do and how you can best do it is crucial to getting the final product you want. Writing, like any other skill, takes practice. The more you do it in the context of different situations–whether it be writing on the job or writing for school or publication–the better you become. If you study and apply the information in this section consistently–refer to it and follow it each time you have to write a paper, you will begin to develop habits that can really improve your ability to get your message across.

Some of you hate to write, but are really good at giving oral reports. With today's computers you can write by speaking–there are many voice-activated programs (e.g., *Dragon Naturally Speaking*). These types of programs can help you learn the basics because you get the hard part of getting your thoughts down on paper done early.

How to Write to Get Results

1. Determine exactly *what* you aim to do with your paper.
   - Communicate (inform, instruct, or persuade)?
     Examples: Essays, term papers, articles, memos, letters, charting.
   - Form values (clarify your own values or explain them to others)?
     Examples: Personal journals, essays, term papers, articles, letters.
   - Learn (sort out and remember thoughts about specific topics rather than communicate)?
     Examples: Personal journals, note-taking.
2. Decide exactly *who* will read your writing and keep this in mind as you write. Change your style accordingly. ***Examples:*** Your approach to writing for your boss or instructor should be different than for a friend, and your approach to writing for lay people must be simpler than 'for nurses.
3. Identify what *content* you need to include to achieve your purpose.
   - What exactly are you writing *about*?
   - Make an outline, jot down topic headings, or draw a mind map (see page 260).
4. Decide what *type* of writing approach will best achieve your purpose (you may have more than one of the following purposes).
   - Expressive: This is what I see, think, and feel.
   - Persuasive: This is what I believe, and this is why you should believe it.
   - Narrative: This is what happened (what I observed and heard) and then … .
   - Informational: This is what I know and how I know it. This is what others know and how I know they know it.
5. Identify one to four outcomes (*observable* results) you hope to achieve (this depends on the length of the paper).

Example Outcome: My teacher will read a paper that explains my beliefs on prolonging life in terminal illness and follows the guidelines she gave us in the assignment.

6. Use headings to let the reader know what's coming up (see the headings throughout this book). Keep paragraphs short and focused on one idea at a time. Once you've written the paragraphs, evaluate how they relate to the headings you used.
   ◆ Have you wandered from the topic?
   ◆ Do you need to change the heading?
   ◆ Can you make the headings more interesting?

7. Keep it simple: Simple terms make it easier to understand. When you find yourself struggling with long sentences or paragraphs, consider whether bullets or numbered points could express the information more easily.
   ◆ See how easy it is to read these short points?
   ◆ Our brains do better with short phrases or sentences than long ones.
   ◆ Bulleted points are actually also easier to write.

8. Use the following to get your point across better.
   ◆ Examples and analogies to make your point and show why your information is relevant.
   ◆ Tables and illustrations to increase understanding.
   ◆ Active voice to keep it simple (for example, *people see different things* is simpler to read than *different things are seen by different people*).
   ◆ Action verbs to engage the reader (e.g., *turn the patient* rather than *the patient is turned*).

9. Develop your own style. Don't be afraid to let your personality come through rather than sticking to strict, formal rules. (Check style requirements first if you're writing a formal paper or for a journal.)

10. Give yourself enough time to write at least two drafts. Critically evaluate your first and final draft (see Box 6-12).

11. Got writer's block? (see Box 6-13).

12. For school papers, use the following strategies as a guide.

10 Strategies for School Papers

1. **Give yourself enough time to complete the following steps:**

Plan: Determine your purpose and theme and set a schedule (don't wait till the last minute or you may have trouble getting the resources you need; for example, the best library books might be gone).

Write: Write your paper according to the plan (you may, however, change the plan somewhat as you write if necessary; the point is to start with some sort of plan).

Revise: Evaluate and improve (get others' input if possible).

Box 6-12 CRITICALLY EVALUATING IMPORTANT ESSAYS,
PAPERS, LETTERS, AND MEMOS

Using a 0–1-scale (0 = I'm not at all satisfied with my product and 10 = I'm very
satisfied), check each category below against your final paper.

— It gives a good first impression of my work.
— The main purpose or objective is clearly stated at the beginning of the paper.
— Major headings are listed, and the paragraphs pertain to the headings.
— The paper shows that I followed instructions for content and format
  carefully (compare paper with assignment).*
— The paper is written specifically for whom I expect to read it.*
— Opinions given are supported by facts.
— If I pull out all the headings and list them on a piece of paper, they show log-
  ical progression.
— I checked spelling.
— I asked someone to critique my first draft.
— I asked someone to proofread my final draft.
— Overall, based on the above, I'm pleased with this work.

*Doesn't apply to letters and memos.

Box 6-13 STRATEGIES FOR GETTING OVER WRITER'S BLOCK

1. **Just get started**, letting your ideas flow onto the paper (or the computer) in
   whatever order they come to you. Sometimes, writing is like exercising. You need
   a warm-up period.
2. **Dictate your ideas** to a tape recorder or buy voice-activated software such as
   Dragon Naturally Speaking so that you can just talk your way through the paper.
3. **Break the paper down into small tasks**. For example, if you can't seem to
   get started on the introduction, go on to address some of your other headings.
   It's not unusual to write the best introduction after you complete your paper.
   Doing easier headings before the introduction reduces your anxiety, helps you
   see progress, and gets your brain in "writing gear."
4. **Talk through your paper.** Say to someone, "I'm stuck on a point for my
   paper. Can you listen so I can explain it to you?" Write down key points as you
   explain them.

Edit: Proofread and correct.

**2. Carefully review your instructor's requirements, including
style requirements (formal, informal, type of citations, etc.).**
Make a checklist of what's most important to do and keep this in a
place where you readily see it (for example, at the front of your notebook or taped to your computer). Refer to the checklist frequently to

make sure you're focusing your paper in such a way that it meets the most important criteria being graded. Stay in touch with your instructor as needed–remember he is there to help you and clarify any questions you have.

Example checklist:

☐ 25% of grade is on description of nursing theory.
☐ 50% of grade is on analysis and application of nursing theory.
☐ 25% of grade is on format (grammar, spelling, bibliography).
☐ Make sure to focus on how the theory can be applied today.
☐ Wants lots of examples.

3. **Start by discovering your thoughts and ideas without being concerned about grammar or spelling.**
   ◆ List key ideas and questions that come to mind. Then review your ideas and ask yourself, What questions or thoughts do these ideas raise? Write these questions and thoughts down, too.
   ◆ Share your thoughts, feelings, and perceptions with friends. Ask them what questions or thoughts are raised for them.
   ◆ Keep a running list of your own ideas and ideas from your readings (be sure to cite your references in your notes or you might forget where the information came from and be accused of plagiarism).
   ◆ Do your bibliography as you go along. When you encounter an interesting reference, immediately write down the full citation.
   ◆ Use mind mapping (see pages 260-262).

4. **Develop one central idea, issue, or theme that you can explain to someone in two or three sentences.**

5. **Make an outline or simply list headings of things you want to cover.** Once you've listed your headings, number them in order of importance. Then decide on a logical flow of headings.

6. **Write the first draft with as few interruptions as possible.** Immersing yourself in a project helps you stay focused and logical. Be realistic–this doesn't mean pulling an all-nighter.

7. **As you write, visualize your instructor in your mind's eye.** Predict what he or she will want to know and provide the information. If you don't want to visualize your instructor, visualize someone else you know who is inquisitive.

8. **Remember the Three T's.**
   Tell them what you're going to tell them (introduction).
   Tell them (body).
   Tell them what you told them (summary).

9. **Once you've written the first draft, revise and improve, preferably a few days later to give yourself a fresh eye.** Revising is as important as writing a first draft: This is when you apply critical

thinking to your own work and challenge yourself to write (and think) more clearly. Revising entails asking yourself questions like:

◆ How well is the central idea of my paper addressed early in the paper? Somewhere early in the paper you should have something like, The purpose of this paper is … or This paper addresses … (use these exact words). It won't be unusual to find a strong statement of this sort buried in the middle of your first draft (probably because your mind was on a roll at that point) or at the end, when you were making your final statements. Move these statements to the introduction.

◆ How does my paper compare with my initial checklist of key points?

◆ How persuasively have I made my points or explained why I came to the conclusions I presented?

◆ How clearly does my summary describe what the paper addressed?

◆ How can I make the introduction and summary catchy or inspiring?

10. **Edit your paper to increase clarity and correct grammar and spelling problems**.

◆ Have someone else proofread your paper. You won't be able to proofread it well because you've looked at it too much.

◆ If you can't get someone else to proofread, read your paper out loud. When you read your paper out loud, you hear your mistakes.

◆ Trim the fat: Get rid of unnecessary words. Wordy sentences muddle your message and dilute its impact. For example, compare the clarity of the following messages (*b* says the same thing as *a*, but extra words are eliminated).

   a. Altogether too many students feel that writing should be taught only to those people who want to go into journalism once they have finished school. What these students don't realize is that their efforts in practicing writing can greatly enhance their general ability to think critically.

   b. Many students feel that writing should be taught only to those who want to go into journalism. What these students don't realize is that writing can enhance critical thinking.

◆ Play ICM (I Caught Me): Check yourself for repetition. We tend to use the same words over and over, making them lose their impact. Sometimes we even write two sentences back to back that actually say the same thing. Compare the clarity of the following statements: I played ICM with *a* below and deleted the number of times I used "think," ending up with the easier-to-read *b*.

   a. When thinking about how to write, think about what's most important. If you focus your thinking on what's most important, you'll improve your thinking and your grades.

b. When writing, stay focused on what's most important. You'll clarify your thoughts and improve your grades.

◆ If using a computer, run a grammar check (but remember, it doesn't pick up everything–you still need a proofreader).

Want to know more about writing with a purpose?

There's a lot of writing help online. For example, check out The Roane State Community College Online Writing Lab. Available at: http://www.rscc.cc.tn.us/owl/owl.html. Accessed 6/27/2002. Here you have the following links: Writing Help, Writing for Nurses, Writing Resources, How to Conduct Web Research, How to Cite Online Sources, Citation Styles, E-mail Etiquette Guidelines, Resume and Job Help, and Search Engines. Also check with your local universities and colleges for online help.

Critical Moments

WRITING HELPS YOU THINK

Once I asked a nurse if he wished he could do his charting by just dictating to a tape recorder. He responded, "Not really. When I write, I think." Then I asked, "What if you could dictate, then print out your notes and read them?" He responded, "Maybe then I'd like it because I could still evaluate my thoughts and see what I missed." When charting, evaluate your thinking–look for flaws and correct them. When pondering something important, put your thoughts down on paper. It helps you stay focused and evaluate thoughts as you write.

WATCH THOSE FAXES, E-MAILS, AND MEMOS!

It's easy to become impulsive with e-mails, faxes, and interdepartmental memos. They are so quick that you tend to send them off before giving them thought and attention they need. Remember that faxes, e-mails, and memos may be subject to more eyes than you intend. Be careful about what you write and how you say it. If you want to be assured of privacy, send it regular mail and mark it private.

Other Perspectives

SWEATING OUT WRITER'S BLOCK

Once I asked someone, "Do you know how to get rid of writer's block?" He replied, "Yeah. You sit in front of the computer and stare at the blank screen until beads of sweat form on your forehead and you sweat it out."

CRITICAL THINKING EXERCISES

1. Brainstorm about a way you can teach about how to get over writer's block. Make a list of your ideas, then pair off with a partner and exchange brainstorming lists.
   - Each of you add to the other person's list of ideas.
   - Switch them back and have the original author circle three or four ideas that are closely related, including what the partner added.
   - As partners, write one or two sentences connecting the ideas.
2. Pick a partner and choose a controversial issue together.
   a. One of you write a short pro paper, supporting the issue, and the other a short con paper, opposing it.
   b. Switch papers. Edit and improve each other's papers, keeping in mind the original purpose of the paper.
3. Keep all of your papers in a portfolio.
   a. Ask if you can improve or revise one of them to meet a course objective. Hand in both the old and new papers.
   b. Evaluate them according to the criteria in the checklist in Box 6-12.
4. Offer to critique and proofread peers' papers. It's great practice for learning what makes a good paper.
5. Keep a journal. Practice letting your thoughts flow.

Recommended Reading

Highfield, M. (2000). Facilitating student publication. *Nurse Author and Editor, 10*(3),4, 7.

Lashley, M., & Wittstadt, R. (1993). Writing across the curriculum: An integrated curricular approach to developing critical thinking through writing. *Journal of Nursing Education, 32*(9),422–424.

Lusardi, P. Research corner: communication: what is the patient's reality? *AACN News, 18*(3) 3,5,12. Retrieved July 2, 2002 from http://www.aacn.org/AACN/aacnnews.nsf/ ff1487bfe89b77df882565a6006cfc3f/4b21707cd865d06d88256a15007947e1?OpenDocument# research

Oermann, M. (2002). *Writing for publication in nursing.* Philadelphia: Lippincott.

Ruggiero, V. (1998). *The art of thinking: A guide to critical and creative thought* (5th ed.). New York: Longman.

Sorrell, J., Brown, H., Cipriano, S., & Kohlenberg, E. (1997). Use of writing portfolios for interdisciplinary assessment of critical thinking outcomes of nursing students. *Nursing Forum, 32*(4), 12–23.

Chapter References

1. Block, P. (1996). *Stewardship: Choosing service over self-interest.* San Francisco: Berrett-Koehler, 29.
2. Ibid., p. 37.
3. Ibid.
4. Henneman, E., & Roche, J. Eight ways to nurture a new student. Retrieved June 2, 2002 from http://community.nursingspectrum.com/MagazineArticles/article.cfm?AID=5948
5. E-mail communication. (June 2002).
6. Covey, S. (1989). *The seven habits of highly effective people.* New York: Simon & Schuster.
7. Rogers, P., & Bocchino, N. L. (1999). Restraint-free care: Is it possible? *American Journal of Nursing, 99*(10),26–33.
8. E-mail communication. (June 2002).
9. Dickenson-Hazard, N. (2001). Block party. *Reflections on Nursing LEADERSHIP, 27*(1), 5.
10. Campion, C. (1998). Embracing our differences. *Nursing Spectrum FL Ed., 8*(14),5.

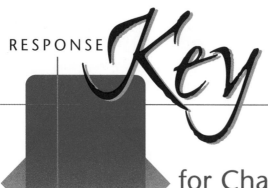

RESPONSE *Key*

for Chapters 1 to 5
Critical Thinking Exercises

Because the practice exercises are open-ended, the following are *example* responses for the practice exercises, not the *only* responses. If you have questions about whether your responses are appropriate, check with your instructor. If a number isn't listed below, it's because giving an example response is inappropriate for that particular exercise.

CHAPTER 1

Example Responses (pages 16 to 18)

1. You must clearly identify the problems, issues, or risks that must be managed to achieve the outcomes.

4. All three terms address confidence in one's own ability to reason well. However, *confidence in reason* also includes having faith that others will reason best when allowed to approach things in their own way.

5. (**a**) Facts are clearly observable and easily validated to be true. Opinions may vary depending on personal perspectives: They may or may not be valid. (**b**) The best way to determine if an opinion is valid is to ask for the facts or evidence that supports the opinion.

9. (**a**) Paraphrase any of the definitions beginning on page 4. (**b**) Thinking is basically any mental activity–it can be aimless and uncontrolled. Critical thinking is controlled, purposeful, and more likely to get needed results. (**c**) Three reasons are listed on pages 4 to 6. (**d**) Critical thinking focuses on achieving outcomes (results).

(**e**) CTIs are short descriptions of behaviors that promote critical thinking (see page 8). (**g**) Both critical thinking and problem solving focus on finding effective solutions. Critical thinking requires a more proactive approach, focusing on predicting, preventing, detecting, and managing problems and on finding ways to improve things, even when they are satisfactory. (**h**) See page 12.

CHAPTER 2

Example Responses (page 38)

2. (**a**) Feelings have a tremendous impact on what and how we think. Those of us who are driven by feelings are likely to have more problems thinking critically, especially when situations are emotionally charged. (**b**) Thinking critically requires that you recognize feelings and their impact on thinking and then use your head to apply logical and ethical reasoning principles. All too often we aren't even aware of deep strong feelings involved in certain situations. Those of us who are able to connect with emotions and give them the attention they deserve–to make them explicit, to accept them, and recognize their influence over thinking–can facilitate more logical, sensible thinking.

3. (**b**) Once you're aware of your thinking style–how your personality and learning preference affects your usual approaches to gaining understanding and making decisions, you can find ways to improve. (**c**) Habits are automatic. We do them without thinking. When we have deeply ingrained habits such as the ones that inhibit critical thinking on pages 30-37, we may believe we're thinking critically but are blind to how our habits inhibit our reasoning. If we create new habits that promote critical thinking like Covey's habits on page 37, we'll be more likely to automatically think critically.

Example Responses (pages 52 to 53)

1. Sometimes the terms goals and outcomes are used interchangeably. However, it's more correct to use goals when stating general intent (what you aim to do) and to use outcomes to clearly describe what you expect others to observe when the goal is observed. *Example goal:* I want to teach Mr. Molinas about diabetes. *Example outcome:* After 3 weeks, Mr. Kline will be able to give his own insulin and state how he will manage his dosage based on his diet, activity level, and glucose monitor readings.

3. In the first situation you'd encourage creative, off-the-top-of-your-head ideas, while in the second situation, because of the risks involved, you'd want sound, evidence-based ideas.

5. Jack and Jill are goldfish, and a cat knocked the fish tank on the floor, shattering it. You could have asked, "Who are Jack and Jill?"

◆ CHAPTER 3

Example Responses (pages 72 to 73)

2. A book can't give all scenarios of what can happen. Clinical situations often don't happen in the logical, sequential way they're described in a book. Simulated and observed experiences can help you acquire and remember key knowledge and skills required for critical thinking.

4. "I don't know" isn't an acceptable answer. A critical thinker who is oriented to satisfying customers would respond, "I'll find out." Finding out will help her broaden her knowledge and help Mr. Vina.

5. In the presence of known problems, you predict the most likely and most dangerous complications and take immediate action to (**a**) prevent them and (**b**) be prepared to manage them in case they can't be prevented. *Example:* If you're going to care for someone with a wired jaw and you aren't familiar with the care of someone with a wired jaw, you'd look it up so that you'd know common and dangerous complications (e.g., in this case, one dangerous complication is aspiration because the person is unable to open his mouth, so you would have wire cutters nearby). You also look for evidence of risk and causative factors (things we know cause problems or put people at risk for problems). You then aim to manage these factors to prevent the problems themselves. *Example:* In the case of the wired jaw, you'd assess for nausea (a risk factor for aspiration). If nausea was present, you'd ask for an antinausea drug, you'd hold food, and you'd keep suction equipment and wire cutters nearby. Finally, you promote health and function by asking the person how he's handling dietary and fluid intake needs, and make suggestions as needed.

6. (**b**) See Goals and Outcomes of Nursing and What Are the Implications on pages 60-61. (**c**) It means that care is directed at reaching specific, observable beneficial results in the client, and that the decisions we make and treatments we plan are based on data or evidence from clinical studies or accepted references. (**d**) Both DT and PPMP focus on treating problems. However, PPMP is more

proactive and focused on prevention and health promotion through early intervention than the DT model.

Example Responses (page 98)

1. The terms clinical judgment, clinical reasoning, and critical thinking are often used interchangeably. You use clinical reasoning and critical thinking to make a clinical judgment. Critical thinking is an umbrella term that includes thinking both in and outside the clinical setting.

2. Clinical judgment often requires thinking on your feet. It also requires knowing when to take your time and contact experts before making a decision. Clinical judgment entails things like knowing what to look for, how to recognize when a patient's status is changing, and what to do about it. It requires theoretical and experiential knowledge and application of standards, ethics, and principles of nursing process.

3. In today's competitive health care arena, the organizations that succeed will be those that best satisfy their customers' needs. We also realize that people deserve to be treated in a timely way by honest, courteous professionals.

4. You could irrigate a nasogastric tube if the facility permitted it, you've received permission from your instructor, you have the required knowledge and level of competence, the procedure is reasonable and prudent, and you're willing to assume accountability for how you perform the procedure and the patient response to the procedure.

5. (**a**) It's unlikely that the off-going nurse has really assessed the family's needs. It's highly unlikely that the family is doing fine. It appears as though the family has had limited involvement in the child's care. (**b**) You need to assess the family's needs and begin to include interventions that meet these needs in the nursing plan (e.g., allow the family to spend more time with the child).

8. (**a**) See Rule (the terms *diagnose* and *diagnosis* have legal implications) on page 77. (**b**) Decision making is guided by ethics codes and national and facility standards and guidelines. (**c**) *Some suggestions:* Write an outcome statement that clearly shows what you'll be able to do when you improve your ability to use good clinical judgment. Identify ways you can increase your theoretical and experiential knowledge. Get actively involved in seeking out learning resources and experiences. Make a commitment to study judiciously and prepare for learning experiences so that you can get the most out of them. Get involved in helping as a community, church, hospital, or nursing home volunteer. Seek out a mentor.

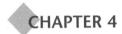

CHAPTER 4

Example Responses (pages 118 to 119)

Moral and Ethical Reasoning Exercises
1. Ask for a family meeting to make the decision, including an ethicist, trusted friends, or clergy to help.
2. Justice, beneficence, accountability.

Nursing Research Exercises
1. (**b**) Get the actual article. Check whether it comes from a refereed journal. Get more articles on the same topic. Check with a research text or find an article addressing how to analyze research studies. Discuss the results with experts and peers.
3. (**b**) These articles are more likely to be reliable.

Example Responses (page 132)

1. A major nursing outcome is to show improved independence and functioning. By teaching people about their health care, we empower them to be independent and healthy.
4. (**b**) Knowing how to memorize efficiently helps you remember the facts you need to think critically (critical thinking requires knowledge). Reasoning, or thinking your way through learning, helps you master and remember information from your own perspective.

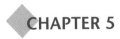

CHAPTER 5

Example Responses (pages 138 to 187)

1. Identifying Assumptions (pages 139 to 142)
1. There's not enough evidence to indicate that the patient needs instruction. Many people are fully knowledgeable about their diet but aren't able to stick to it.
2. You might waste your time teaching information the patient already knows. You might alienate the patient: Who likes to be taught things they already know? The patient gets the message that you don't understand the problem—that you jump to conclusions.
3. ***Scenario One.*** (**a**) She seems to have assumed that she can *create* a positive attitude for Jeff by talking about advances in diabetic care. (**b**) She needed to assess Jeff's *human response* to learning he's a diabetic. Jeff may be well aware of advances in diabetic care but is still

having trouble coming to terms with having to regulate his diet and take insulin for the rest of his life. She didn't *assess* before *acting.* (**c**) Jeff probably thinks Anita is a know-it-all because she didn't take the time to find out what his point of view on the situation was. It's a real turn-off when someone starts trying to change your attitude before he or she finds out what your attitude is.

    Scenario Two. (**a**) She seems to have assumed the mother can read and that the mother will let her know if she has questions. (**b**) If the mother can't read or is embarrassed to ask questions, the child may have inadequate care from his mother. If harm results from the nurse's failure to determine the mother's understanding, the nurse may be accused of negligence.

    Scenario Three. (**a**) That he would have the desired response to the drug without any adverse reactions. (**b**) It's likely that she was concerned that Mr. Schmidt wouldn't respond to the diuretic as expected–that he might experience an adverse reaction. (**c**) She probably thought the physician wouldn't like it if she challenged his judgment.

2. *Assessing Systematically and Comprehensively (pages 143 to 146)*

1. The body systems approach to assessment (Fig. 3-3, page 82) is probably the best method. Or you may choose the head-to-toe approach, clustering signs and symptoms of medical problems after you perform the assessment.
2. A nursing model approach (Box 3-7, page 82).
3. *Scenario One.* (**a**) Assess the extent of Pearl's voluntary movement (can she wiggle her toes?); color of toes and skin around cast edges; whether Pearl feels numbness or tingling in her foot or leg; whether there is any edema of the leg or toes; the quality of the dorsalis pedis pulse; whether Pearl perceives a needle prick as being sharp; whether her toes are warm or cool. (**b**) Assessing each of the above helps you detect early signs of circulatory problems, nerve compression, or skin irritation: If you find one area that begins to exhibit abnormal assessment findings (e.g., edema), you should increase the frequency and intensity of assessment of other areas (e.g., skin color). Specific relevance of each area of assessment follows: checking movement, numbness, and sensation monitors for nerve compression. Checking for color, edema, pulse quality, and warmth monitors circulation and skin condition. (**c**) Check circulation by assessing the dorsalis pedis pulse quality and capillary refill in toes; check for nerve compression by asking her to wiggle her toes and ask whether there is any numbness or tingling. If these are satisfactory, you might choose to put a warm sock over the toes;

encourage her to wiggle her toes frequently to increase the circulation, and continue to monitor her dorsalis pedis pulse, toe temperature, and toe sensation closely.

Scenario Two. (**a**) You'd look up digoxin in a reference, and then assess as follows. To assess for therapeutic effect, check to see if Mr. Wu's serum digoxin level is within therapeutic range (0.8– 2 ng/ml). Determine status of cardiac symptoms, as compared with baseline (status of apical/radial pulse rate and rhythm, lung sounds, urine output, edema, activity tolerance). To assess for adverse reactions, check Mr. Wu for signs and symptoms of any of the adverse reactions listed in the drug reference. You'd also assess for contraindications and toxicity/overdose, as follows. To assess for contraindications, check Mr. Wu for signs and symptoms of any of the contraindications listed in the drug reference. Most common contraindications for digoxin include serum potassium levels <3.5 mEq/L (increases the risk of toxicity); pulse rate less than 60 or physician-prescribed parameters; clinical signs of toxicity/overdose. To assess for toxicity/overdose, check Mr. Wu for signs and symptoms of toxicity/overdose. Most common signs and symptoms of digoxin toxicity include serum digoxin level >2 ng/ml; atrioventricular block (PR interval >0.24 sec); progressive bradycardia, nausea, vomiting, visual disturbances (blurring, snowflakes, yellow-green halos around images). (**b**) If no therapeutic effect is achieved by giving a drug or if the person is experiencing adverse reactions, you need to question whether there needs to be a change in dosage or whether the drug should be continued at all. If you identify contraindications to giving the drug, you need to withhold the drug. If you identify signs of toxicity/overdose, it's especially important to withhold the drug because you'd be adding to the toxicity/overdose problem.

Scenario Three. (**a**) Vital signs: Take temperature, pulse, respira- tions, and blood pressure. *Eye opening:* Call Gerome's name. Tell him to open his eyes. If no response, pinch him. *Best motor response:* Ask him to move each extremity. Use a pin prick or pinch him and see if he can tell you where he feels it. If no response, pinch him and note whether he flexes his extremity to withdraw from pain, flexes in spasm, or extends his extremity. *Best verbal response:* Ask him what his name is, where he is, and what day it is. Pupillary reaction: Determine size of each pupil in millimeters before flashing a light into it. Then flash a light into each pupil and observe whether it constricts briskly. Purposeful limb movement: Check each extremity by asking Gerome to move it, observing for muscle contraction (attempts to move), ability to lift extremity, and ability to lift extremity even though you try to hold it down. *Limb sensation:* Prick each limb with a sterile needle and ask Gerome what he feels (this may be unnecessary for Gerome, since he has a head injury rather than a spinal cord injury). *Seizure activity:* Observe for muscle twitching. *Gag reflex:* Place a clean tongue blade in the back of Gerome's throat and see if it triggers gagging. (**b**) By assessing all of these parameters, signs and symptoms of increased intracranial pressure can be detected early. Signs and symptoms of increased intracranial pressure are: decreasing level of consciousness; increasing restlessness; irritability and confusion; stronger headache; nausea and vomiting; increasing speech problems; pupillary changes (dilated and nonreactive or constricted and nonreactive pupils); cranial nerve dysfunction; increasing muscle weakness, flaccidity, or coordination problems; seizures; decerebrate posturing (muscles stiff and extended, head retracted); and decorticate posturing (muscles rigid and still, with arms flexed, fists clenched, and legs extended)–the latter two are both late signs of increased intracranial pressure. (**c**) Monitor other parameters of neurologic assessment closely for other signs of increased intracranial pressure. If there are no other changes and you can indeed arouse Gerome, you don't need to be immediately concerned; however, you should increase the frequency of assessment of all parameters until you're comfortable that the increased somnolence is merely a sign of the combined effects of fatigue and existing brain swelling (rather than increasing brain swelling). If you have ANY QUESTIONS about how to proceed, report the increased somnolence to your supervisor. (**d**) Check other neurologic parameters closely and report and record findings immediately; increase the frequency of assessment. (**e**) If the baseline pulse was rapid, this may be a normal finding. However, you should closely assess all the other assessment parameters to check for other reportable signs and symptoms. If the pulse is dropping to 60 beats per minute, closely monitor all the other assessment parameters and report the findings immediately (may be a sign of life-threatening increase in intracranial pressure).

3. Checking Accuracy and Reliability of Data (Validation) (page 147)
1. Talk with Mrs. Molinas and explore her feelings and concerns.
2. You may be able to turn on his blood glucose monitor and check it (some monitors automatically show the previous blood glucose level. If not, you can ask Mr. Nola to take it again now (quietly observe his technique). If he is proficient at performing a check for blood glucose, it's likely his previous result was correct. If the second reading is significantly different from the previous reading, consider whether there is a relationship between the change in

blood sugar reading and recent food intake or peak insulin levels. I would consider the blood sugar reading the patient took with you observing as being most valid.

3. Take it in the right arm. Take it again in 15 minutes.

4. Explore with Mr. McGwire why he thinks he got his foot ulcers. Ask him to tell you what he does to avoid getting foot ulcers. He may be very knowledgeable about diabetic care and foot ulcers and still be getting these ulcers.

4. *Distinguishing Normal from Abnormal/Identifying Signs and Symptoms (page 149)*

1. (**a**) If you assumed this was an oral temperature, you should have "S" here. You may have placed a question mark here, which is actually a more correct response. You need to ask, *"How was this temperature taken (orally? rectally? tympanic?")*. (**b**) If you assumed the patient never has rales, you should have an "S" here. You may have placed a question mark here, which is actually a more correct response. You need to ask questions like, *"What do the patient's lungs sound like when he's in his usual state of health? What is the respiratory rate? How far up the back can you hear the rales? Are there just a few rales or copious rales? When the patient coughs, do the rales clear?"* (**c**) You may have put an "S" here, but you really need to ask *if this is a normal pattern for the person and why the person only sleeps 3 hours at a time (e.g., it's not unusual for mothers of newborns to sleep only 3 hours at a time because of feeding schedules).* (**d**) S. (**e**) O or question mark. This is usually a normal finding, but you may have placed a question mark because you wanted to know such things as *whether there's any drainage, whether the area is hot to touch, and whether the patient is afebrile.* (**f**) O. This is normal for a 2-year-old. (**g**) S. (**h**) You may have placed an "S" here, but a better response is a question mark. Ask, *"What are the bathing practices of a person of this culture?"* (**i**) S. This is likely to be a normal finding, since the dialysis takes over the work of the kidney. (**j**) S or question mark. The pulse is somewhat slow but might be normal for someone who is young and athletic or older and on cardiac medication. You may have wanted to ask, *"What is this person's normal pulse?"* or *"Is the person taking any cardiac medications that slow the heart rate?"*

2. The italicized words in the answers to the previous exercise here provide examples of what else you might have wanted to know.

5. *Making Inferences (Drawing Valid Conclusions) (pages 150-151)*

1. I suspect this information indicates infection of some sort.

2. I suspect this information indicates financial problems.

3. I suspect this information indicates that the patient has trouble sticking to his diet.
4. I suspect this information indicates that the child wants to be sure his mother approves of his answer, or perhaps he is afraid.
5. I suspect this information indicates there is some medical reason for the grandmother's confusion.

6. Clustering Related Cues (Data) (page 152)

Scenario One. (**a**) Stung by a bee on the ear an hour ago; ear has no stinger, is red and swollen; no rash or wheezing; normal pulse and respirations. (**b**) Afraid he might die; wants to have a popsicle and watch TV. (**c**) Didn't make sure she had parents' phone number down (investigate whether this was lack of knowledge or oversight); doesn't know first aid for a bee sting.

Scenario Two. (**a**) 41 years old; acute abdominal pain; vomiting for 2 days and unable to keep any food down; abdomen distended; no bowel sounds; scheduled to go to the operating room at 2 PM; pain suddenly getting worse; vital signs unchanged, except pulse is increased by approximately 30 beats/min. (**b**) 41-year-old businessman; hates everything about hospitals; scheduled to go to the operating room at 2 PM; worried because his brother died in the hospital after a car accident; suddenly experiencing severe pain.

7. Distinguishing Relevant from Irrelevant (pages 154 to 155)

Scenario One. (**a**) May be relevant because buspirone hydrochloride can cause confusion in the elderly. (**b**) May be relevant because it may be a sign of infection, which can cause confusion in the elderly. (**c**) May be relevant because it's indicative of previous cardiovascular disease, which is a risk factor for cerebrovascular accident (stroke), which may be the cause of the confusion. (**d**) May be relevant because dehydration in the elderly can cause electrolyte imbalance and confusion. (**e**) Not relevant. (**f**) Not relevant.

Scenario Two. (**a**) Probably relevant. It takes time to adjust to a diabetic regimen. (**b**) Not relevant (not abnormal). (**c**) May be relevant (may feel constipation is caused by new diet). (**d**) May be relevant because she has to prepare meals for others, increasing temptation. (**e**) Very probably relevant. Someone who likes to cook usually takes joy in eating a variety of foods. (**f**) Relevant. She needs to eat even less than she will when her weight is within normal limits. (**g**) Not relevant (has nothing to do with sticking to a diabetic diet).

8. Recognizing Inconsistencies (page 156)

Scenario One. (**a**) It doesn't make sense that she has only just started coming to prenatal clinic but has been going to birthing classes. If she hasn't had prenatal care until now, you wonder whether she's really happy about the baby coming or realizes the importance of prenatal visits. You may also wonder why her mother, rather than her boyfriend, came to the clinic visit. (**b**) Check her records to see if there's any mention of receiving prenatal care somewhere else for the earlier part of her pregnancy; ask her where she's been going to birthing classes; ask how her boyfriend and mother feel about the baby coming.

Scenario Two. Her age is inconsistent with risk factors for a myocardial infarction (MI). The big picture here—her age, absence of pain, and previously normal electrocardiogram—is inconsistent with the big picture of an MI. *Occasionally* people don't have pain when they have an MI, but usually there are other risk factors and signs and symptoms present. Her signs and symptoms are more consistent with those of a panic attack.

9. *Identifying Patterns (page 158)*
   (**a**) Impaired Respiratory Function. Signs and symptoms of respiratory function problems are present. (**b**) Normal Coping Pattern. There are no signs or symptoms of abnormal coping pattern. (**c**) Pattern of Potential (Risk) for Impaired Bowel Elimination. There are risk factors for constipation but no signs and symptoms. (**d**) Normal Sleep-Rest Pattern. Considering the person works nights, there are no signs and symptoms of an abnormal sleep-rest pattern. (**e**) Potential (Risk) for Ineffective Sexual-Reproductive Pattern. There are risk factors for Ineffective Sexual-Reproductive Pattern.

10. *Identifying Missing Information (page 159)*
    (**a**) What are the person's *other* vital signs (pulse, blood pressure, temperature)? Is there a history of smoking? Is the person smoking now? How long has this pattern persisted? What does the person feel is contributing to this pattern? How does the person tolerate activity? (**b**) How does the husband feel about helping her? (**c**) Who is the major caregiver? What factors are contributing to the lack of roughage in his diet and his inadequate fluid intake? What's the patient's (or caregiver's) knowledge of how to prevent altered bowel elimination? Why does the patient spend most of his time in bed? How motivated is the patient to do the things necessary to prevent altered bowel elimination? (**d**) Does the person feel he's getting adequate rest? Are any sleeping aids being taken? If so, what are they? (**e**) What are the woman's feelings about having herpes? What does the woman know about herpes transmission? How does she

feel about telling prospective partners about the herpes? How does the patient plan to prevent herpes transmission?

11. *Promoting Health by Identifying and Managing Risk Factors (page 161)*

1. Do you have any family history of health problems? What's your ethnic background? Do you smoke? What do your usual meals consist of? Do you exercise regularly and get enough rest? How do you manage stress? Do you drink alcohol or take drugs that aren't prescribed? Are you sexually active? Do you wear your seat belt? What do you do to stay healthy?

2. Her age puts her at risk for osteoporosis. The history of falls together with the risk of osteoporosis put her at high risk for fractures. You need to look closely at why she is falling (e.g., balance problems? coordination problems? weakness or fatigue? vision problems? home hazards?). You should also assess calcium intake, which needs to be adequate to prevent osteoporosis.

3. Even though this is a social interaction, rather than professional nurse-patient interaction, keep in mind that because you're a nurse, he's likely to listen. Reinforce that he has a good question–that we all live longer now and that it's good to do things to increase the likelihood of living longer and healthier. Give some examples, like the importance of staying active and eating well. Stress the importance of annual exams that include blood studies to monitor things like cholesterol, blood sugar, and prostate specific antigen. Suggest doing this annual exam around a specific time (birthday, Christmas, etc.) so that he remembers.

12. *Diagnosing Actual and Potential (Risk) Problems (pages 165 to 166)*

    Scenario One. Potential for (or Risk for) Violence related to agitation and previous history of striking caregivers.

    Scenario Two. Potential complications: hemorrhage, shock, vomiting with aspiration, pneumonia, infection, paralytic ileus.

    Scenario Three. Hopelessness related to new diagnosis of terminal cancer as evidenced by statements of hopelessness and withdrawn behavior (sleeps most of the time, doesn't want to talk to anyone). Powerlessness is also an acceptable response. There is a fine line between these two diagnoses.

    Scenario Four. History of smoking or lung disease, whether the fractures are stable (risk for punctured lung), whether he has pain that is preventing him from coughing and clearing his lungs (risk for pneumonia).

13. Setting Priorities (pages 170 to 171)

1. (**b**) (*a* is likely to be dealt with informally or at home. *c* is likely to be covered by protocols and standards for care of colostomies.)
2. **Scenario One.** Reporting the chest pain should be your immediate priority. Myocardial infarction and pulmonary embolus, both serious problems, are potential complications of thrombophlebitis.
    Scenario Two. 1. (**a**) 3. (**b**) 2 or 3. (**c**) 2 or 3. **2.** No response provided. **3.** (**b**) This isn't a problem that must be addressed to achieve the major outcomes. It's unrealistic to try to resolve this problem in 2 days. Rather, be a good listener, provide support, and encourage him to seek support from family or counselors.

14. Determining Client-Centered Expected Outcomes (page 174)

1. Client will maintain intact skin, free of signs of redness or irritation.
2. After suctioning, mouth, nose, and lungs will be clear.
3. After the health team conference, the client will express feelings about powerlessness and relate increased sense of power over his situation as evidenced by statements that he is allowed to make as many choices about his own care as possible.
4. After irrigation, Foley catheter will be patent and draining urine.
5. Endotracheal tube will be out by (date).
6. Will demonstrate increased activity tolerance as evidenced by ability to walk the length of the hall and back by (date).

15. Determining Specific Interventions (pages 177 to 178)

1. (**a**) Monitor fluid intake every shift. Keep iced tea (patient's preference) at the bedside on ice. Encourage drinking at least 3 quarts during the day and 1quart at night. Reinforce the importance of maintaining adequate hydration. Record fluid intake. (**b**) Monitor anxiety level. Encourage her to express feelings and concerns. Fully explain all procedures. (**c**) Monitor comfort level. After applying heat for 30 minutes, assist with range of motion exercises 3 times a day.
2. **Scenario. a.** (**1**) It's quite likely the children won't report finding ticks, increasing the likelihood that the mother won't know when the children may have been bitten. It also increases the likelihood that the ticks won't be properly disposed of. I doubt that there will be benefits from using this approach (punishment). (**2**) It's possible that they may go looking for ticks, increasing the likelihood of being bitten. It's also possible that this approach might work, but the risks outweigh the benefits. **b.** Determine children's understanding of the severity of the consequences of tick bites and the importance of finding ways to avoid them. Initiate teaching as indicated. Explain to the children that they can best help by asking for insect repellent to

be applied before going outside, reporting ticks found on themselves and on each other, and avoiding tall grassy areas. Start a rule that the children can't go outside without first applying insect repellent. Have the mother praise good behavior (e.g., asking for insect repellent) verbally, rather than offering rewards. Instruct the mother not to offer rewards for finding ticks.

16. Note: Skill Number 16 *(pages 178 to 179)* has no exercises.

17. *Determining a Comprehensive Plan/Updating the Plan*
    (pages 181 to 182)
  1. (**a**) Not achieved. (**b**) Achieved. (**c**) Partially achieved; focus teaching toward mother's needs.
  2. ***Scenario.*** *Discharge outcome:* Will be discharged home with husband able to demonstrate administration of epinephrine by 6/29. *Nursing diagnosis no. 1:* Deficient knowledge (husband): Epinephrine administration. *Expected outcome:* Husband will relate knowledge of action and side effects of epinephrine and when to give epinephrine and demonstrate subcutaneous injection technique. *Interventions:* Provide husband with literature about epinephrine administration. Assess husband's knowledge of epinephrine action, side effects, and administration. Also determine preferred learning style. Reinforce what he already knows; teach gaps in knowledge using the husband's preferred learning style. Record husband's progress toward expected outcome after each teaching session. *Nursing diagnosis no. 2:* Altered Comfort (itching feet) related to hives as evidenced by hives over feet. *Expected outcome:* Patient will experience decreased itching as evidenced by statements of increased comfort. *Interventions:* Assist patient to place feet in cool water prn. Medicate as ordered prn for itching. *Note:* You may have chosen another diagnosis, such as *Ineffective Coping,* for Mrs. Edmunds, in the hope that you can help her cope with the possibility of learning how to give her own injections. However, in the interest of time, *teaching the husband* is first priority.
  3. You've identified a care variance. According to the predicted care, she should be voiding normal. Report the problem to the physician to determine appropriate approach.
  4. Expected outcomes: actual and potential problems (those that must be addressed to reach the overall outcomes; specific interventions designed to achieve the outcomes; evaluation statements (progress notes).

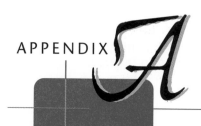

APPENDIX **A**

Mind Mapping: Getting in the "Right" State of Mind

WHAT IS MIND MAPPING?

Mind mapping (sometimes called concept mapping) uses the right brain (creative hemisphere) to enhance ability to understand information and solve problems: You combine writing and drawing. Unlike outlining, which uses the left brain (logical hemisphere), mind mapping is flexible, has few rules, and is easy to learn and teach. Figure A-1 shows a mind

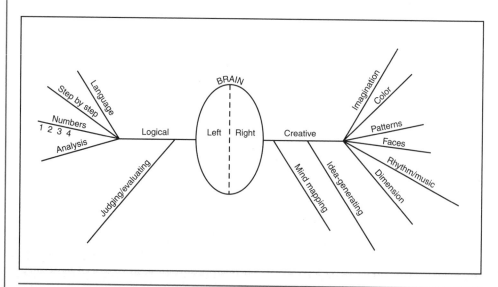

Figure A-1 ◆ Mind map of how the brain works.

Adapted from Menthey, M., & Miller, D. (1991). Tools for leaders, tools for managers. *Nursing Management, 22,* 2–21, with permission of Springhouse Corporation.

map of how the brain works. The boxes on the next page compare right and left brain function and give steps for how to mind map.

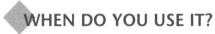

WHEN DO YOU USE IT?

You can use it for a variety of purposes. Following are some of the most common:
◆ Taking notes/learning new content
◆ Writing papers/preparing presentations
◆ Preparing for exams
◆ Promoting idea generation (brainstorming)
◆ Facilitating group problem solving

WHAT ARE THE BENEFITS?

General benefits and specific group benefits follow:

General Benefits

◆ Quicker than regular note-taking
◆ Highlights key ideas/gets rid of the irrelevant
◆ Helps you quickly gather, review, and recall large amounts of information
◆ Increases brainpower available for learning and problem solving by reducing energy used on concerns about structure and documentation
◆ Encourages you to identify relationships and be creative
◆ Helps you retain what you learn because you "play with the information" in your own way as you make your map

Group Benefits

◆ Promotes communication (keeps everyone focused on the main issues)
◆ Facilitates problem solving (generates more ideas, helps group suspend judgment)
◆ Makes ideas and relationships clear

HOW DOES IT PROMOTE CRITICAL THINKING?

Mind mapping facilitates the "productive phase" of critical thinking–the phase when you need to gather relevant information, identify relationships, and produce new ideas. After you complete this productive phase, you can get in touch with your left brain talents and move to the "judgment phase"–you can evaluate what your mind has produced, make judgments about its accuracy and usefulness, and make refinements.

APPENDIX A

LEFT VERSUS RIGHT HEMISPHERE FUNCTION

Left Brain (Logical, Judging, Evaluating)	Right Brain (Creative, Idea Generating)
Deals with:	Deals with:
Language	Images/imagination
Logic	Colors/geometry
Linearity (step-by-step approaches)	Pattern, face, and map recognition
Numbers and sequence	Rhythm/music
Analysis	Dimension

EIGHT STEPS FOR MIND MAPPING TO PROMOTE CRITICAL THINKING

1. **Put central theme or concept** in the center, bottom, or top of the page and draw a circle around it (see an example mind map below).
2. **Place the main ideas relating to the concept** on lines (or in circles) around the central theme.
3. **Add details** by putting them on lines (or in circles) connecting them to the main ideas.
4. **Use key words or simple pictures** only; keep it legible.
5. **Make sure no idea stands alone**. If you can't connect an idea with something on the page, it's irrelevant to the central theme.
6. **Don't allow yourself to slow down** over concerns about where to place words (this is your left brain habit trying to dominate). Rather, let your ideas flow and use lines to show connections.
7. **Use colors** to highlight the most important ideas.
8. **Once you've completed your mind map**, get in touch with your left brain talents (judging and evaluating) and evaluate what you've produced. **Revise as needed**.

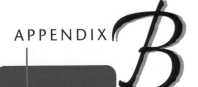

American Nurses Association Standards for Practice and Code of Ethics

AMERICAN NURSES ASSOCIATION STANDARDS FOR PRACTICE*

Standards of Care (Use of the Nursing Process)

Standard I Assessment: The nurse collects patient health data.

II Diagnosis: The nurse analyzes assessment data in determining diagnoses.

III Outcome Identification: The nurse identifies expected outcomes individualized to the patient.

IV Planning: The nurse develops a plan of care that prescribes interventions to attain expected outcomes.

V Implementation: The nurse implements the interventions identified in the plan of care.

VI Evaluation: The nurse evaluates the patient's progress toward attainment of outcomes.

Standards of Professional Performance (Professional Behavior)

Standard I Quality of Care: The nurse systematically evaluates the quality and effectiveness of nursing practice.

II Performance Appraisal: The nurse evaluates his/her own nursing practice in relation to professional practice standards and relevant statutes and regulations.

---

*Reprinted with permission from American Nurses Association (1998). Standards of Clinical Nursing Practice, 2nd Ed. © 1998 nursesbooks.org, the publishing program of ANA. 600 Maryland Avenue, SW, Suite 100W, Washington, DC 20024-2571. American Nurses Publishing. (Please note: These standards apply only until such time in mid-2003 when they are superseded by a revised set of standards. Monitor the ANA web site, http://www.nursingworld.org, for developments.)

III Education: The nurse acquires and maintains current knowledge in nursing practice.

IV Collegiality: The nurse interacts with, and contributes to the professional development of, peers and other healthcare providers as colleagues.

V Ethics: The nurse's decisions and actions on behalf of patients are determined in an ethical manner.

VI Collaboration: The nurse collaborates with the patient, significant others, and healthcare providers in providing patient care.

VII Research: The nurse uses research findings in practice.

VIII Resource Utilization: The nurse considers factors related to safety, effectiveness, and cost in planning and delivering patient care.

CODE OF ETHICS FOR NURSES*

1. The nurse, in all professional relationships, practices with compassion and respect for the inherent dignity, worth and uniqueness of every individual, unrestricted by considerations of social or economic status, personal attributes, or the nature of health problems.

2. The nurse's primary commitment is to the patient, whether an individual, family, group, or community.

3. The nurse promotes, advocates for, and strives to protect the health, safety, and rights of the patient.

4. The nurse is responsible and accountable for individual nursing practice and determines the appropriate delegation of tasks consistent with the nurse's obligation to provide optimum patient care.

5. The nurse owes the same duties to self as to others, including the responsibility to preserve integrity and safety, to maintain competence, and to continue personal and professional growth.

6. The nurse participates in establishing, maintaining, and improving healthcare environments and conditions of employment conducive to the provision of quality health care and consistent with the values of the profession through individual and collective action.

7. The nurse participates in the advancement of the profession through contributions to practice, education, administration, and knowledge development.

---

*Retrieved July 6, 2002 from http://nursingworld.org/ethics/chcode.htm. To order *Code of Ethics for Nurses with Interpretive Statements* (2001) go to http://nursingworld.org/anp/pdescr.cfm?cnum=5.#CEN21.

8. The nurse collaborates with other health professionals and the public in promoting community, national, and international efforts to meet health needs.
9. The profession of nursing, as represented by associations and their members, is responsible for articulating nursing values, for maintaining the integrity of the profession and its practice, and for shaping social policy.

APPENDIX B

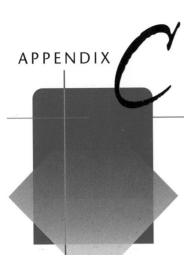

Example Critical Pathway

Clinical Pathway ■	**CARE PATH NAME: TOTAL ABDOMINAL HYSTERECTOMY**	
	□ With Burch	□ Without Burch

DRG: 353-358   ELOS: 2 Days
Expected Disposition: Home

Focus	Preadmission	Day of Surgery
LABORATORY/ TESTS/ PROCEDURES	□ Blood work □ <40 years Hct □ >40 years SMA 6, CBC □ EKG if >40 years □ CXR if >60 years □ Type and screen	
CONSULTS/ REFERRALS/	□ Anesthesia Consult □ Nursing Consult	
PHYSICAL ASSESSMENT	□ H & P obtained	□ VS per post-op routine □ Routine post-op assessment □ I/O
DIAGNOSIS:		
ACTIVITY	□ Ad lib	□ Dangle at bedside or OOB to chair
TREATMENTS	□ Instruction on IS □ Review of procedure	□ IS/C&DB Q 1 h WA □ Foley □ SCD's □ Drains: **BURCH ONLY:** □ Suprapubic Catheter

Collaborative Problem List
1. Discharge Planning
2. Pain/Comfort Management
3. Coping Response to
   Surgery/Diagnosis
4. _____

Post-Op Day 1	Post-Op Day 2
☐ CBC	
☐ Primary RN	
☐ VS Q shift	☐ VS Q shift
☐ Q shift assessment	☐ Q shift assessment
☐ I/O	☐ I/O
☐ Weight	☐ Weight
☐ Fever assessment (if temp >39° C)	☐ Fever assessment (if temp >38.5° C)
☐ Exam	☐ Exam
☐ Cultures of surgical area	☐ Cultures of surgical area
☐ CBC with diff	☐ CBC with diff
☐ Blood cultures	☐ Blood cultures
☐ OOB to chair	☐ Ambulate QID
☐ IS/C&DB Q 1 h WA	☐ IS/C&DB Q 1 h
☐ D/C Foley	☐ D/C Drains:
☐ SCD's	**BURCH ONLY:**
☐ Drains:	☐ Suprapubic Catheter
BURCH ONLY:	☐ Monitor postvoid residuals
☐ Suprapubic Catheter	☐ Begin clamp routine 24 h after surgery if no hematuria

APPENDIX C

Continued

Clinical Pathway ■ **CARE PATH NAME: TOTAL ABDOMINAL HYSTERECTOMY**
(*Continued*)

Focus	Preadmission	Day of Surgery
DIET	☐ NPO pre-op	☐ Ice chips ☐ Clear liquids
MEDICATIONS		☐ PCA protocol ☐ Epidural protocol ☐ IV pain meds ☐ IV antibiotics: ☐ IVF:
DISCHARGE PLANNING/ TEACHING	☐ Discharge Planning Review: 　☐ Pre-op checklist 　☐ Advanced directives 　☐ Client care path pamphlet ☐ Determine services needed 　☐ Client lives alone 　☐ Client lives with others 　　Support person: 　　Phone number:	☐ Client lives alone ☐ Client lives with others 　Support person: 　Phone Number:
INDIVIDUALIZED CARE FOCUS		
INTERMEDIATE OUTCOMES	☐ Client able to explain home-going plan ☐ Client able to describe pro-cedure(s) to be performed ☐ Client states she has partici-pated in decision making and plan	☐ Afebrile ☐ Client states pain is ade-quately controlled ☐ Client shows no evidence of post-op complications

Discharge Outcomes:	Met

1. Abdominal incision approximated and healing
2. Has minimal, odorless vaginal discharge
3. Able to describe/perform pericare
4. Has functional pattern for bladder and bowel
5. Maintains adequate nutritional intake
6. Pain controlled by oral medication
7. States use of homegoing medications
8. Describes plan for follow-up care
9. Describes feeling about effects of surgery on health and sexuality
10. Identifies support systems and resources available to her after discharge
11. Afebrile or Temp <38° C with normal WBC
12. **BURCH ONLY:** Able to demonstrate clamp routine

APPENDIX C

Post-Op Day 1	Post-Op Day 2
☐ Advanced as tolerated	☐ House diet
☐ D/C PCA at 08:00	☐ PO meds
☐ D/C Epidural	☐ D/C HL
☐ IV pain meds to PO	
☐ IVF:	
☐ Heplock when taking PO	
Provide Homegoing Instructions:	☐ Review home-going
☐ Hysterectomy PI-128	instructions
☐ "Women and AIDS" pamphlet	
☐ Breast self exam pamphlet	
☐ Hormone replacement therapy	
☐ Instruct on pericare	
BURCH ONLY:	
☐ Clamp Routine PI Sheets	
	☐ Ambulates independently
☐ Able to void without difficulty	☐ Has had a bowel movement and/or
☐ Afebrile or temp <38° C with	passed flatus
normal WBC	☐ Tolerates house diet
☐ Tolerating PO fluids	☐ Client able to describe procedure(s)
☐ Ambulates with assistance	performed
☐ Client states pain is ade-	☐ Client able to describe pericare
quately controlled with PO	☐ Client able to explain all discharge
Pain medication	instructions
	BURCH ONLY:
	☐ Able to measure and record
	postvoid residuals

Not Met	Comments	Date/Initials

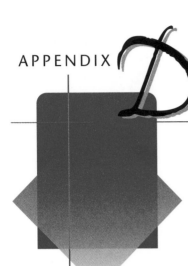

NANDA Nursing Diagnoses*

TAXONOMY II: DOMAINS, CLASSES, AND DIAGNOSES

Domain 1. Health Promotion: the awareness of well-being or normality of function and the strategies used to maintain control of and enhance that well-being or normality of function

> **Class 1. Health Awareness:** recognition of normal function and well-being

> **Class 2. Health Management:** identifying, controlling, performing and integrating activities to maintain health and well-being

> > **Approved Diagnoses**
> > Effective individual therapeutic regimen management
> > Ineffective individual therapeutic regimen management
> > Ineffective family therapeutic regimen management
> > Ineffective community therapeutic regimen management
> > Health seeking behaviors (specify)
> > Ineffective health maintenance
> > Impaired home maintenance

*Source: Handout from First Biennial Conference of the NANDA, NIC & NOC Alliance (NNN: Working Together for Quality Nursing Care). Chicago. April 10–13, 2002.

Domain 2. Nutrition: the activities of taking in, assimilating, and using nutrients for the purposes of tissue maintenance, tissue repair, and the production of energy

Class 1. Ingestion: taking food or nutrients into the body

Approved diagnoses
Ineffective infant feeding pattern
Impaired swallowing
Imbalanced nutrition: less than body requirements
Imbalanced nutrition: more than body requirements
Risk for imbalanced nutrition: more than body requirements

Class 2. Digestion: the physical and chemical activities that convert foodstuffs into substances suitable for absorption and assimilation

Class 3. Absorption: the act of taking up nutrients through body tissues

Class 4. Metabolism: the chemical and physical processes occurring in living organisms and cells for the development and use of protoplasm, production of waste and energy, with the release of energy for all vital processes

Class 5. Hydration: the taking in and absorption of fluids and electrolytes

Approved Diagnoses
Deficient fluid volume
Risk for deficient fluid volume
Excessive fluid volume
Risk for fluid volume imbalance

Domain 3. Elimination: secretion and excretion of waste products from the body

Class 1. Urinary System: process of secretion and excretion of urine

Approved Diagnoses
Impaired urinary elimination
Urinary retention
Total urinary incontinence
Functional urinary incontinence
Stress urinary incontinence
Urge urinary incontinence
Reflex urinary incontinence
Risk for urge urinary incontinence

Class 2. Gastrointestinal System: excretion and expulsion of waste products from the bowel

Approved Diagnoses
Bowel incontinence
Diarrhea
Constipation
Risk for constipation
Perceived constipation

Class 3. Integumentary System: process of secretion and excretion through the skin

Class 4. Pulmonary System: removal of by-products of metabolic products, secretions, and foreign material from the lung or bronchi

Approved Diagnoses
Impaired gas exchange

Domain 4. Activity/Rest: the production, conservation, expenditure, or balance of energy resources

Class 1. Sleep/Rest: slumber, repose, ease, relaxation, or inactivity

Approved Diagnoses
Disturbed sleep pattern
Sleep deprivation

Class 2. Activity/Exercise: moving parts of the body (mobility), doing work, or performing actions often (but not always) against resistance

Approved Diagnoses
Risk for disuse syndrome
Impaired physical mobility
Impaired bed mobility
Impaired wheelchair mobility
Impaired transfer ability
Impaired walking
Deficient diversional activity
Wandering
Dressing/grooming self care deficit
Bathing/hygiene self care deficit
Feeding self care deficit
Toileting self care deficit
Delayed surgical recovery

Class 3. Energy Balance: a dynamic state of harmony between intake and expenditure of resources

Approved Diagnoses
Disturbed energy field
Fatigue

Class 4. Cardiovascular/Pulmonary Responses: cardiopulmonary mechanisms that support activity/rest

Approved Diagnoses
Decreased cardiac output
Impaired spontaneous ventilation
Ineffective breathing pattern
Activity intolerance
Risk for activity intolerance
Dysfunctional ventilatory weaning response
Ineffective tissue perfusion (specify type: renal, cerebral, cardiopulmonary, gastrointestinal, peripheral)

Domain 5. Perception/Cognition: the human information processing system including attention, orientation, sensation, perception, cognition, and communication

Class 1. Attention: mental readiness to notice or observe

APPENDIX D

Approved Diagnoses
Unilateral neglect

Class 2. Orientation: awareness of time, place, and person

Approved Diagnoses
Impaired environmental interpretation syndrome

Class 3. Sensation/Perception: receiving information through the senses of touch, taste, smell, vision, hearing, and kinesthesia and the comprehension of sense data resulting in naming, associating, and/or pattern recognition

Approved Diagnoses
Disturbed sensory perception (specify: visual, auditory, kinesthetic, gustatory, tactile)

Class 4. Cognition: use of memory, learning, thinking, problem-solving, abstraction, judgment, insight, intellectual capacity, calculation, and language

Approved Diagnoses
Deficient knowledge (specify)
Acute confusion
Chronic confusion
Impaired memory
Disturbed thought processes

Class 5. Communication: sending and receiving verbal and non-verbal Information

Approved Diagnoses
Impaired verbal communication

Domain 6. Self-Perception: awareness about the self

Class 1. Self-Concept: the perception(s) about the total self

Approved Diagnoses
Disturbed identity

Powerlessness
Risk for powerlessness
Hopelessness
Risk for loneliness

Class 2. Self-Esteem: assessment of one's own worth, capability, significance, and success

Approved Diagnoses
Chronic low self-esteem
Situational low self-esteem
Risk for situational low self-esteem

Class 3. Body Image: a mental image of one's own body

Approved Diagnoses
Disturbed body image

Domain 7. Role Relationships: the positive and negative connections or associations between persons or groups of persons and the means by which those connections are demonstrated

Class 1. Caregiving Roles: socially expected behavior patterns by persons providing care who are not health care professionals

Approved Diagnoses
Caregiver role strain
Risk for caregiver role strain
Impaired parenting
Risk for impaired parenting

Class 2. Family Relationships: associations of people who are biologically related or related by choice

Approved Diagnoses
Interrupted family processes
Dysfunctional family processes: alcoholism
Risk for impaired parent/infant/child attachment

Class 3. Role Performance: quality of functioning in socially expected behavior patterns

Approved Diagnoses
Effective breastfeeding
Ineffective breastfeeding
Interrupted breastfeeding
Ineffective role performance
Parental role conflict
Impaired social interaction

Domain 8. Sexuality: sexual identity, sexual function, and reproduction

    Class 1. Sexual Identity: the state of being a specific person in regard to sexuality and/or gender

    Class 2. Sexual Function: the capacity or ability to participate in sexual activities

        Approved Diagnoses
        Sexual dysfunction
        Ineffective sexuality patterns

    Class 3. Reproduction: any process by which new individuals (persons) are produced

Domain 9. Coping/Stress Tolerance: contending with life events/life processes

    Class 1. Post-trauma Responses: reactions occurring after physical or psychological trauma

        Approved Diagnoses
        Relocation stress syndrome
        Risk for relocation stress syndrome
        Rape-trauma syndrome
        Rape-trauma syndrome: silent reaction
        Rape-trauma syndrome: compound reaction
        Post-trauma syndrome
        Risk for post-trauma syndrome

    Class 2. Coping Responses: the process of managing environmental stress

        Approved Diagnoses
        Fear
        Anxiety

Death anxiety
Chronic sorrow
Ineffective denial
Anticipatory grieving
Dysfunctional grieving
Impaired adjustment
Ineffective individual coping
Disabled family coping
Compromised family coping
Defensive coping
Ineffective community coping
Readiness for enhanced family coping
Readiness for enhanced community coping

Class 3. Neuro-behavioral Stress: behavioral responses reflecting nerve and brain function

Approved Diagnoses
Autonomic dysreflexia
Risk for autonomic dysreflexia
Disorganized infant behavior
Risk for disorganized infant behavior
Readiness for enhanced organized infant behavior
Decreased intracranial adaptive capacity

Domain 10. Life Principles: principles underlying conduct, thought, and behavior about acts, customs, or institutions viewed as being true or having intrinsic worth

Class 1. Values: the identification and ranking of preferred modes of conduct or end states

Class 2. Beliefs: opinions, expectations, or judgments about acts, customs, or institutions viewed as being true or having intrinsic worth

Approved Diagnoses
Readiness for enhanced spiritual well-being

Class 3. Value/Belief/Action Congruence: the correspondence or balance achieved between values, beliefs, and actions

Approved Diagnoses
Spiritual distress
Risk for spiritual distress
Decisional conflict (specify)
Noncompliance (specify)

Domain 11. Safety/Protection: freedom from danger, physical injury or immune system damage, preservation from loss, and protection of safety and security

Class 1. Infection: host responses following pathogenic invasion

Approved Diagnoses
Risk for infection

Class 2. Physical Injury: bodily harm or hurt

Approved Diagnoses
Impaired oral mucous membrane
Risk for injury
Risk for perioperative positioning injury
Risk for falls
Risk for trauma
Impaired skin integrity
Risk for impaired skin integrity
Impaired tissue integrity
Impaired dentition
Risk for suffocation
Risk for aspiration
Ineffective airway clearance
Risk for peripheral neurovascular dysfunction
Ineffective protection

Class 3. Violence: the exertion of excessive force or power so as to cause injury or abuse

Approved Diagnoses
Risk for self-mutilation
Self-mutilation
Risk for other-directed violence
Risk for self-directed violence
Risk for suicide

Class 4. Environmental Hazards: sources of danger in the surroundings

Approved Diagnoses
Risk for poisoning

Class 5. Defensive Processes: the processes by which the self protects itself from the non-self

Approved Diagnoses
Latex allergy response
Risk for latex allergy response

Class 6. Thermoregulation: the physiologic process of regulating heat and energy within the body for purposes of protecting the organism

Approved Diagnoses
Risk for imbalanced body temperature
Ineffective thermoregulation
Hypothermia
Hyperthermia

Source: Handout from First Biennial Conference of the NANDA, NIC & NOC Alliance (NNN: Working Together for Quality Nursing Care). Chicago. 2002.

APPENDIX D

Glossary

advanced practice nurse A nurse who, by virtue of credentials (usually completion of a master's program and certification), has a wide scope of authority to act (may include treating medical problems and prescribing medications).

air embolism An air bubble that gets into the bloodstream. Can be fatal.

analysis A mental process in which one seeks to get a better understanding of the nature of something by carefully separating the whole into smaller parts. For example, if you want to know more about someone's physical health, you examine each organ and system separately.

anaphylactic shock Extreme hypotension caused by an allergic reaction; requires immediate treatment or can be fatal.

assessment tool A printed or computerized form used to ensure that key information is gathered and recorded during assessment.

assumption Something that's taken for granted without proof. (Compare with *hypothesis* and *inference*.)

attitude A way of acting, feeling, or thinking that shows one's disposition, opinion, etc. (e.g., a threatening attitude).

baseline data Information that describes the status of a problem before treatment begins.

benchmark A standard or point in measuring quality. In health care, benchmarks are determined by analyzing the data collected over a period of time.

best practices A term referring to ways certain problems are best prevented and managed from an outcome and cost perspective.

care variance When a patient hasn't achieved activities or outcomes by the time frame noted on a critical path.

caring behavior Behavior that shows understanding and respect for another's perceptions, feelings, needs, and desires.

circumstances The conditions or facts attending an event or having some bearing on it.

classify To arrange or group together data according to categories, thereby increasing understanding because relationships become more obvious.

client-centered outcome (1) A statement that describes the benefits the client is expected to experience from nursing care. (2) A statement or phrase that describes what the client or patient is expected to be able to do when the plan of care is terminated. For example, "Will be discharged home able to walk independently using a walker by 8/24."

clinical judgment (1) Nursing opinion(s) made about a person's, family's, or group's health at a certain point in time. (2) Nursing decisions made about things like what to assess, what health data suggest, what to do first, and who should do it.

clinical reasoning The process used to make a clinical judgment.

collaborative actions Nursing actions prescribed by a physician or facility protocol. For example, administering IVs. (Compare with *independent nursing actions*.)

competence The quality of having the necessary knowledge, skill, and attitude to perform an action.

context The circumstances in which a particular event occurs.

critical Characterized by careful and exact evaluation; crucial.

Critical Thinking Indicator™ (CTI)™ Short description of behavior that demonstrates the knowledge, characteristics, and skills that promote critical thinking.

cues See *data*.

data Pieces of information about health status (e.g., vital signs).

database assessment Comprehensive data collected when the client first enters the health care facility to gain information about all aspects of the health status.

data base form See assessment tool.

deductive reasoning Drawing specific conclusions from general principles and rules. For example, since it's true that bacteria are killed by antibiotics, bacterial infection requires treatment with antibiotics. (Compare with *inductive reasoning*.)

defining characteristics The signs and symptoms usually associated with a specific nursing diagnosis.

definitive diagnosis The most specific, most correct diagnosis.

definitive interventions The most specific actions required to prevent, resolve, or control a health problem.

diagnose To identify and name health problems after careful analysis of evidence from an assessment.

diagnostic error When a health problem has been overlooked or incorrectly identified.

diagnostic reasoning A method of thinking that involves specific, deliberate use of critical thinking to reach conclusions about health status.

GLOSSARY

diagnostic statement A phrase that clearly describes a diagnosis; includes the problem name, related (risk) factors, and any evidence confirming the diagnosis.

diaphoretic The condition of being sweaty, usually suspected to be a sign of a health problem (e.g., shock, disease).

disposition One's customary frame of mind or manner of response.

diuretic A drug given to enhance kidney function, thereby increasing fluid elimination from the body.

efficiency The quality of being able to produce a desired effect safely, with minimal risks, expense, and unnecessary effort.

emboli More than one embolus. (See *embolus*.)

embolus A clot that has moved through one vessel and lodged in another, reducing or totally blocking blood supply to tissues usually nourished by the vessels involved. (Compare with *thrombus*.)

empathy Understanding another's feelings or perceptions but not sharing the same feelings or point of view. (Compare with *sympathy*.)

empiric Relying solely on practical experience, ignoring science.

epidemiology The body of knowledge reflecting what is known about a specific health state.

esthetics A sense of what is pleasing to the eye.

ethics The study of the general nature of morals and of the specific moral choices to be made by individuals in relationships with others.

etiology The cause or contributing factors of a health problem.

expected outcome See *client-centered outcome*.

expedite To make something happen in a quick fashion.

explicit Clearly and specifically expressed or described.

focus assessment Data collection that aims to gain specific information about only one aspect of health status.

guidelines Documents that delineate how care is to be provided in specific situations.

habits of inquiry Habits that enhance the ability to search for the truth (e.g., following rules of logic).

human responses Reactions of individuals or groups to health care concerns. For example, a woman may react to being told she is diabetic by feeling overwhelmed and unable to cope, or she may react by wanting to learn more about diabetes.

humanistic A way of thought or action concerned with the interests or ideals of people.

hypothesis (1) A hunch. (2) An assertion subject to verification or proof. (Compare with *assumption* and *inference*.)

imply To suggest by logical necessity.

independent nursing actions Nursing actions performed independently, without need for physician's orders or facility protocols. For example, ensuring adequate oral intake to prevent dehydration. (Compare with *collaborative actions*.)

independent nursing interventions See *independent nursing actions*.

indicator A criterion for evaluating progress toward a goal.

inductive reasoning Drawing *general* conclusions by observing a few *specific* members of a class. For example: "Since everyone I ever knew with a bacterial infection required an antibiotic, and Jane has a bacterial infection, Jane requires an antibiotic." (Compare with *deductive reasoning*.)

infer To suspect something or to attach meaning to information. For example, if someone is frowning, we may infer that he or she is worried.

inference Something we suspect to be true, based on a logical conclusion after examination of the evidence. (Compare with *assumption* and *hypothesis*.)

intervention Something done to prevent, cure, or control a health problem (e.g., turning someone every 2 hours is an intervention to prevent skin breakdown).

intubation The process of inserting a tube into an individual's bronchus to facilitate breathing.

intuition Knowing something without evidence.

irrigate To flush a tube (with normal saline solution or water) to keep it patent.

life processes Events or changes that occur during one's lifetime (e.g., growing up, getting married, losing someone).

logic A system of reasoning that leads to valid conclusions.

malpractice The negligent conduct of a person acting within his professional capacity.

measurable Capable of being clearly observed so that the quality or quantity of something can be determined.

medical domain Actions a physician is legally qualified to perform.

mentor A knowledgeable, insightful, and trusted person who helps someone else clarify thinking.

moral Concerned with the judgment of whether a human action or character is right or wrong.

myocardial infarction Partial or complete occlusion of one or more of the coronary arteries, causing death of coronary tissue.

nasogastric tube A tube inserted through the nose, down the esophagus, and into the stomach.

negligence Failure to provide the degree of care that someone of ordinary prudence would provide under the same circumstances. To claim negligence, it is necessary that there be a duty owed by one person to another, that the duty be breached, and that the breach cause harm.

nursing actions Something done by a nurse to achieve an outcome.

nursing intervention Action taken by a nurse to produce a nursing outcome.

nursing domain Actions a nurse is legally qualified to perform.

objective data Information that you can clearly observe or measure. For example, a pulse of 140 beats per minute.

outcome The expected result of interventions.

outcome measure A change, or absence of change, in a diagnosis.

paradigm (pa'-ra-dim) A model or way of doing things.

patent Open, so as to allow the flow of fluid or air.

phenomena Factors influencing humans that are concerns of nursing at a point further along in time dimension.

policies See *guidelines*.

potential diagnosis A health problem that may occur because of certain risk factors present (e.g., someone who's on prolonged bed rest has a potential [or risk] for Impaired Skin Integrity).

potential problem See *potential diagnosis*.

preceptor An experienced, more qualified nurse assigned by a facility to facilitate learning for a less experienced nurse.

proactive (comes from *act before*) A way of thinking and behaving that accepts responsibility for one's actions and takes initiative to plan ahead to anticipate and prevent problems before they happen.

procedures See *guidelines*.

protocols See *guidelines*.

pulmonary embolus A clot that has blocked off circulation and oxygenation to lung tissue. Considered to be life-threatening.

QA See *quality assessment*.

QI See *quality improvement*.

qualified Having the competence and authority to perform an action.

quality The degree to which patient care services increase the probability of achieving desired outcomes with the decreased probability of undesired outcomes.

quality assessment (QA) Ongoing studies designed to evaluate quality of patient care and services. Just as assessment is the first step of the nursing process, QA is the first step of QI (quality improvement).

quality care Health care services that increase the probability of achieving desired results with decreased probability of undesired results.

quality improvement (QI) Ongoing studies designed to identify ways to promote achievement of desired outcomes in a timely, cost-effective fashion while decreasing the risks for undesired outcomes.

rales Abnormal breath sounds (crackles) caused by the passage of air through bronchi containing fluid. This sign is frequently associated with congestive heart failure.

related factor See *risk factor*.

response A reaction of an organism or person to a specific mechanism.

risk factor Something known to contribute to (or be associated with) a specific problem. (See also *etiology*.)

risk nursing diagnosis Human response to health conditions or life processes that may develop in a vulnerable individual, family, or community. Supported by risk factors that contribute to increased vulnerability.[1]

signs Objective data that cause you to suspect a health problem.

somnolent Overly sleepy; difficult to arouse.

standards of care See *guidelines*.

standard of nursing care The degree of skill, care, and diligence exercised by members of the nursing profession practicing in the same or a similar locality. Many states refer to standards in their nurse practice acts.

subjective data Information the patient states or communicates; the patient's perceptions. For example, "My heart feels like it's racing."

sympathy Sharing the same feelings as another. (Compare with *empathy*.)

symptoms Subjective data that cause you to suspect a health problem.

synthesis The process of putting pieces of information together to make a whole. For example, nurses put individual signs and symptoms together to make a diagnosis.

thrombi More than one thrombus. (See *thrombus*.)

thrombus A clot that threatens blood supply to tissues. If the clot moves, it becomes an embolus.

tubal ligation Surgery performed to sterilize a woman by cutting and suturing her fallopian tubes.

validation The process of gathering more data to determine whether the information or data you've already collected are factual or true.

validity The extent to which something can be believed to be factual and true.

variance in care See *care variance*.

wellness diagnosis A clinical judgment about an individual, family, or community in transition from a specific level of wellness to a higher level of wellness.[2]

---

[1]North American Nursing Diagnosis Association. *Nursing diagnosis: Definitions and classifications 2001–2002.* Philadelphia: Author.
[2]Ibid.

COMPREHENSIVE

Bibliography

Adams, B. (1999). Nursing education for critical thinking: An integrative review. *Journal of Nursing Education, 38*(3),111–118.

Adams, J. (2002). Exceeding customer expectations. *Advance for Nurses,* (2FL) *24,* 27–28.

Adams, M., Whitlow, J., Stover, L., & Johnson, K. (1996). Critical thinking as an educational outcome: An evaluation of current tools of measurement. *Nurse Educator, 21*(3),23–31,110–118.

Alfaro-LeFevre, R. (2002). *Applying nursing process: Promoting collaborative care* (5th ed.). Philadelphia: J.B. Lippincott.

Alfaro-LeFevre, R. (2001). A right brain approach to critical thinking. Retrieved July 3, 2002 from http://nsweb.nursingspectrum.com/cfforms/GuestLecture/CriticalThinking.cfm

Alfaro-LeFevre, R. (2000). Don't worry! Be happy! Harmonize diversity through personality sensitivity. *Nursing Spectrum, 10*(16FL),14–17. Retrieved July 3, 2002 from http://nsweb.nursingspectrum.com/ce/ce236.htm

Alfaro-LeFevre, R. (2001). Evaluating critical thinking: How do you read minds? Retrieved July 3, 2002 from http://community.nursingspectrum.com/MagazineArticles/article.cfm?AID=4164

Alfaro-LeFevre, R. (2000). Improving your ability to think critically. Retrieved July 3, 2002 from http://nsweb.nursingspectrum.com/ce/ce168.htm

Alfaro-LeFevre, R. (2001). Thinking critically about your assignments. *Nurse Educator, 26*(1),15–16.

Allen, D., Bowers, B., & Diekelmann, N. (1989). Writing to learn: A reconceptualization of thinking and writing in the nursing curriculum. *Journal of Nursing Education, 28,*6–11.

Alters, S., & Schiff, W. (2003). *Essential concepts for healthy living* (3rd ed.). Boston: Jones and Bartlett.

Alters, S., & Schiff, W. (2003). *Applying concepts for healthy living: A workbook* (3rd ed.). Boston: Jones and Bartlett.

American Association of Critical Care Nurses. (1998). *Discovering your beliefs about healthcare choices (facilitator training manual): A guide to living wills and medical powers of attorney.* Aliso Viejo, CA: Author.

American Association of Critical Care Nurses. *The synergy model of certified practice.* Retrieved June 4, 2002 from http://www.certcorp.org/certcorp/certcorp.nsf/edcfc72ba47aaa708825666b0064bdcf/08482aa8ec2a5b6388256 66b00654be7?OpenDocument.

American Nurses Association. (1991). *Standards of clinical nursing practice.* Washington, DC: Author.

American Nurses Association. (1991). *Position statement on cultural diversity in nursing practice.* Kansas City, MO: Author.

American Nurses Association. (1995). *A social policy statement.* Washington DC: Author.

American Nurses Association. (2001). *Code of ethics for nurses with interpretive statements.* Washington DC: Author.

American Philosophical Association. (1990). *Critical thinking: A statement of expert consensus for purposes of educational assessment and instruction.* The Delphi Report: Research findings and recommendations prepared for the committee on pre-college philosophy. (ERIC Document Reproduction Services. No. ED 315–423).

Andrews, M., & Boyle, J. (1999). *Transcultural concepts in nursing care* (3rd ed.). Philadelphia: Lippincott Williams & Wilkins.

Angel, B., Duffey, M., & Belyea, M. (2000). An evidence-based project for evaluating strategies to improve knowledge acquisition and critical-thinking performance in nursing students. *Nurse Educator, 39*(5),219–228.

Arnold, E., & Boggs, K. (1999). *Interpersonal relationships: Professional communication skills for nurses* (3rd ed.). Philadelphia: W.B. Saunders.

Australian Nursing Council Inc. (1993). *Code of ethics for Australian nurses.* Canberra, Australia: Author.

Bandman, E., & Bandman, B. (1995). *Critical thinking in nursing* (2nd ed.). Norwalk, CT: Appleton & Lange.

Barger, R. *A summary of Lawrence Kohlberg's stages of moral development.* Retrieved July 17, 2002 from http://www.nd.edu/~rbarger/kohlberg.html.

Benner, P. (2001). *From novice to expert.* Upper Saddle River, NJ: Prentice Hall.

Benner, P., Tanner, C., & Chesla, C. (1996). *Experience in nursing practice: Caring, clinical judgment and ethics.* New York: Springer.

Block, P. (1996). *Stewardship: Choosing service over self-interest.* San Francisco: Berrett-Koehler.

Bloom, B. (Ed.). (1956). *Taxonomy of educational objectives. Handbook 1, Cognitive domain.* New York: McKay.

Boud, D., & Feletti, G. (1991). *The challenge of problem-based learning.* New York: St. Martin's Press.

Boychuk, J. E. D. (1999). Catching the wave: Understanding the concept of critical thinking. *Journal of Advanced Nursing, 29*(3),577–583.

Brigham, C. (1993). Nursing education and critical thinking: Interplay of content and thinking. *Holistic Nurse Practice, 7*(3),48–54.

Brookfield. S. (1987). *Developing critical thinkers.* San Francisco: Jossey-Bass.

Brown, H., & Sorrell, J. (1993). Use of clinical journals to enhance critical thinking. *Nurse Educator, 18*(5),16–18.

Burfitt, S., Greiner, D., & Miers, L. (1993). Professional nurse caring as perceived by critically ill patients: A phenomenologic study. *American Journal of Critical Care, 2*(6),489–499.

Buzan, T. (1991). *Use both sides of your brain.* New York: Fawcett Columbine.

Canadian Nurses Association. (1985). *Ethics code for nurses.* Ottawa: Author.

Campion, C. (1998). Embracing our differences. *Nursing Spectrum FL Ed., 8*(14),5–6.

Carpenito, L. (2002a). *Handbook of nursing diagnosis* (9th ed.). Philadelphia: Lippincott Williams & Wilkins.

Carpenito, L. (2002b). *Nursing diagnosis: Application to clinical practice* (9th ed.). Philadelphia: Lippincott Williams & Wilkins.

Case, B. (1998). *Developing competence: Critical thinking, clinical judgment and technical ability,* In Kelly, Karen. *Nursing Staff Development: Current Competence, Future Focus* (2nd ed.). Philadelphia: Lippincott-Raven.

Celia, L., & Gordon, P. (2001). Using problem-based learning to promote critical thinking in an orientation program for novice nurses. *Journal for Nurses in Staff Development, 17*(1),12–17. Retrieved July 13, 2002 from http://216.251.241.177/ce/test/article.cfm?id=0AA85AC8%2DEE2D%2D11D4%2D83E0%2D00508B605149.

Clark, H., & Wearing, J. (2002). Regulation of registered nursing: The Canadian perspective. *Reflections on Nursing LEADERSHIP, 27*(4),26–27.

Coehn, E. (2000). *Nursing case management: From essentials to advanced practice applications* (3rd ed.). St. Louis: Mosby.

Covey, S. (1989). *The seven habits of highly effective people.* New York: Simon & Schuster.

Crawford, L. (2002). Regulation of registered nursing: The American perspective. *Reflections on Nursing LEADERSHIP, 27*(4),28–29.

De Bono, E. (1985). *Six thinking hats: The power of focused thinking.* Boston: Little, Brown.

DeCastillo, S. (1999). *Strategies, techniques, and approaches to thinking.* Philadelphia: W.B. Saunders.

Deep, S., & Sussman, L. (1995). *Smart moves for people in charge: 30 checklists to help you be a better leader.* Reading, MA: Addison-Wesley.

Dickenson-Hazard, N. (2001). Block party. *Reflections on Nursing LEADERSHIP, 27*(1),5.

Dickenson-Hazard, N. (1990). The psychology of successful test taking. *Pediatric Nursing, 16,*66–67.

Dickenson-Hazard, N. (1989). Anatomy of a test question. *Pediatric Nursing, 15,* 480–481.

Dickenson-Hazard, N. (1989). Making the grade as a test taker. *Pediatric Nursing, 15,*302–304.

DiVito-Thomas, P. (2000). Identifying critical thinking behaviors in clinical judgments. *Journal of Nursing Staff Development, (16)*3,174–180.

Dobbin, K. (2001). Applying learning theories to develop teaching strategies for the critical care nurse: Don't limit yourself to the formal classroom lecture. *Critical Care Nursing Clinics of North America, 13*(1),1–11.

Doble, R., Curley, M., Hession-Laband, E., Marino, B., & Shaw, S. (2000). The synergy model in practice. *Critical Care Nurse, 20*(3),86–91.

Donald, J. (2002). *Learning to think: Disciplinary perspectives.* San Francisco: Jossey-Bass.

Edge, R., & Groves, J. (1999). Ethics of health care: *A guide for clinical practice.* Albany, NY: Delmar.

Ennis, R. (1987). A taxonomy of critical thinking dispositions and abilities. In J.B. Baron, J.J. Sternberg (Eds.), *Teaching thinking skills: Theory and practice.* New York: Freeman.

Ennis, R. (1990). Experience, education, and nurses' ability to make clinical judgments. *Nursing and Health Care, 11*(6),290–294.

Ennis, R., Millman, J., & Tomoko, T. (1985). *Cornell critical thinking tests level X and level Z manual* (3rd ed.). Pacific Grove, CA: Midwest Publications.

Facione, P., & Facione, N. (1994). *The California critical thinking skills test.* Millbrae, CA: California Academic Press.

Facione, P., & Facione, N. (1992). *California critical thinking disposition inventory.* Millbrae, CA: California Academic Press.

Facione, N., Facione, P., & Sanchez, C. (1994). Critical thinking disposition as a measure of competent clinical judgment: The development of the California Critical Thinking Disposition Inventory. *Journal of Nursing Education, 33*(8), 345–351.

Fonteyn, M. (1998). *Thinking strategies for nursing practice.* Philadelphia: Lippincott-Ravin.

Fonteyn, M. (1991). Implications of clinical reasoning studies for critical care nursing. *Focus, 18*(4),322–327.

Fry, S. Adequacy of workplace resources to identify ethical issues: Perceptions of RNs in five areas of practice. Retrieved July 17, 2002 from http://www.bc.edu/bc_org/avp/son/ethics/abstracts/ab04.html.

Fry, S. (2001). The development and psychometric evaluation of the ethical issues scale. *Journal of Nursing Scholarship, Third Quarter, 278–277.*

Gardner, H. (1993). *Multiple intelligences*. New York: Basic Books.

Geissler, E. (1999). *Pocket guide to cultural assessment* (2nd ed.). St. Louis: Mosby.

Glaser, E. (1941). *An experiment in the development of critical thinking*. New York: Bureau of Publications, Teachers College, Columbia University.

Glass, N., & Walter, R. (2000). An experience of peer mentoring with student nurses: Enhancement of personal and professional growth. *Journal of Nursing Education, 39*(4),155–160.

Goleman, D. (1995). *Emotional intelligence*. New York: Bantam Books.

Good, V., & Schulman, C. (2000). Employee competency pathways. *Critical Care Nurse, 20*(3),75–85.

Gordon, M. (2002). *Manual of Nursing Diagnosis* (10th ed.). St. Louis: Mosby.

Gorin, S., & Arnold, J. (1998). *Health promotion handbook*. St. Louis: Mosby.

Grossman, S., & Valiga, T. (2000). *The New Leadership Challenge: Creating the Future of Nursing*. Philadelphia: F.A. Davis.

Halpern, D. (1984). *Thought and knowledge*. Hillsdale, NJ: Lawrence Erlbaum Associates.

Hand, E. (2002). Surviving Clinical Competencies: Taking the "Immunity Challenge," *Critical Care Nurse, 22*(1),87–88.

Hansten, R., & Washburn, M. (2001). Intuition in professional practice: Executive and staff perceptions. *Journal of Nursing Administration, 30*(4),185–188.

Hartman, T. (1998). *The color code*. New York: Scribner.

Haynor, P. (1998). Meeting the challenge of advance directives. *American Journal of Nursing, 98*(3),26–32.

Hendricks, L. (2001). Leadership competencies are found in everyday skills and activities. *AACN News, 18*(4),10.

Ignatavicius, D., & Workman, L. (2002). *Medical-surgical nursing: Critical thinking for collaborative care*. Philadelphia: WB Saunders.

Ignatvicius, D. (2001). Six critical thinking skills for at-the-bedside success. *Nursing Management, 32*(1),37–39.

Johnson, M., & Maas, M. (2000). Nursing outcomes classification (2nd ed.). St. Louis: Mosby.

Johnstone, M. (1999). *Bioethics: A nursing perspective* (3rd ed.). Sydney, Australia: WB Saunders/Bailliere Tindall.

Joint Commission on Accreditation of Healthcare Organizations. (2001). *Accreditation Manual for Hospitals*. Oakbrook Terrace, IL: Author.

Joint Commission on Accreditation of Healthcare Organizations. Revisions to Joint Commission Standards in Support of Patient Safety and Medical/Health Care Error Reduction. Retrieved July 3, 2002 from http://www.jcaho.org./standard/fr_ptsafety.html.

Joint Commission on Accreditation of Healthcare Organizations. (2000). *JCAHO and HCFA: Understanding the requirements for hospitals*. Oakbrook Terrace, IL: Author.

Katooka-Yahiro, M., & Saylor, C. (1994). A critical thinking model for nursing judgment. *Journal of Nursing Education, 33*(8),351–356.

Kenney, E. (1998). Creating fulfillment in today's workplace: A guide for nurses. *American Journal of Nursing, 98*(5),44–48.

Kohlberg, L. (1976). Moral stages and moralization: The cognitive-developmental approach. In T. Likona (Ed.), *Moral development and behavior: Theory, research, and social issues.* New York: Holt, Rinehart, & Winston.

Lamond, D., & Thompson, C. (2000). Intuition and analysis in decision making and choice. *Journal of Nursing Scholarship, 32*(3),411–414.

Lashley, M., & Wittstadt, R. (1993). Writing across the curriculum: An integrated curricular approach to developing critical thinking through writing. *Journal of Nursing Education, 32*(9),422–424.

Lehmkuhl, D., & Lamping, D. (1993). *Organizing for the creative person.* New York: Crown Publishers, Inc.

Levenson, J., & Pettrey, L. (1994). Controversial decisions regarding treatment and DNR: An algorithmic guide for the uncertain in decision-making ethics. (GUIDE). *American Journal of Critical Care, 3*(2),87–91.

Lower, J. (2002). Developing a unit-based code of conduct. *Advance for Nurses* (FL ed.), *2*(2),29–31.

Luckman, J. (1999). *Transcultural communication in nursing.* Albany, NY: Delmar.

Mastal, M. (2000). Making the grade. *Nursing Spectrum* (FL. Ed.), *10*(30),8–9.

McClosky, J., & Bulechek, G. (2000). *Nursing interventions* (3rd ed.). St. Louis: Mosby.

McGovern, M., & Valiga, T. (1997). Promoting the cognitive development of freshmen nursing students. *Journal of Nursing Education, 36*(1),229–235.

Meyers, C. (1986). *Teaching students to think critically.* San Francisco: Jossey-Bass.

Musinski, B. (1999). The educator as a facilitator: A new kind of leadership. *Nursing Forum, 34*(1),21–29.

Norman, G. (1988). Problem-solving skills, solving problems, and problem-based learning. *Medical Education, 22,*279–286.

North American Nursing Diagnosis Association. *Nursing Diagnosis: definitions and classifications 2001–2002.* Philadelphia: Author.

Ouellette, F. (1988). A textbook coding tool, part 1: Assessing elements that promote analytic abilities. *Nurse Educator, 13*(5),8–13.

Paul, R. (1995). *Critical thinking: How to prepare students for a rapidly changing world.* Santa Rosa, CA: Foundation for Critical Thinking.

Paul, R., & Elder, L. (2002). *Critical thinking: Tools for taking charge of your learning and your life.* Upper Saddle River, NJ: Prentice Hall.

Provost, P., et al. (2001). Efficient Clinical Practice. *American Journal of Critical Care, 10*(6),376–382.

Robinson, A. (1993). *What smart students know: Maximum grades, optimum learning, minimum time.* New York: Crown Trade Paperbacks.

Rogers, S. What nurses can do about end-of-life care. Retrieved July 17, 2002 from http://www.advancefornurses.com/CE_Tests/eolCare.html.

Ross, B. (2002). Critical Thinking–Part I: The Eight Elements of Reasoning. Retrieved July 3, 2002 from http://www.onlinece.net/courses.asp?course=124&action=view.

Ross, B. (2002). Critical Thinking–Part II: Resolving Ethical Dilemmas. Retrieved July 3, 2002 from http://www.onlinece.net/courses.asp?course=125&action=view.

Ruggerio, V. (1998). *The art of thinking: A guide to critical and creative thought* (5th ed.). New York: Addison Wesley Longman.

Saarmann, L., Freitas, L., Rapps, J., & Riegel, B. (1992). The relationship of education to critical thinking ability and values among nurses: Socialization into professional nursing. *Journal of Professional Nursing, 8*(1),26–34.

Scanlan, J., Care, W., & Gessler, S. (2001). Dealing with the unsafe student in clinical practice. *Nurse Educator, 26*(1),23–27.

Scheffer, B., & Rubenfeld, M. (2000). A consensus statement on critical thinking in nursing. *Journal of Nursing Education, 39*(8),352–359.

Schuster, P. (2000). Concept mapping: Reducing clinical care plan paperwork and increasing learning. *Nurse Educator, 25*(2),76–81.

Senge, P. (1990). *The fifth discipline.* New York: Doubleday.

Secretary's Commission on Achieving Necessary Skills. (1992). *Learning a living: A blueprint for high performance, a SCANS report for America 2000.* The U.S. Department of Labor.

Sides, M., & Korchek, N. (1997). *Nurses' guide to successful test-taking* (3rd ed.). Philadelphia: J.B. Lippincott.

Silver, J., & Winland-Brown, J. (2000). Power asymmetry and patient autonomy. *American Journal of Critical Care, 9*(5),360–361.

Sorrell, J., Brown, H., Cipriano, S., & Kohlenberg, E. (1997). Use of writing portfolios for interdisciplinary assessment of critical thinking outcomes of nursing students. *Nursing Forum, 32*(4),12–23.

Spence, H., Laschinger, S., Finegan, J., Shamian, J., & Casier, S. (2000). Organizational trust and empowerment in restructured healthcare settings: Effects on staff nurse commitment. *Journal of Nursing Administration, 30*(9),413–425.

Steinke, E. (2001). Ease the strain of evaluating research reports. *AACN News, 18*(7),4.

Stevens, K. (1999). *Evidence-based teaching: Current research in nursing education.* New York: NLN Press.

Stevens, K. (2000). Mentoring on the cutting edge. *Reflections on Nursing LEADERSHIP, 26*(1),31–32,46.

Stevens, K., & Valiga, T. (2001). The national agenda for nursing education research. *Nursing and Health Care Perspectives, 20*(5),178–179.

Snyder, M. (1993). Critical thinking: A foundation for consumer-focused are. *The Journal of Continuing Education in Nursing, 24*(5),206–210.

Stine, J. (2000). *Super brainpower: 6 keys to unlocking your hidden genius.* Paramus, NJ: Prentice Hall.

Tanner, C. (1999). Evidenced-based practice: Research and critical thinking. *Journal of Nursing Education, 38*(3),99.

Tanner, C. (1983). Research on clinical judgment. In W.L. Holzemer (Ed.), *Review of research in nursing education.* Thorofare, NJ: Charles B. Slack.

Taylor, C., Lillis, C., & Lamone, P. (2001). *Fundamentals of nursing: The art and science of nursing care (4th ed.).* Philadelphia: Lippincott Williams & Wilkins.

Toliver, J. (1988). Inductive reasoning: Critical thinking skills for clinical competence. *Clinical Nurse Specialist, 2*(4),174–179.

Tompson, C., & Rebeschi, L. (1999). Critical thinking skills of baccalaureate nursing students at program entry and exit. *NLN Journal: Nursing & Health Care Perspectives, 20*(5),248–254.

Tschikota, S. (1993). The clinical decision-making processes of student nurses. *Journal of Nursing Education, 32*(9),387.

Vaca, K., Vaca, B., & Daake, C. (1998). Review of nursing home regulations. *MEDSURG Nursing, 7*(3),165–171.

Valiga, T., & Bruderle, E. (1997). *Using the arts and humanities to teach nursing: A creative approach.* New York: Springer.

Villaire, M. (1996). The synergy model of certified practice: Creating safe passage for patients. *Critical Care Nurse, 16*,95–99.

Wailey D. (1995). *Empires of the mind: Lessons to lead and succeed in a knowledge-based world.* New York: William Morrow and Co.

Watson, G., & Glaser, E. (1980). *Watson-Glaser critical thinking appraisal manual.* Cleveland, OH: Psychological Corporation.

Weirda, L., & Natzke, C. (2000). Students' collaborative clinical experience. *Journal of Nursing Education, 39*(4),183–184.

Weisinger, H. (1998). *Emotional intelligence at work.* San Francisco: Jossey-Bass.

Wilkinson, J. (2001). *Nursing process and critical thinking.* (3rd ed.). Paramus, NJ: Prentice Hall.

Williams, M. (2001). Make building leadership skills a journey. *AACN News, 18*(4),10.

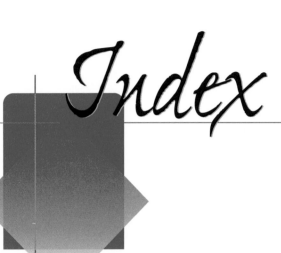

Index

Page numbers followed by b refer to boxes; page numbers followed by f refer to figures; page numbers followed by t refer to tables.

A

A Patient's Bill of Rights, 105
Acceptance, in adapting to change, 191
Accommodators, in conflict management, 209b
Accountability, in ethical reasoning, 105
Accuracy, of information, 45
Activities of daily living, 78
Advance Directives, 106, 108b
Age, critical thinking ability and, 30, 30t
American Nurses Association Standards for
    Practice, 263–264
Analytical thinking, 11
Anger, in adapting to change, 191
Anticipation, 44
Anxiety, 30t, 34
Assertive behavior, vs. aggressive behavior, 206b
Assessment
    approach to, 142–146
    database, definition of, 138
    definition of, 142
    focus, definition of, 138
    neurologic focus, guide for, 145–146,
        262f–263f
    in nursing process, 73–74, 75b, 82f
    tools for, pre-established, 142–143, 183f–186f
Assumptions
    definition of, 128
    identification of, 138–142
Autonomy, in ethical reasoning, 105
Avoiders, in conflict management, 209b

B

Bad news, communication of, 194–196
Baseline data, definition of, 138
Behavior(s)
    assertive vs. aggressive, 206b
    demonstrating intellectual skills/
        competencies, 47t
    demonstrating knowledge, 46t
    enhancing and impeding interpersonal
        relationships, 229b
    patterns of, critical thinking and, 48–49
Beneficence, in ethical reasoning, 105
Biases, 30t, 31
Big picture focus, 44
Bill of Rights, for patient, 107
Brain
    left vs. right hemisphere function of, 262
    mind mapping and, 260–262, 260f

C

Care-based approach, to ethics, 110t
Care plan, 75–76
    development of, 180–182
Case management, 71b
Causative factor, definition of, 137
Change
    methods of, 193b
    navigating and fascilitating, 190–193, 193b
    resistance to, 36

Character
  critical thinking, developing, 49–50
  critical thinking and, 50–51, 50f
Characteristics, defining, definition of, 138
Charting, critical thinking and, 95–96
Choosing-only-one habit, 36
Chronically ill, care of, concern for, 70b
Clinical judgment
  assessment tools and, pre-established,
    142–143, 183f–186f
  clustering related cues in, 151–153
  creativity in, 85–86, 87b
  critical thinking and, 56
  decision making and, 88–90, 89f
  determining care plan in, 180–182
  determining interventions in, 175–178
  determining outcomes in, 171–174, 173b–174b
  developing, 83–95
  diagnosing actual and potential problems in,
    161–166
  effective, development of, 90–95, 93b–94b
  evaluating and correcting thinking in,
    178–179, 179b
  identifying and managing risk factors in,
    159–161
  identifying missing information in, 158–159
  identifying patterns in, 156–158
  identifying relevant information in, 153–155
  identifying signs and symptoms in, 148–149
  intuition in, 84–85, 87b
  logic in, 84–85
  making inferences in, 149–151
  nursing process as tool for, 74, 75b
  recognizing inconsistencies in, 155–156
  scope of decisions and, 86
  setting priorities in, 167–171, 168b
  skills in, practicing, 134–186
  validating data and, 146–148
Clinical outcomes, 69
Clinical practice guidelines (CPGs), 68b
Clinical reasoning, 13
Code of Ethics for Nurses, 264–265
Collaboration, encouraging, 70b
Collaborative problem solvers, in conflict man-
  agement, 209b
Collaborative thinking, 13
Comfort, 78
Common good approach, to ethics, 110t
Common sense, critical thinking and, 6
Communication skills, 30t, 32, 32b–33b
Community needs, services driven by, 71b
Compare and contrast, 45
Complaints, constructive response to, 196–199
Complications, common, 79b–80b
Compromisers, in conflict management, 209b

Computer use, trends in, 71b
Confidentiality, in ethical reasoning, 105
Conflict, management of, 207–213, 208t,
  209b–210b
  personal style of, 209b
Conflict resolution skills, in learning to think
  critically, 49–50
Conformity, 36
Consumer, services driven by, 71b
Counseling, as responsibility, 71b
Covey, Stephen, 37
Creativity, in clinical judgment, 85–86, 87b
Critical paths, 71b, 75, 266–269
Critical thinker
  attitudes of, 8b
  characteristics of, 6–9
  influences on, 25, 29–38
  intellectual traits of, 10t–11t
  personal influences on, 23, 25, 25b, 26b–27b,
    30–34
  situational influences on, 30t, 34–35
  summary of, 15
Critical thinking
  barriers to, 35–37
  definition of, 56–59, 93t
  descriptions of, 4, 10t–11t
  evaluation of, 178–179
  evaluation own potential for, 14f
  mentoring and, 28–29
  mind mapping for, 260–262, 260f
  in nursing, 5, 56–60
  purpose of, 2–3
  skills for, 46–48, 46t–47t, 48b. See also
    Critical thinking skills.
  strategies for, 40–45
  synonym for, 4
  ten key questions for, 40–42
  vs. thinking, 3–4
Critical thinking indicators (CTIs), 7–9, 8b
  intellectual skills as, 46–47
  knowledge as, 46–47
Critical thinking skills. See also Workplace
  skills.
  evaluating thinking in, 178–179
Criticism, constructive response to, 204–207
Cues
  definition of, 138
  related, clustering of, 151–153
Cultural needs, 70b
Culture, thinking and, 25, 28

D

Data
  absence of, 158–159

accuracy of, checking, 146–148
baseline, definition of, 138
definition of, 137
effective use of, 233–238
grouping of, 151–153
inconsistencies in, 155–156
objective, definition of, 137
patterns in, 156–158
relevance of, 153–155
subjective, definition of, 137
validating, 146–148
Database assessment, definition of, 138
Databases, health-related, 234b
Deadlines, 35
Decision making, 32, 88–89, 89f
clinical judgment and, 88–90, 89f
ethical and moral, 103–105
moral and ethical, approach to, 110t
Defining characteristics, definition of, 138
Definitive diagnosis, definition of, 137
Delegating in clinical setting, 169b
Denial, in adapting to change, 191
Depression, in adapting to change, 191
Diagnosis(es)
definitive, definition of, 137
medical, 79b–80b
nursing
accountability for, 76–77
definition of, 78
legal implications of, 77
NANDA, 270–279
nursing responsibilities related to,
77–81
in nursing process, 73–74, 75b, 76–81
in rehabilitation nursing, 79b
risk, definition of, 137
Dislikes, 30t, 31
Durable Power of Attorney for Health Care
(DPAHC), 108b
Dynamic nursing process, 73–74

E

Early evaluation, 33
Educated guesses, for test taking,
128b
Elderly, care of, concern for, 70b
Emotional intelligence, 30t, 31
Empowered relationships, developing,
199–203, 201t
Environmental distractions, 35
Errors, 45
constructive response to, 221–223
prevention of, 218–227
Ethical dilemmas, growth of, 70b

Ethical reasoning
definition of, 103
principles of, 105
steps in, 108–109
10 key questions in, 111b
Ethics, 102
Evaluation, 30t, 33, 34, 72
in nursing process, 73–74, 75b
Evaluative style, 34
Evidence-based care, 67–69, 68b
Experience, 30t, 33
Expert thinking, vs. novice thinking,
61–64, 63t

F

Face-saving habit, 36
Fair-mindedness, 30, 30t
Fairness approach, to ethics, 110t
Fatigue, 30t, 34
Feedback, giving and taking, 204–207
Fidelity, in ethical reasoning, 105
Flaws, in thinking, 45
Focus, loss of, in adapting to change, 191
Focus assessment, definition of, 138
Forcers, in conflict management, 209b
Functional outcomes, 69

G

Goals vs. outcome, 38–39
Gordon's functional health patterns, 82b

H

Habits
as critical thinking barriers, 35–37
of highly effective people, 37
Hartman Personality Profile, 26b–27b
Health, promotion of, 78
Health care, trends in, 70b–71b
Healthy People 2010, critical thinking and, 71b
Home care, increase in, 70b
Human potential, maximization of, 13
Human responses, 78

I

Implementation, in nursing process, 73–74,
75b
Inconsistencies, 138
recognizing, 155–156
Infer, definition of, 138
Inference(s), 149–151
definition of, 138

Information. *See also* Data.
  missing, identifying, 158–159
Injury, risk for, 78
Inquiry habits, 45
Insight, 9
Intellectual skills
  behaviors demonstrating, 47t
  indicators of, 46–47
Intelligence, emotional, 30t, 31
Interaction error, 222
Interpersonal skills, 13, 30t, 32
Interventions, determination of, 175–178
Intuition, 43
  in clinical judgment, 84–85, 87b
Irrelevancy, of information, 153–155

J

Judgment, clinical. *See* Clinical judgment.
Judgmental style, 30t, 34
Justice, in ethical reasoning, 105
Justice approach, to ethics, 110t

K

Knowledge
  behaviors demonstrating, 46t
  as critical thinking indicator, 46–47
Knowledge deficits, 78
Knowledge error, 222

L

Leaders, team, 228–229
Learning, 30t, 34, 123–125
  memorizing for, 123–125
  test taking and, 125–129, 127b, 128b,
    130b–131b
Learning error, 222
Learning preferences, strategies for, 24t
Learning style, 22–28
Living Will, 108b
Logic, 43
  in clinical judgment, 84–85

M

Managed care, 71b
Management, vs. treatment, 66
Managing, in PPMP approach to problems,
  65–66, 66t, 67
Maslow's Hierarchy of Human Needs, setting
  priorities according to, 168b
Medication errors, prevention of,
  218–227

Medication regimens, tailoring of, for
  individual, 78
Members, team, 230–2321
Memorization, 123–125
Mental slip, 221–222
Mentoring, 28–29
Mind mapping, 260–262, 260f
Mine-is-better habit, 36
Mistakes, 44
  constructive response to, 221–223
  prevention of, 218–227
Mnemonic, in learning, 124
Monitoring patient, 77
Moral development, 30, 30t
Moral dilemma, 104
Moral distress, 104
Moral reasoning
  definition of, 103
  steps in, 108–109
  10 key questions in, 111b
Moral uncertainty, 104
Motivating factors, 30t, 34–35
Myers-Briggs Type Indicator, 25b

N

Needs, human, Maslow's Hierarchy of, setting
  priorities according to, 168b
Negative information, communication of,
  194–196
Negotiation, 211b
Neurologic focus assessment guide, 145–146,
  262f–263f
Novice thinking, vs. expert thinking, 61–64, 63t
Nursing
  goals of, 60
  health care trends and, 70b–71b
  outcome-focused, 60–61
  predictive model approach to, 64–67
Nursing diagnosis(es), 73–74, 75b, 76–81
  accountability for, 76–77
  definition of, 78
  legal implications of, 77
  NANDA, 270–279
  nursing responsibilities related to, 77–81
Nursing process, 31
  changes in, 73–82, 75b, 76f
  dynamic, 73–74

O

Objective data, definition of, 137
Organization
  of information, 45
  of work in time management, 215–217

Outcome-focused thinking, 38–40
Outcome-focused writing, 238–245
Outcomes
  clinical, 69
  of conflict, 208t
  expected, client-centered, determination of,
      171–174, 173b–174b
  functional, 69
  goals vs., 38–39
  in nursing, 60–61
  protective factor, 69
  quality of life, 69
  risk reduction, 69
  satisfaction, 70
  symptom severity, 69
  therapeutic alliance, 70
  use of service, 70

P

Pain, management of, 78
Paraphrasing, 45
Partnerships
  empowered
    building, 28–29
    development of, 199–203, 201t
  nurturing, 70b
Patient's Bill of Rights, 107
Patients' rights, 70b
Personal learning style, 22–28
Personality types, 23, 25, 25b, 26b–27b
Planning, in nursing process, 73–74, 75b
Positive reinforcement, 34
Potential problem, definition of, 137
PPMP approach to problems, 65–66,
    66t, 67
Practice guidelines, 88–90
Predicting, in PPMP approach to problems,
    65–66, 66t, 67
Predictive model, in nursing, 64–67
Prejudices, 30t, 31
Prevention, 78
  in PPMP approach to problems, 65–66,
      66t, 67
Priorities
  ranking of, in time management,
      215
  setting, 167–181, 168b
Problem, potential, definition of, 137
Problem solvers, collaborative, in conflict
    management, 209b
Problem solving, 11, 30t, 31
Problems
  actual, diagnosing, 161–165, 164b
  potential, diagnosing, 161–163, 164b, 165

Professional standards, 263–264
Promoting, in PPMP approach to problems,
    65–66, 66t, 67
Protective factor outcomes, 69

Q

Quality improvement, research and, 115–118
Quality of life outcomes, 69
Questions
  for critical thinking, 40–42
  test, 127b

R

Reading skills, 30t, 34
Reasoning, 4, 56
  clinical, 13
  ethical
    steps for, 108–109
    10 key questions in, 111b
  moral
    steps for, 108–109
    10 key questions in, 111b
Reflection, 9
Related factor, definition of, 137
Relationships, parental vs. empowered, 201t
Relevance, of information, 153–155
Reliability, of information, checking, 146–148
Research, 112–118
  article evaluation for, 113–114, 114b
  by beginning nurse, 112–113
  definition of, 112
  principles of, 31
  for quality improvement, 115–118
  use of, 115–118, 116b–117b
Resources, awareness of, 30t, 34
Responsibility, taking, in learning to think
    critically, 49
Results-oriented thinking, 38–40
Rights approach, to ethics, 110t
Risk diagnosis, definition of, 137
Risk factor(s)
  definition of, 137
  identification and management of, 159–161
Risk reduction outcomes, 69
Risks, awareness of, 30t, 34

S

Satisfaction outcomes, 70
Scientific method, 12–13
Self-confidence, 30t, 31
Self-deception, 37
Self-focusing, 35

Signs
 definition of, 137–138
 identification of, 148–149
Skills
 critical thinking, 46–48, 46t–47t, 48b. *See
  also* Critical thinking skills.
 workplace, 188–245. *See also* Workplace
  skills.
Small picture focus, 44
Smoothers, in conflict management, 209b
Standards
 of Care, 263
 evidence-based, 71b
 of Professional Performance, 263–264
Standards of Nursing Practice, 105
Stereotyping, 36–37
Stress, 30t, 34
Subjective data, definition of, 137
Symptom severity outcomes, 69
Symptoms
 definition of, 137–138
 identification, 148–149
System error, 222–223

T

Teaching, 120–125. *See also* Learning.
 of others, 120–121, 121b–122b
 as responsibility, 71b
 of selves, 123–125
Team
 building, 227–233, 229b, 230b
 working as, in learning to think critically,
  49–50
Teamwork, creation of, 227–233, 229b, 230b
Technical skills, practicing, in learning to think
  critically, 50
Technology, overreliance on, errors from, 222
Ten key questions, for critical thinking, 40–42
Test taking, 125–129, 127b, 128b, 130b–131b
 educated guesses for, 128b
 preparatory questions for, 126
 question structure for, 126, 127b
Therapeutic alliance outcomes, 70
Thinking. *See also* Critical thinking.
 critical thinking vs., 3–4
 cultural influences on, 25, 28
 evaluating and correcting, 178–179, 179b
 novice vs. expert, 61–64, 63t
 out loud, 44
 personality and, 23, 25, 25b, 26b–27b
 trends influencing, 70b–71b

upbringing and, 25
Threats, emerging, 70b
Time limitations, 35
Time management, 213–218
Treatment
 management vs., 66
 tailoring of, for individual, 78
Trial and error, 43
Tunnel vision, 36

U

Upbringing, thinking and, 25
Use of service outcomes, 70
Utilitarian approach, to ethics, 110t

V

Value, proving, 70b
Veracity, in ethical reasoning, 105
Virtue approach, to ethics, 110t
Vision, tunnel, 36

W

Well-being, promoting, 78
Wellness centers, 71b
What-else question, 44
What-if question, 44
What-if strategies, 13
Will, Living, 108b
Workplace skills, 188–245. *See also* Critical
  thinking skills.
 communicating bad news as, 194–196
 complaint handling as, 196–199
 developing empowered partnerships as,
  199–203, 201t
 giving feedback as, 204–205, 206b
 managing conflict as, 207–213, 208t,
  209b–210b
 navigating and facilitating change as,
  190–193, 193b
 preventing mistakes as, 218–227
 taking criticism as, 204, 205, 206–207
 team building as, 227–233, 229b, 230b
 time management as, 213–218
 using information as, 233–238
 writing as, 238–245
Writer's block, overcoming, 241b, 244
Writing, 30t, 33
 evaluation of, 241b
 outcome-focused, 238–245

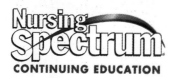

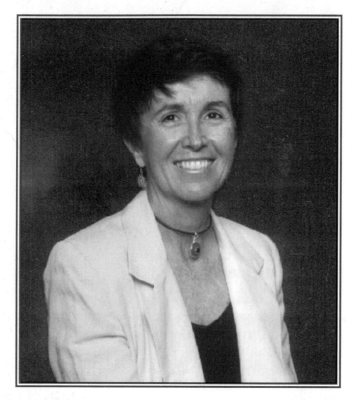

Rosalinda Alfaro-LeFevre is the president of Teaching Smart/Learning Easy, in Stuart, Florida. She has more than 20 years' clinical nursing experience and has taught in baccalaureate and associate degree programs. A Sigma Theta Tau "Best Pick" recipient, she is known for making difficult content easy to understand. Her work has been translated into six languages. Born in Buenos Aires, Argentina to a British mother and Argentine father, Rosalinda came to the United States via Canada as a child. Although Rosalinda says she's an American at heart, she points out that she has been blessed with multicultural experiences, presenting nationally and internationally, and enjoying close relationships with her family in Spain, Argentina, and the United Kingdom.